Managing Complications of Foot & Ankle Surgery

Editor

J. CHRIS COETZEE

FOOT AND ANKLE CLINICS

www.foot.theclinics.com

Consulting Editor
MARK S. MYERSON

September 2014 • Volume 19 • Number 3

ELSEVIER

1600 John F. Kennedy Boulevard • Suite 1800 • Philadelphia, Pennsylvania, 19103-2899

http://www.theclinics.com

FOOT AND ANKLE CLINICS Volume 19, Number 3
September 2014 ISSN 1083-7515, ISBN-13: 978-0-323-32323-9

Editor: Jennifer Flynn-Briggs
Developmental Editor: Yonah Korngold

Foot and Ankle Clinics (ISSN 1083-7515) is published quarterly by Elsevier, Inc., 360 Park Avenue South, New York, NY 10010-1710. Months of issue are March, June, September, and December. Periodicals postage paid at New York, NY, and additional mailing offices. Subscription price per year is $315.00 (US individuals), $421.00 (US institutions), $155.00 (US students), $360.00 (Canadian individuals), $506.00 (Canadian institutions), $215.00 (Canadian students), $460.00 (foreign individuals), $506.00 (foreign institutions), and $215.00 (foreign students). To receive student/resident rate, orders must be accompanied by name of affiliated institution, date of term, and the *signature* of program/residency coordinator on institution letterhead. Orders will be billed at individual rate until proof of status is received. Foreign air speed delivery is included in all *Clinics* subscription prices. All prices are subject to change without notice. **POSTMASTER:** Send address changes to *Foot and Ankle Clinics*, Elsevier Health Sciences Division, Subscription Customer Service, 3251 Riverport Lane, Maryland Heights, MO 63043. **Customer Service: 1-800-654-2452 (US and Canada). From outside of the United States and Canada, call 314-447-8871. Fax: 314-447-8029. E-mail: JournalsCustomerService-usa@ elsevier.com (for print support); JournalsOnlineSupport-usa@elsevier.com (for online support).**

Reprints. For copies of 100 or more, of articles in this publication, please contact the Commercial Reprints Department, Elsevier Inc., 360 Park Avenue South, New York, NY 10010-1710. Tel.: 212-633-3874; Fax: 212-633-3820; E-mail: reprints@elsevier.com.

Contributors

CONSULTING EDITOR

MARK S. MYERSON, MD
Director, The Institute for Foot and Ankle Reconstruction, Mercy Medical Center, Mercy Hospital, Baltimore, Maryland

EDITOR

J. CHRIS COETZEE, MD
Orthopedic Foot and Ankle Surgeon, Minnesota Orthopedic Sports Medicine Institute at Twin Cities Orthopedics, Edina, Minnesota

AUTHORS

Prof. ROGER M. ATKINS, MA (Oxon), MB BS (London), DM (Oxon), FRCS (England)
Consultant Orthopaedic Surgeon, Bristol Royal Infirmary, Bristol, United Kingdom

PIERRE BAROUK, MD
Foot and Ankle Surgery Center, Sport's Clinic, Bordeaux-Mérignac, France

STEPHEN K. BENIRSCHKE, MD
Professor, Department of Orthopaedics, University of Washington, Seattle, Washington

MICHAEL E. BRAGE, MD
Associate Professor, Department of Orthopaedics, University of Washington, Seattle, Washington

MICHAEL BUTLER, MA, MB BS, FRCS (Tr & Orth)
Consultant Orthopaedic Surgeon, Department of Trauma and Orthopaedics, Royal Cornwall Hospital, Truro, Cornwall, United Kingdom

MICHAEL J. COUGHLIN, MD
Director, Saint Alphonsus Coughlin Foot and Ankle Clinic, Boise, Idaho; Clinical Professor of Orthopaedic Surgery, University of California, San Francisco, San Francisco, California

MATTHEW D. CRAWFORD, MD
Orthopaedic Resident, Department of Orthopaedic Surgery, Duke University Medical Center, Durham, North Carolina

MARK DAVIES, FRCS (Tr & Orth)
London Foot and Ankle Centre, Hospital of St John and St Elizabeth, London, United Kingdom

ERIN M. DEAN, MD
Crystal Clinic Orthopaedic Center, Hudson, Ohio

JESSE F. DOTY, MD
Instructor, Department of Orthopaedic Surgery, University of Tennessee College of Medicine, Chattanooga, Chattanooga, Tennessee

PAUL T. FORTIN, MD
Associate Professor, Department of Orthopaedic Surgery, Oakland University William Beaumont, School of Medicine, Royal Oak, Michigan

ERIC GIZA, MD
Associate Professor of Orthopaedic Surgery; Chief, Foot and Ankle Surgery, Department of Orthopaedics, University of California, Davis, Sacramento, California

NIKOLAOS GOUGOULIAS, MD, PhD, CCT (Orth)
Consultant Orthopaedic Foot and Ankle Surgeon, Department of Trauma and Orthopaedics, Frimley Park Hospital NHS Foundation Trust, Surrey, United Kingdom

JOHN S. GOULD, MD
Professor of Surgery/Orthopaedic, Division of Orthopaedic Surgery, Section of Foot and Ankle, University of Alabama at Birmingham (UAB), Birmingham, Alabama

JUSTIN GREISBERG, MD
Associate Professor of Orthopaedic Surgery, Columbia University, New York, New York

ERIC R. JAMES, MD
Fellow in Foot and Ankle Surgery, Foundation for Athletic and Reconstructive Research, Houston, Texas

HYUK JEGAL, MD
Foot and Ankle Service, KT Lee's Orthopedic Hospital, Seoul, Republic of Korea

NATHAN J. KIEWIET, MD
Drisko, Fee & Parkins Orthopaedics, PC, Independence, Missouri

KYUNG TAI LEE, MD, PhD
Foot and Ankle Service, KT Lee's Orthopedic Hospital, Seoul, Republic of Korea

THOMAS H. LEE, MD
Attending Physician, Orthopedic Foot and Ankle Center, Westerville, Ohio

BENJAMIN J. LINDBLOOM, MD
Resident, Department of Orthopaedic Surgery, University of Texas Health Science Center at Houston, Houston, Texas

WILLIAM C. McGARVEY, MD
Associate Professor, Chief of Foot and Ankle Surgery and Residency Program Director, Department of Orthopaedic Surgery, University of Texas Health Science Center at Houston; Fellowship Program Director, Foundation for Athletic and Reconstructive Research, Houston, Texas

CAIO NERY, MD
Associate Professor, Department of Orthopedics and Traumatology, UNIFESP - Federal University of Sao Paulo, Sao Paulo, Brazil

MAURICE O'FLAHERTY, MB BCh, BaO, MSc Sports Med, FRCSEd (Tr & Orth)
Foot and Ankle Fellow; Department of Trauma and Orthopaedics, Royal Surrey County Hospital and Frimley Park Hospital, Surrey, United Kingdom

YOUNG UK PARK, MD, PhD
Clinical Assistant Professor, Division of Foot and Ankle Surgery, Department of
Orthopaedic Surgery, Ajou University School of Medicine, Suwon, Gyeonggi-do,
Republic of Korea

STEPHEN W. PARSONS, MA, BS, FRCS, FRCS (Ed)
Consultant Orthopaedic Surgeon, Department of Trauma and Orthopaedics,
Royal Cornwall Hospital, Truro, Cornwall, United Kingdom

JAYMIN PATEL, BS
School of Medicine, University of California, Davis, Sacramento, California

DAVID R. RICHARDSON, MD
Department of Orthopaedic Surgery and Biomedical Engineering, University of
Tennessee-Campbell Clinic, Memphis, Tennessee

ANTHONY SAKELLARIOU, MBBS, BSc, FRCS (Orth)
Consultant Orthopaedic Foot and Ankle Surgeon, Department of Trauma and
Orthopaedics, Frimley Park Hospital NHS Foundation Trust, Surrey, United Kingdom

DISHAN SINGH, MBChB, FRCS (Orth)
Foot and Ankle Department, Royal National Orthopaedic Hospital, Brockley Hill,
Stanmore, Middlesex, United Kingdom

MATTHEW SOLAN, FRCS (Tr & Orth)
Surrey Foot and Ankle Clinic, Mount Alvernia Hospital; Royal Surrey County Hospital,
Guildford, Surrey, United Kingdom

CLARE F. TAYLOR, BM, MRCS
Orthopaedic Registrar, Department of Trauma and Orthopaedics, Royal Cornwall
Hospital, Truro, Cornwall, United Kingdom

MATTHEW TOMLINSON, MBChB, FRACS
Consultant Foot and Ankle Surgeon, Mercy Ascot Hospitals, Counties Manukau Health,
Auckland, New Zealand

PHILIP VAUGHAN, MBBS, FRCS (Tr & Orth)
Foot and Ankle Department, Royal National Orthopaedic Hospital, Brockley Hill,
Stanmore, Middlesex, United Kingdom

LOWELL WEIL Jr, DPM, MBA
President and Fellowship Director, Weil Foot and Ankle Institute; Partner, Foot and Ankle
Business Innovations, Des Plaines, Illinois

Contents

The Failed First Metatarsophalangeal Joint Implant Arthroplasty   343

Justin Greisberg

> Chronic pain in a first metatarsophalangeal implant arthroplasty can be early or late, and may be due to infection or implant failure. Although excisional arthroplasty can be considered, the most predictable result will come from arthrodesis. Conversion of a failed implant arthroplasty to fusion will usually require structural bone graft, with slower healing times than primary fusion.

Pain After Cheilectomy of the First Metatarsophalangeal Joint: Diagnosis and Management   349

Matthew Tomlinson

> Cheilectomy is commonly performed for osteoarthritis of the first metatarsophalangeal joint and generally has a successful outcome and high rate of patient satisfaction over the short to medium term. Despite the relatively good results achieved in most cases, a proportion of patients have ongoing pain after cheilectomy. This article outlines the potential causes of ongoing pain, including progression of osteoarthritis, neuralgic symptoms, and transfer metatarsalgia. Management strategies for treating the ongoing symptoms are discussed.

Deceptions in Hallux Valgus: What to Look for to Limit Failures   361

Kyung Tai Lee, Young Uk Park, Hyuk Jegal, and Thomas H. Lee

> The treatment of hallux valgus depends on multiple factors, including clinical examination, patient considerations, clinical findings, radiographic assessment, and surgeon preference. Appropriate procedure selection and proper technique will usually result in good-to-excellent outcomes. Complications following hallux valgus correction include recurrence, transfer metatarsalgia, avascular necrosis, hallux varus, and nonunion and malunion of metatarsal osteotomies. In order to decrease the risks of complication, a precise and meticulous physical examination should be conducted preoperatively. In addition, a surgeon should select appropriate osteotomies to correct complex hallux valgus deformities. As a general principle, the severity of deformity dictates treatment options.

Iatrogenic Hallux Varus Treatment Algorithm   371

Matthew D. Crawford, Jaymin Patel, and Eric Giza

> Iatrogenic hallux varus is a relatively rare complication of corrective hallux valgus surgery that has multiple pathologic facets. It requires a comprehensive assessment that focuses on joint flexibility, joint integrity, soft

tissue balance, and bony deformity. A step-wise treatment approach is used to address all elements of the deformity. The literature on hallux varus treatments consists mainly of retrospective case series, with several proposed procedures addressing various degrees of deformity. Comparison of these procedures is a challenging endeavor and each case should be considered on an individual basis.

The terms crossover toe and lesser metatarsophalangeal joint instability both describe a deterioration of the soft tissue structures that give stability to the lesser MTP joints. Initial treatment regimens focused on indirect repair of the instability without addressing the primary pathology. A staging system of the clinical examination and a grading system of the surgical findings are now available to help surgeons classify and treat the plantar plate insufficiency. Improved imaging techniques and direct surgical repair techniques through a dorsal approach have changed the treatment and possibly the results of this difficult condition.

Recurrent metatarsalgia has a multifactorial etiology. The analysis of the cause is critical in planning appropriate treatment. Understanding etiology helps understand the mechanism of prevention, which is the best treatment. Recurrent metatarsalgia is often due to poor technique or poor understanding of the underlying problem. In hallux valgus surgery, recurrent metatarsalgia can be a problem of position of the first metatarsal after an inappropriate or poorly done first metatarsal osteotomy or a problem of gastrocnemius tightness not previously recognized. The best treatment is to restore the normal anatomy but that is not always possible, and surgery on affected rays could be the solution.

Disorders of the hallux sesamoids can be a source of considerable pain and disability. Inappropriate or inept removal can lead to further disability and pain. Surgical intervention should only follow careful accurate assessment, appropriate investigation, and failure of conservative treatments.

Interdigital neuromas are a common cause of forefoot pain, and approximately 80% of patients require surgical excision for symptom relief. Although 50% to 85% of patients obtain relief after primary excision, symptoms may recur because of an incorrect diagnosis, inadequate resection, or adherence of pressure on a nerve stump neuroma. The symptom relief rate after reoperation is similar to that after primary excision. A plantar longitudinal incision provides optimal exposure, and transposition of the nerve stump into bone or muscle and avoids traction or pressure on the nerve ending that can result in a painful stump neuroma. Preoperative counseling is essential to align patient expectations with potential outcomes.

Recurrence of tarsal tunnel syndrome after surgery may be due to inadequate release, lack of understanding or appreciation of the actual anatomy involved, variations in the anatomy of the nerve(s), failure to execute the release properly, bleeding with subsequent scarring, damage to the nerve and branches, persistent hypersensitivity of the nerves, and preexisting intrinsic damage to the nerve. Approaches include more thorough release, use of barrier materials to decrease adherence of the nerve to surrounding tissues to avoid traction neuritis, excisions of neuromas using conduits, and consideration of nerve stimulators and systemic medications to deal with persistent neural pain.

Concomitant hindfoot and midfoot deformity is common. Hindfoot fusion is associated with prolonged recovery and significant disability. Further surgery is often required to obtain a plantigrade foot. Understanding normal structural and kinematic relationships between the midfoot and hindfoot, as well as recognizing common combined patterns of midfoot and hindfoot deformity, can minimize the unanticipated consequences of hindfoot fusion. Treatment of residual or resultant midfoot deformity requires a thorough analysis of the deformity and familiarity with a variety of operative techniques for correction.

Triple arthrodesis is a powerful corrector of hindfoot deformity related to trauma, rheumatoid arthritis, and long-standing peritalar subluxation with posterior tibial tendon dysfunction. To avoid the common postoperative complications related to triple arthrodesis, one must be meticulous in preoperative evaluation as well as surgical technique. Presented are some tips and tricks to avoid the common complications and provide the patient with a plantigrade, stable foot, as well as some salvage options for triple arthrodesis in a malunited position.

Metatarsal fractures are those most frequently encountered in the foot. More than half of these are of the 5th metatarsal. The incidence is increasing, along with the activity levels of the general population. Fractures of the 5th metatarsal require careful evaluation and classification to ensure selection of the optimum treatment plan. Distal fractures rarely require fixation, even when displacement is wide. Cases of established nonunion or refracture require fixation.

The surgical treatment of calcaneal malunion is technically very demanding and requires a careful assessment of the exact cause of the problem. A number of different surgeries are available depending on the precise cause of symptoms. The results are reasonable and justify surgery in an otherwise disabled group of patients. Calcaneal malunion surgery should not be performed by the occasional surgeon, as the price of error is usually amputation.

Although a painful accessory navicula and a pes planus often coexist, they are not necessarily causally related, and each condition should be assessed and treated individually. A child or adolescent will notice the rubbing of an accessory navicula against footwear as the foot and boney swelling grows. The cause of persistent local pain such as inadequate bony resection, scar pain, irritation of the tibialis posterior tendon, and so forth should be sought and addressed; management will depend on the specific presentation and previous procedure performed. The cause of the ongoing pain should be investigated.

Patients with a preexisting hindfoot deformity, who undergo resection (with or without soft tissue interposition) of a tarsal coalition, may present with recurrent pain and worsening planovalgus deformity. This is due to the secondary effect of soft tissue contractures (lateral ligaments, peroneal tendons, calf muscles) "pulling" the foot into more valgus. Physiotherapy and insoles may help some patients. Depending on the flexibility of the hindfoot and the presence or otherwise of joint degeneration, joint-preserving corrective procedures or corrective joint fusions may be needed. Gastrocnemius, Achilles, and/or peroneal tendon releases may be required, to avoid equinus or further recurrence.

Osteomyelitis of the foot and ankle is a common, potentially devastating condition with diagnostic and treatment challenges. Understanding the epidemiology and pathogenesis of osteomyelitis can raise clinical suspicion and guide testing and treatments. History and physical examination, laboratory studies, vascular studies, histologic and microbiologic analyses, and various imaging modalities contribute to diagnosis and treatment. Treatment including empiric broad-spectrum antibiotics and surgery should take a multidisciplinary approach to optimize patient factors, ensure eradication of the infection, and restore function. Optimization of vascular status, soft tissues, limb biomechanics, and physiologic state of the patient must be considered to accelerate and ensure healing.

FOOT AND ANKLE CLINICS

NOW AVAILABLE FOR YOUR iPhone and iPad

Preface

Managing Complications of Foot and Ankle Surgery

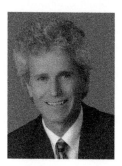

J. Chris Coetzee, MD
Editor

This issue of *Foot and Ankle Clinics of North America* is dedicated to the management of complications in foot and ankle surgery.

Complications are never easy to talk about, but it is an integral part of any surgeon's practice. I am convinced that 90% of the mental energy spent in my practice is worrying about my own patients with complications and trying to figure out how best to deal with the problem at hand.

I am not sure if it is due to the personality of surgeons, or maybe the fear of being ridiculed, or in no small measure, the fear of litigation, but discussion and management of complications in the literature are amazingly sparse.

I would therefore like to personally thank all the contributors to this publication for doing a remarkable job in shedding light on how to deal with some of the more common complications that we see. I know that there is not a lot of literature about these problems, so I asked highly experienced surgeons to step out of their comfort zone and give us advice on how to manage these problems.

Moving forward, I would like to challenge researchers, young and old, to publish their complications and how they dealt with them. I am more interested in the 5% to 10% of patients that did not do well with a given procedure than the 90% to 95% that did well. They do not need ongoing care; it is the failures that need attention. Hopefully, this issue of *Foot and Ankle Clinics of North America* might convince more people to share their experiences and knowledge about dealing with complications.

On that note, the AOFAS has a biannual Complications Course that is probably the most intense, compact, and dynamic encounter that any surgeon could hope for. It is highly recommended to attend.

Foot Ankle Clin N Am 19 (2014) xiii–xiv
http://dx.doi.org/10.1016/j.fcl.2014.06.017
1083-7515/14/$ – see front matter © 2014 Published by Elsevier Inc.

foot.theclinics.com

Finally, I would like to thank my childhood friend, and longtime wife, for supporting me for so many years in everything I do. She makes complications of any sort easier to live with!

J. Chris Coetzee, MD
Minnesota Orthopedic Sports Medicine Institute
at Twin Cities Orthopedics
4010 West 65th Street
Edina, MN 55435, USA
Website: http://www.tcomn.com

E-mail address:
jcc@tcomn.com

if the radiograph shows excessive loosening and osteophyte around the implant (a radiographic "failure"), yet the patient was quite satisfied until an acute change, that patient might be just fine with an excision only (**Fig. 1**).

FIRST MTP ARTHRODESIS

- With a failed MTP implant, conversion to fusion will give the most predictable result. Fusion is an appropriate option for any failed MTP implant and is especially appropriate for the patient who was never satisfied with the implant arthroplasty from the beginning.
- When an MTP implant is removed, there will be some degree of bone loss. If the full metatarsal head is preserved (with a failed hemiarthroplasty of the proximal phalanx), direct fusion of the phalanx to the metatarsal is possible without structural graft. However, in a total joint arthroplasty, or whenever there is any significant loss of first metatarsal length, an interposition graft is needed to restore first ray length. If the ray is fused short, transfer metatarsalgia will be a problem.
- It is difficult to obtain union on both sides of a structural graft. Allograft bone is easily available, but it is relatively expensive and may have a lower union rate. Autograft traditionally is harvested from the iliac crest and may carry some morbidity and inconvenience. It is possible to harvest an adequate structural graft from the proximal tibial metaphysis (**Fig. 2** and see later discussion).

PREOPERATIVE PLANNING

- Even if there is no sign or suspicion for infection, it is a good idea to obtain an erythrocyte sedimentation rate and a C-reactive protein level test before surgery for a failed MTP implant.
- If there is some suspicion for infection, joint aspiration for culture can be performed.

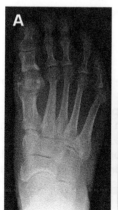
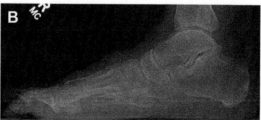

Fig. 1. (A) This 67-year-old man underwent first MTP arthroplasty 7 years ago with a hinged rubber prosthesis. He was completely satisfied with his function, with no pain, until a couple months ago, when he developed increasing pain and swelling of the joint. Note on the anteroposterior view, the implant, which has subsided well into the cortex of the first metatarsal. (B) The patient was found at surgery to have an infection, probably acquired during a recent transient bacteremia. He was treated with an aggressive debridement and several weeks of antibiotics. The joint was treated with an excisional arthroplasty, with no attempt to place any interposition material. By 1 month after surgery, he felt as good as he had before the infection developed.

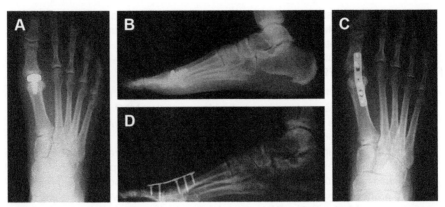

Fig. 2. (*A, B*) A 44-year-old woman had first metatarsal hemiarthroplasty for hallux rigidus. She had persistent pain in the joint from the beginning. (*C, D*) At revision surgery 2 years after arthroplasty, the implant was removed and the joint was fused with a small structural graft from the proximal tibia. A precontoured plate with low-profile screws held the fusion, and she healed by 3 months postoperatively. Newer models of dorsal plates have more options for screw placement than this linear plate.

- Weight-bearing radiographs should be obtained. If the first metatarsal will be much shorter than the second after implant removal, transfer metatarsalgia may be a problem; arthrodesis with an interposition bone graft is the most predictable solution.
- Dorsiflexion (elevation) of the first metatarsal can be appreciated on the lateral radiograph. Dorsiflexion could be due to previous osteotomies or may be present as metatarsus primus elevatus (an elevated first ray), one of the proposed causes of hallux rigidus. Plantarflexion of the first ray, through either an osteotomy or a fusion at the metatarsocuneiform joint, may be needed.
- MTP implants do not require brand-specific equipment to remove, but a selection of thin osteotomes may be helpful.

SURGICAL TECHNIQUE

- An ankle block, or other regional anesthesia, can be helpful for both intraoperative and postoperative anesthesia/analgesia.
- The patient is positioned supine, and the foot and potential bone graft site are prepared. With a thigh tourniquet, the entire leg can be prepared, including the proximal tibia for potential bone graft, as well as the iliac crest.
- The previous surgical incision is used. Most commonly, this will be dorsal, with deep dissection just medial to the extensor hallucis longus tendon. If the previous incision is dorsomedial, be careful to identify or at least not injure the dorsomedial cutaneous nerve, a terminal branch of the superficial peroneal. Painful neuromas can result.
- The joint capsule is opened longitudinally to facilitate later repair, and cultures should be taken as a routine.
- Removal of the previous implant is usually not too difficult. Frequently, the implant is not well fixed to the bone, so a bit of work with a thin osteotome can dislodge it. It may be trapped in fibrous tissue, so circumferential dissection at the edge of the implant is necessary.
- If performing an excisional arthroplasty, then the procedure is mostly done at this point. The ends of the bones can be gently contoured to a smooth surface, or a

ball of soft tissue ligament can be sewn in as an interposition graft. The author prefers to use no interposition material.

- When proceeding with arthrodesis, the bone ends are then prepared by removing any soft tissue. The ends are freshened up by perforating with a small drill after scraping with osteotomes and curettes. Removal of the implant will leave both the metatarsal and the phalanx with a concavity. The interposition graft will fit into the recess on both ends.
- The metatarsal often is healthy after debridement, but the proximal phalanx seems to have less intra-osseous blood flow in these cases. In the author's experience, nonunions (when they occur) tend to be at the graft-phalanx junction.
- The rough dimensions of the graft are then measured. The graft will need to be oblong, like a football, or possibly cubic. It is fairly easy to harvest a 1-cm cube of graft from the proximal lateral tibial metaphysis, just proximal to the anterior compartment musculature, and well distal to the knee joint. A 2- to 3-cm transverse skin incision is made, and the anterior compartment muscle is identified. By staying right at the top edge of the muscle, the surgeon can be sure not to violate the knee joint. A narrow saw blade defines the borders of the graft, and a narrow curved osteotome carves it out. The graft is unicortical, but the metaphyseal bone is usually fairly dense, and more cancellous graft can be harvested from the proximal tibia through the same hole.
- Grafts larger than 1 cm should probably come from the anterior iliac crest. An incision over the crest is made, and an effort should be made not to injure the lateral femoral cutaneous nerve, although it is difficult to identify and protect. The graft can be harvested from the inner table only or can include both tables to be tricortical. Alternately, iliac crest allograft can be used, but allograft may have a higher nonunion rate (not proven either way), and the nonunion rate is high enough with autograft.
- The graft is wedged into place in the first MTP joint, positioning the first toe in slight dorsiflexion. Although authors often cite 15° of extension, a useful trick is to place a flat object (perhaps a metal tray lid from the screw set) under the bottom of the foot. The proximal phalanx should sit a few millimeters above the flat surface, but not so high as to rub on shoes.
- It is smart to add some cancellous autograft at the ends of the structural graft. Then rigid fixation is achieved with a dorsal plate. There are many brands of first MTP fusion plates, often with small or mini screws. Some are locking plates. Many are lower profile than standard screws and plates, which may reduce the incidence of hardware prominence later.
- Because the plate is placed on the dorsal side of the joint, it is mechanically suboptimal; under weight-bearing, the joint is pushed into extension, and a dorsal plate is less able to resist deforming forces. Unfortunately, although a plantar plate is mechanically better, it is not feasible to place a plate on the plantar side. Intramedullary/intra-osseous fixation may be mechanically superior to dorsal bridging plates and may be used more in the future.
- Although technically difficult, a 3.5-mm screw can be placed before dorsal plate application from the plantar medial first metatarsal head, across the graft, and into the proximal phalanx. It often may not be possible to place this screw.
- Following fixation and intraoperative imaging to confirm alignment, layered closure is performed. The joint capsule is closed to protect against dehiscence, and the skin is closed with careful technique. Leg elevation is emphasized for the first few weeks until wounds are sealed. To protect the fusion, the patient is kept non-weight-bearing on the leg for 8 to 10 weeks. Postoperative computed

tomographic scanning may be more accurate than traditional radiographs for assessing healing.

OUTCOMES

- Several studies have shown successful fusion rates from 80% to 100%.[4–7]
- Nonunions can be treated with cancellous bone graft and revision plate application, or possibly lag screws.
- A common complication is prominent dorsal hardware, but the plate should not be removed until there is adequate incorporation of the graft.
- Wound dehiscence and secondary infection of the graft are a difficult problem. Perhaps the best strategy is careful soft tissue closure at fusion surgery. If the wound dehisces, the plate and structural graft will usually be exposed and secondarily infected.
- Although it might be possible to treat with local wound care and suppressive antibiotics, it probably is most effective to remove the plate and any nonviable graft bone and treat similar to an infected prosthesis, as outlined above (excision vs antibiotic-cement spacer with plan for revision fusion with graft).

REFERENCES

1. Cracchiolo A 3rd, Swanson A, Swanson GD. The arthritic great toe metatarsophalangeal joint: a review of flexible silicone implant arthroplasty from two medical centers. Clin Orthop Relat Res 1981;(157):64–9.
2. Kampner SL. Total joint prosthetic arthroplasty of the great toe–a 12-year experience. Foot Ankle 1984;4(5):249–61.
3. Raikin SM, Ahmad J, Pour AE, et al. Comparison of arthrodesis and metallic hemiarthroplasty of the hallux metatarsophalangeal joint. J Bone Joint Surg Am 2007; 89(9):1979–85.
4. Brodsky JW, Ptaszek AJ, Morris SG. Salvage first MTP arthrodesis utilizing ICBG: clinical evaluation and outcome. Foot Ankle Int 2000;21(4):290–6.
5. Hecht PJ, Gibbons MJ, Wapner KL, et al. Arthrodesis of the first metatarsophalangeal joint to salvage failed silicone implant arthroplasty. Foot Ankle Int 1997;18(7): 383–90.
6. Machacek F Jr, Easley ME, Gruber F, et al. Salvage of the failed Keller resection arthroplasty. Surgical technique. J Bone Joint Surg Am 2005;87(Suppl 1(Pt 1)): 86–94.
7. Myerson MS, Schon LC, McGuigan FX, et al. Result of arthrodesis of the hallux metatarsophalangeal joint using bone graft for restoration of length. Foot Ankle Int 2000;21(4):297–306.

Pain After Cheilectomy of the First Metatarsophalangeal Joint

Diagnosis and Management

Matthew Tomlinson, MBChB, FRACS

KEYWORDS

- Hallux rigidus • Cheilectomy • First metatarsophalangeal joint • Complications
- Postoperative pain • Revision surgery • First metatarsophalangeal arthrodesis

KEY POINTS

- Significant postoperative pain occurs in about 10% of patients after cheilectomy.
- Inadequate resection of bone can lead to ongoing symptoms.
- Care should be taken to avoid injury to cutaneous nerves to the great toe during surgery.
- Progression of osteoarthritis occurs in most patients and can lead to ongoing pain.
- When ongoing pain occurs owing to progression of arthritis, arthrodesis is the procedure of choice based on current evidence.
- If transfer metatarsalgia occurs, gait rehabilitation and offloading insoles may help.
- Patients should be counseled preoperatively on the risks of postoperative pain and the possible need for revision surgery after cheilectomy.

INTRODUCTION

Dorsal cheilectomy for osteoarthritis of the first metatarsophalangeal joint (MTPJ; hallux rigidus) was first described by Nilsonne[1] in 1930. Only 2 cases were reported and only temporary relief of symptoms was noted. Similarly, Bonney and MacNab[2] found disappointing results in the 9 patients in their series. It was not until 1959 that DuVries[3] described a comprehensive procedure that combined debridement of the first MTPJ utilizing a dorsal approach with synovectomy, debridement of all loose bodies and osteophytes on both sides of the joint and a capsular release.

This type of procedure offers theoretic advantages over other operative procedures for hallux rigidus such as fusion or joint replacement because of its relative simplicity

Disclosure: The authors have nothing to disclose.
Department of Orthopaedic Surgery, Mercy Ascot Hospitals, Counties Manukau Health, Private Bag 93311, Otahuhu, Auckland, New Zealand
E-mail address: mtomlinson@middlemore.co.nz

Foot Ankle Clin N Am 19 (2014) 349–360
http://dx.doi.org/10.1016/j.fcl.2014.06.002
1083-7515/14/$ – see front matter © 2014 Elsevier Inc. All rights reserved.

foot.theclinics.com

and its ability to maintain or increase joint range of motion, but without the need for a long period of immobilization or limited weight bearing. Other perceived advantages are the maintenance of relatively normal joint structure and function and the relative ease of conversion to other procedures such as fusion or arthroplasty in the event of failure or ongoing pain.[4–9]

Further to the development of isolated cheilectomy as a treatment method, Bonney and MacNab[2] and Moberg[10] have described the use of a dorsal closing wedge osteotomy of the proximal phalanx that can be used in combination with a cheilectomy to try and improve dorsiflexion range of motion.

More recently, arthroscopic[11,12] or percutaneous[13] debridement techniques have been described, although sufficient numbers of patients have not yet been analyzed to make any firm conclusions as to whether the less invasive techniques offer any significant advantages over traditional open techniques.

Recently, a number of studies have attempted to analyze the results of cheilectomy with or without proximal phalangeal osteotomy as reported in the literature and generally high rates of patient satisfaction and improved function have been noted.[8,14–16] McNeil and assocaites[16] performed an evidence-based analysis of the efficacy for operative treatment of hallux rigidus and out of 135 published articles found a lack of quality, level I, randomized, controlled trials on which to base treatment recommendations. There was poor evidence (grade C) in support of cheilectomy as well as most other treatment methods. Only first metatarsophalangeal (MTP) arthrodesis achieved a grade B recommendation. Roukis[14] performed a systematic review of isolated cheilectomy by analyzing the available literature and found an overall revision rate of 8.8% of 706 cheilectomies. In a separate review, the same author looked at articles describing the results of cheilectomy performed in association with a Moberg proximal phalangeal osteotomy and found an overall revision rate of 4.8% in 374 cheilectomies.[15] Of the reviewed studies, the authors noted that the methodology was generally poor, with most studies providing only level II or in most cases level IV evidence for treatment recommendations.

Currently, the most accepted and widely used classification of hallux rigidus is the Coughlin-Shurnas classification,[7] which includes radiologic degrees of osteoarthritis combined with subjective clinical findings including the presence or absence of mid range pain and joint range of motion (**Table 1**).

The degree of arthritic change in the first MTPJ that can be managed with cheilectomy with or without proximal phalangeal osteotomy remains controversial; some authors recommend the surgery for only Coughlin-Shurnas grade I and II disease,[6,17–20] but others for more severe grades of the disease.[7,21–23]

Many causes of persistent pain after cheilectomy have been described. It should be noted that not all patients with persistent pain go on to have revision surgery such as a fusion,[18] some opting to live with the pain or seek nonoperative treatment. Revision rates therefore may not accurately reflect the number of patients with persisting pain.

Although the success rate of cheilectomy has been shown to be in the order of 72% to 90%, Harrison and coworkers[18] found that pain scores improved in only 59% of their patients as measured on the Manchester-Oxford Foot questionnaire score, a part-specific outcome score that assesses foot pain and function.[24] According to the review of cheilectomy plus proximal phalangeal osteotomy done by Roukis,[15] pain was completely relieved in only 24.6% of patients, improved in 64.6% and unchanged or worse in 10.8% of procedures.

Described causes of persistent pain after cheilectomy include progression of osteoarthritis,[6,7,17,21] persistent dorsal impingement,[25] over-resection and instability,[25]

Table 1
Coughlin–Shurnas grading system for hallux rigidus (both radiographic and clinical findings)

Grade	Dorsiflexion	Radiographic Findings*	Clinical Findings
0	40°–60° and/or 10%–20% loss compared with normal side	Normal	No pain; only stiffness and loss of motion on examination
1	30°–40° and/or 20%–50% loss compared with normal side	Dorsal osteophyte is main finding, minimal joint space narrowing, minimal periarticular sclerosis, minimal flattening of metatarsal head	Mild or occasional pain and stiffness, pain at extremes of dorsiflexion and/or plantar flexion on examination
2	10°–30° and/or 50%–75% loss compared with normal side	Dorsal, lateral, and possibly medial osteophytes giving flattened appearance to metatarsal head, no more than one quarter of the dorsal joint space involved on lateral radiograph, mild-to-moderate joint space narrowing and sclerosis, sesamoids not usually involved	Moderate-to-severe pain and stiffness that may be constant; pain occurs just before maximum dorsiflexion and maximum plantarflexion on examination
3	≤10° and/or 75%–100% loss compared with normal side; notable loss of metatarsophalangeal plantarflexion as well (often ≤10° of plantar flexion)	Same as in grade 2, but with substantial narrowing, possibly periarticular cystic changes, more than one quarter of the dorsal joint space involved on lateral radiograph, sesamoids enlarged and/ or cystic and/or irregular	Nearly constant pain and substantial stiffness at extremes of range of motion but not mid range
4	Same as in grade 3	Same as in grade 3	Same as grade 3 but there is definite pain at mid range of passive motion

* Weight bearing and anteroposterior and lateral radiographs are used.
From Coughlin MJ, Shurnas PS. Hallux rigidus. Grading and long-term results of operative treatment. J Bone Joint Surg Am 2003;85:2072–88.

chondrolysis,[7] avascular necrosis of the metatarsal head,[26] recurrence of dorsal osteophyte,[5,6,17] delayed wound healing,[27,28] postoperative infection,[7,17,21,29] symptomatic implants,[21] dysesthesia of the dorsal medial cutaneous nerve,[13,17,28,30] delayed union or nonunion of a proximal phalangeal osteotomy, painful arthritis of the hallux interphalangeal joint (IPJ),[31] reflex sympathetic dystrophy,[6] second metatarsalgia,[21,30] and deep venous thrombosis.[21] The most common causes of revision surgery seem to be persistent pain owing to failure of the cheilectomy procedure to relieve the painful joint and progression of osteoarthritis. Technical considerations are also important with both under-resection and over-resection potentially leading to ongoing problems. Further damage to the articular surface at the time of surgery may also lead to accelerated arthritic change.

FAILURE TO RELIEVE SYMPTOMS

Early failure of cheilectomy despite an adequate resection can lead to a lack of relief of first MTP joint pain from the time of surgery and the need for early revision surgery. Some authors have noted a higher rate of failure in patients with higher grades of disease,[7,25] whereas others have not[9,17,21] and pain does not necessarily correlate with radiographic severity.[6] Coughlin and Shurnas[7] have described 2 cases of unexpected and rapid chondrolysis within 1 year of surgery after cheilectomy. Both cases were revised to an arthrodesis.

The use of antiinflammatory medications, analgesics, and intraarticular steroid injections after cheilectomy has not been studied, but it would seem justified to try pharmacologic treatments before considering revision surgery, while hoping for ongoing symptoms to improve.

Several authors have recognized that patients who have mid range pain on clinical examination (Coughlin-Shurnas grade 4) are more likely to require revision to a fusion[7,17] and on that basis recommend fusion as the surgical treatment of choice from the beginning rather than performing a cheilectomy. O'Malley and colleagues,[21] however, showed in their review that the addition of a proximal phalangeal osteotomy gave acceptable results, even in grade 4 disease. Until a prospective, randomised, comparative trial is performed, the question of proximal phalangeal osteotomy will remain unanswered. Patients whose pain is not relieved by cheilectomy and who require early revision to a fusion can be disappointed at the need for a second procedure and all patients undergoing cheilectomy should be warned of the possibility of requiring a second procedure if the cheilectomy is unsuccessful (Fig. 1).

If an arthrodesis is required relatively early after unsuccessful cheilectomy, lack of bone stock can be an issue, particularly if a generous cheilectomy has been performed at the index procedure. The usual recommendation for resection of the dorsal metatarsal head is 25% to 30%. If 30% or more of the joint surface has been resected, there is less bone stock available for achieving a successful arthrodesis and surgeons should consider the need for more stable fixation, such as a dorsal first MTP fusion plate[32] and supplementary bone grafting. Bone graft can be readily harvested from

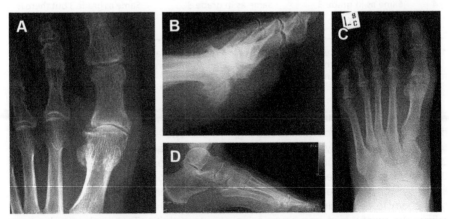

Fig. 1. (*A, B*) Anteroposterior, lateral preoperative x-rays. (*C, D*) Postcheilectomy weight-bearing x-rays at 10 months. Coughlin grade 3 hallux rigidus treated with cheilectomy. The patient had no relief of pain and underwent revision to a fusion at 13 months. Bone resection was not sufficient and was less than 25% of the joint surface.

the calcaneus[33] or proximal tibia[34] for this purpose. Loss of bone stock may also make implant arthroplasty difficult or impossible.

The time it takes for symptoms to settle after cheilectomy varies.[5] Some patients have almost complete relief of symptoms within a very short period of time and can return to a wide range of activities within a few weeks, but others require much longer for symptoms to resolve and more time for rehabilitation. It is essential that patients suffering pain after cheilectomy be given an adequate amount of time for the pain to settle before revision surgery is recommended to allow postoperative inflammation to resolve. This process can take up to 1 year.

PROGRESSION OF OSTEOARTHRITIS

Most authors recognize that progression of osteoarthritis occurs in patients with hallux rigidus despite cheilectomy.[7,9,17,23,25,35–38] This does not necessarily correlate with poor clinical outcomes, because many patients with progression of osteoarthritis still report satisfactory outcomes after cheilectomy.[6] If osteoarthritis does progress over time and symptoms become severe again, the same treatment options are available for a revision procedure as were available for the index procedure; that is, patients can be treated with either a fusion, an arthroplasty, or a repeat cheilectomy, depending on clinical and radiologic findings. The results of repeat cheilectomy are not well-documented,[39] but anecdotally patients can be significantly improved (**Fig. 2**).

More commonly, progression of arthritis leads to an indication for an arthrodesis, because stiffness becomes a significant issue and cheilectomy and arthroplasty are less likely to be effective when the first MTP joint has a very limited range of motion. In studies with longer term follow-up, the incidence of conversion from cheilectomy to arthrodesis ranges from 0% to 25%[6,7,9,21,22,40] and up to 62.5% of patients with grade 4 disease.[7] Arthrodesis was the only intervention for hallux rigidus that received a B grade treatment recommendation in the recent evidence based analysis by McNeil

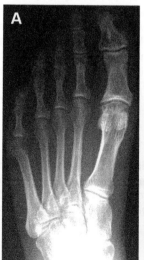
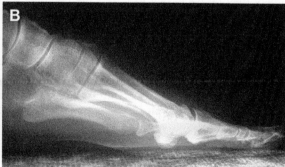

Fig. 2. (*A, B*) At 8 years after cheilectomy for hallux rigidus, a dorsal osteophyte has formed again. The patient has an above-the-knee amputation of the contralateral limb and depends on motion of the metatarsophalangeal joint for ambulation. A revision cheilectomy was performed and a good clinical outcome was achieved.

and colleagues,[16] with other types of surgery receiving only C grade recommendations based on current literature.

Other procedures described for the treatment of progressive arthritis after cheilectomy include Keller arthroplasty,[25,31,37] implant arthroplasty,[25,37,41–43] and insertion of a silastic implant.[25,43] Keller arthroplasty provides an alternative to arthrodesis in patients who are more elderly or who would have difficulty with limited weight bearing owing to comorbidities, although patients considering a Keller arthroplasty should be counseled about the risks of cock-up toe deformity and transfer metatarsalgia. The role of implant arthroplasty has not been fully elucidated in the setting of revision of a cheilectomy and long-term results are unknown.

INFECTION

Pain owing to infection after cheilectomy is uncommon. Deep infection after cheilectomy in the form of septic arthritis or osteomyelitis is rare. Brodsky and associates[29] described 1 case treated successfully with debridement, antibiotics, and arthrodesis utilizing an interpositional, autologous iliac crest bone graft. Superficial infection has been described by a number of authors and the incidence can be expected to be in the order of 6% to 8%.[7,17,21] Superficial infections and delayed wound healing can be expected to respond to appropriate, systemic antibiotic administration and local wound care.

NERVE INJURY

A number of different approaches have been described for cheilectomy of the first MTPJ, including most commonly the dorsal,[7,9,19,23,36,44] dorsomedial,[6,21] and medial approaches.[17,35] The dorsal medial cutaneous branch of the superficial peroneal nerve is vulnerable to injury with all of these approaches and should be protected during surgery (**Fig. 3**). The dorsomedial approach to the first MTPJ is the most likely approach to lead to damage of this nerve.[45] Dysesthesia in this nerve is not uncommon after cheilectomy although, provided the nerve is intact, it usually recovers. Large osteophytes over the dorsal aspect of the first MTPJ may cause pressure symptoms of this nerve branch even preoperatively and care should be taken when resecting osteophytes not to damage the nerve. The deep peroneal nerve branches to the first web space can also be vulnerable in a similar fashion. If these nerve branches are damaged or transected, a painful neuroma can form and if symptoms do not resolve surgery may be necessary to resect the neuroma and bury the nerve in bone or muscle.[46]

IPJ ARTHRITIS

IPJ arthritis is relatively common in patients with hallux rigidus because of increased load placed across the joint as a result of stiffness of the first MTPJ. Symptoms in the IPJ may persist after cheilectomy,[31] although in general terms cheilectomy would be expected to have a protective effect on the IPJ compared with fusion because of the greater postoperative range of motion.

TRANSFER METATARSALGIA

Lateral weight transfer can occur as a result of any painful condition affecting the hallux, because the patient subconsciously or consciously avoids weight bearing through the painful area of the toe. Transfer metatarsalgia is therefore a possible preoperative symptom in patients being treated for hallux rigidus.[28] Relief of pain

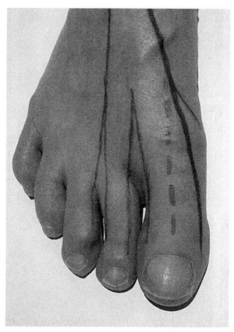

Fig. 3. The dorsal medial cutaneous branch of the superficial peroneal nerve (position indicated by the *solid line* medially on the toe) is vulnerable to injury during approaches to the first metatarsophalangeal joint. The position of the incision for a dorsal approach is indicated by the *dashed line*.

postoperatively should result in improvement of transfer metatarsalgia symptoms, but if pain persists postoperatively then transfer symptoms may persist or develop anew. Many patients will walk more toward the lateral side of the foot after surgery to protect the surgical site and if this habit is not corrected with rehabilitation techniques, transfer metatarsalgia may develop (**Fig. 4**).

Any shortening or elevation of the first ray may also lead to transfer metatarsalgia, particularly in patients who have a short first ray or a long second or third ray.[47] Shortening does not normally occur after cheilectomy, but care should be taken to avoid any shortening or elevation of the first ray if additional procedures such as proximal phalangeal osteotomy are performed.

SESAMOIDITIS

Sesamoiditis can occur in patients with hallux rigidus as a result of osteoarthritis of the sesamoid–first metatarsal articulation or in patients with a dorsiflexed first MTPJ as a result of painful inhibition of plantar flexion of the joint. Activation of the windlass mechanism leads to increased point loading through the sesamoid area. Dorsiflexion of the first MTPJ is not as common as lack of dorsiflexion, but can occur in patients who have central cartilage lesions rather than dorsal lesions. Postoperative sesamoiditis can occur for similar reasons, as noted by O'Malley and colleagues.[21]

SYMPTOMS RELATED TO PROXIMAL PHALANGEAL OSTEOTOMY

Nonunion, delayed union,[27] and symptomatic implants[21] can all lead to persistent symptoms after proximal phalangeal osteotomy, which some authors recommend in

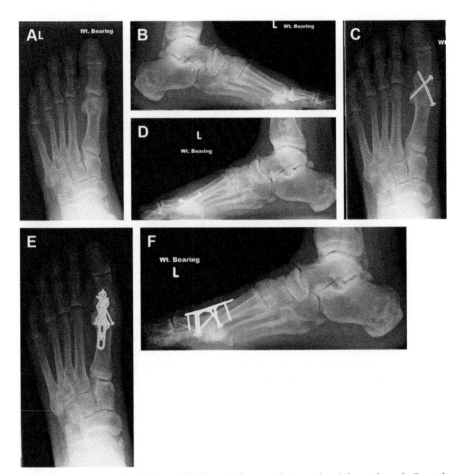

Fig. 4. (*A–F*) This man had bilateral hallux rigidus, grade 4 on the right and grade 3 on the left. He underwent successful fusion on the right side and cheilectomy on the left that never relieved his pain despite good postoperative analgesia and rehabilitation. After 8 months, he elected to proceed with arthrodesis. He developed a nonunion requiring revision and bone grafting. The joint fused but he has ongoing dysesthesia in the dorsal medial cutaneous nerve and transfer metatarsalgia.

association with cheilectomy.[21,30,43] A dorsal closing wedge osteotomy can provide an increase in dorsiflexion of the great toe, although this occurs at the expense of plantar flexion.[21] The role of proximal phalangeal osteotomy remains controversial, but Roukis found a relatively low rate of revision (4.8%) in the 11 studies included in his review.[15] More recently, O'Malley and colleagues[21] analyzed 81 patients with advanced hallux rigidus after cheilectomy with proximal phalangeal osteotomy with a minimum of 2 years follow-up. Thirty-one toes were graded as grade 3 and 50 as grade 4. Sixty-nine patients (85.25%) were either satisfied or very satisfied with the procedure whereas 12 patients (14.8%) were dissatisfied. The reasons for dissatisfaction were not fully explained, but 4 patients underwent eventual fusion at between 1 and 7 years postoperatively.

It seems likely, therefore, that the addition of a proximal phalangeal dorsal closing wedge osteotomy to the cheilectomy procedure may improve dorsiflexion range of motion, but it may also increase the possibility of complications in relation to the procedure. High-quality, prospective, comparative studies between cheilectomy alone and cheilectomy with proximal phalangeal osteotomy are lacking and so a firm treatment recommendation cannot be made at present.

OTHER CAUSES OF PAIN

Reflex sympathetic dystrophy (chronic regional pain syndrome) can occur after any limb surgery and the cheilectomy procedure is no exception.[6,48] When a nerve injury is present, symptoms may be very difficult to control and consultation with a specialist pain service is recommended. Burying of the involved nerve may be necessary to control symptoms.

Avascular necrosis of the metatarsal head is a rare complication of cheilectomy. Brosky and colleagues[26] described the case of a 51-year-old man treated 1 year after isolated cheilectomy for hallux rigidus with an arthrodesis using calcaneal bone graft and a bone substitute with stem cells.

TREATMENT RECOMMENDATIONS

To minimize the possibility of a poor result after cheilectomy, patients should be screened clinically and radiographically to ensure that cheilectomy is the appropriate procedure. Patients who have severe joint stiffness and mid range pain clinically, or where there is gross destruction of the normal joint architecture, are not suitable candidates for cheilectomy. Several technical considerations should be taken into account during the cheilectomy procedure. An approach should be used that minimizes the chance of damage to the peripheral nerve branches to the toe and either a dorsal or medial approach is safest. There is insufficient evidence to recommend a percutaneous or arthroscopic approach at this stage, but these techniques show promise and may reduce the incidence of pain and stiffness postoperatively. Adequate resection of bone, usually down to the level of intact articular cartilage but not exceeding 30% of the joint surface, is advisable. Osteophytes should be debrided from the joint margins on the metatarsal head and base of the proximal phalanx and consideration should be given to drilling or microfracture of central cartilage lesions below the level of the osseous resection.

Patients should be counseled before surgery on the possibility of ongoing symptoms and the possible need for revision surgery, either in the short or long term. If patients have an expectation that revision surgery may be required, they are more likely to accept a poor outcome after cheilectomy and the need for a second procedure.

Postoperatively, adequate pain relief, elevation of the limb, and early gentle range of motion exercises are likely to reduce the incidence of early recurrent pain and stiffness. After wound healing, a graduated return-to-function program can be instituted with an emphasis on return of motion range and normal heel–toe walking pattern.

If pain becomes a significant issue after the procedure, it is important for the treating surgeon to determine the likely cause of the pain. Infection, nerve injury, and mechanical factors such as seamoiditis and metatarsalgia can be diagnosed through appropriate examination and investigations and treated as necessary. If mechanical causes of pain such as transfer metatarsalgia are identified, orthotic management is appropriate initially.

Persistent pain owing to failure of the operation to relieve pain or progression of arthritis can be managed initially with a stiff-soled shoe and analgesic or antiinflammatory medication. Intraarticular steroid injection is another possibility at this time, but evidence is lacking for its efficacy.

Reassurance that symptoms may settle with time can be given and provided that symptoms do settle this approach can be continued. If symptoms worsen with time, particularly after 6 to 12 months, it is unlikely that resolution of symptoms will occur. In these circumstances, arthrodesis can be offered as an alternative treatment, particularly if stiffness is an additional problem. For late recurrence of dorsal osteophytes, a revision cheilectomy can be considered as an alternative to arthrodesis if some joint motion and radiographic joint space remain. If there is significant involvement of the IPJ with associated stiffness of that joint, alternatives to arthrodesis such as joint replacement arthroplasty or Keller procedure can be considered, although evidence is lacking to support the use of these techniques.

SUMMARY

Despite the relatively good results that are reported for cheilectomy for hallux rigidus, a significant proportion of patients have ongoing pain after the procedure. Symptoms may settle with time, but if they do not the treating surgeon must consider the likely causes of persistent symptoms and treat the patient accordingly, with a combination of medications, special shoes, or orthotic devices and appropriate rehabilitation therapy. If symptoms persist in the longer term, further surgery may be necessary in the form of an arthrodesis or arthroplasty. Arthrodesis is the most reliable salvage procedure for pain relief and restoration of function under most circumstances. Patients should be warned of that possibility before the index procedure.

REFERENCES

1. Nilsonne H. Hallux rigidus and its treatment. Acta Orthop Scand 1930;1:295–303.
2. Bonney G, Macnab I. Hallux valgus and hallux rigidus: a critical survey of operative results. J Bone Joint Surg Br 1952;34B(3):366–85.
3. Duvries H. Surgery of the foot. Philadelphia: Mosby; 1959.
4. Yee G, Lau J. Current concepts review: hallux rigidus. Foot Ankle Int 2008;29(6): 637–46.
5. Mann RA, Clanton TO. Hallux rigidus: treatment by cheilectomy. J Bone Joint Surg Am 1988;70(3):400–6.
6. Mulier T, Steenwerckx A, Thienpont E, et al. Results after cheilectomy in athletes with hallux rigidus. Foot Ankle Int 1999;20(4):232–7.
7. Coughlin MJ, Shurnas PS. Hallux rigidus. Grading and long-term results of operative treatment. J Bone Joint Surg Am 2003;85A(11):2072–88.
8. Deland JT, Williams BR. Surgical management of hallux rigidus. J Am Acad Orthop Surg 2012;20(6):347–58.
9. Feltham GT, Hanks SE, Marcus RE. Age-based outcomes of cheilectomy for the treatment of hallux rigidus. Foot Ankle Int 2001;22(3):192–7.
10. Moberg E. A simple operation for hallux rigidus. Clin Orthop Relat Res 1979;(142):55–6.
11. Iqbal MJ, Chana GS. Arthroscopic cheilectomy for hallux rigidus. Arthroscopy 1998;14(3):307–10.
12. Debnath UK, Hemmady MV, Hariharan K. Indications for and technique of first metatarsophalangeal joint arthroscopy. Foot Ankle Int 2006;27(12):1049–54.
13. Mesa-Ramos M, Mesa-Ramos F, Carpintero P. Evaluation of the treatment of hallux rigidus by percutaneous surgery. Acta Orthop Belg 2008;74(2):222–6.
14. Roukis TS. The need for surgical revision after isolated cheilectomy for hallux rigidus: a systematic review. J Foot Ankle Surg 2010;49(5):465–70.

15. Roukis TS. Outcomes after cheilectomy with phalangeal dorsiflexory osteotomy for hallux rigidus: a systematic review. J Foot Ankle Surg 2010;49(5):479–87.
16. McNeil DS, Baumhauer JF, Glazebrook MA. Evidence-based analysis of the efficacy for operative treatment of hallux rigidus. Foot Ankle Int 2013;34(1):15–32.
17. Easley ME, Davis WH, Anderson RB. Intermediate to long-term follow-up of medial-approach dorsal cheilectomy for hallux rigidus. Foot Ankle Int 1999; 20(3):147–52.
18. Harrison T, Fawzy E, Dinah F, et al. Prospective assessment of dorsal cheilectomy for hallux rigidus using a patient-reported outcome score. J Foot Ankle Surg 2010;49(3):232–7.
19. Geldwert JJ, Rock GD, McGrath MP, et al. Cheilectomy: still a useful technique for grade I and grade II hallux limitus/rigidus. J Foot Surg 1992;31(2):154–9.
20. Lau JT, Daniels TR. Outcomes following cheilectomy and interpositional arthroplasty in hallux rigidus. Foot Ankle Int 2001;22(6):462–70.
21. O'Malley MJ, Basran HS, Gu Y, et al. Treatment of advanced stages of hallux rigidus with cheilectomy and phalangeal osteotomy. J Bone Joint Surg Am 2013; 95(7):606–10.
22. Bussewitz BW, Dyment MM, Hyer CF. Intermediate-term results following first metatarsal cheilectomy. Foot Ankle Spec 2013;6(3):191–5.
23. Mackay DC, Blyth M, Rymaszewski LA. The role of cheilectomy in the treatment of hallux rigidus. J Foot Ankle Surg 1997;36(5):337–40.
24. Dawson J, Coffey J, Doll H, et al. A patient-based questionnaire to assess outcomes of foot surgery: validation in the context of surgery for hallux valgus. Qual Life Res 2006;15(7):1211–22.
25. Hattrup SJ, Johnson KA. Subjective results of hallux rigidus following treatment with cheilectomy. Clin Orthop Relat Res 1988;(226):182–91.
26. Brosky TA 2nd, Menke CR, Xenos D. Reconstruction of the first metatarsophalangeal joint following post-cheilectomy avascular necrosis of the first metatarsal head: a case report. J Foot Ankle Surg 2009;48(1):61–9.
27. Wingenfeld C, Abbara-Czardybon M, Arbab D, et al. Cheilectomy and Kessel-Bonney procedure for treatment of initial hallux rigidus. Oper Orthop Traumatol 2008;20(6):484–91 [in German].
28. Waizy H, Czardybon MA, Stukenborg-Colsman C, et al. Mid- and long-term results of the joint preserving therapy of hallux rigidus. Arch Orthop Trauma Surg 2010;130(2):165–70.
29. Brodsky JW, Ptaszek AJ, Morris SG. Salvage first MTP arthrodesis utilizing ICBG: clinical evaluation and outcome. Foot Ankle Int 2000;21(4):290–6.
30. Blyth MJ, Mackay DC, Kinninmonth AW. Dorsal wedge osteotomy in the treatment of hallux rigidus. J Foot Ankle Surg 1998;37(1):8–10.
31. Kilmartin TE. Phalangeal osteotomy versus first metatarsal decompression osteotomy for the surgical treatment of hallux rigidus: a prospective study of age-matched and condition-matched patients. J Foot Ankle Surg 2005;44(1):2–12.
32. Flavin R, Stephens MM. Arthrodesis of the first metatarsophalangeal joint using a dorsal titanium contoured plate. Foot Ankle Int 2004;25(11):783–7.
33. Mahan KT. A new modified technique for harvest of calcaneal bone graft in surgery on the foot and ankle. Foot Ankle Int 1999;20(1):68.
34. Whitehouse MR, Lankester BJ, Winson IG, et al. Bone graft harvest from the proximal tibia in foot and ankle arthrodesis surgery. Foot Ankle Int 2006; 27(11):913–6.
35. Mann RA. Intermediate to long term follow-up of medial approach dorsal cheilectomy for hallux rigidus. Foot Ankle Int 2000;21(2):156.

36. Keogh P, Nagaria J, Stephens M. Cheilectomy for hallux rigidus. Ir J Med Sci 1992;161(12):681–3.
37. Beertema W, Draijer WF, van Os JJ, et al. A retrospective analysis of surgical treatment in patients with symptomatic hallux rigidus: long-term follow-up. J Foot Ankle Surg 2006;45(4):244–51.
38. Nawoczenski DA. Nonoperative and operative intervention for hallux rigidus. J Orthop Sports Phys Ther 1999;29(12):727–35.
39. Budhabhatti SP, Erdemir A, Petre M, et al. Finite element modeling of the first ray of the foot: a tool for the design of interventions. J Biomech Eng 2007;129(5): 750–6.
40. Nawoczenski DA, Ketz J, Baumhauer JF. Dynamic kinematic and plantar pressure changes following cheilectomy for hallux rigidus: a mid-term followup. Foot Ankle Int 2008;29(3):265–72.
41. Olms K, Dietze A. Replacement arthroplasty for hallux rigidus. 21 patients with a 2-year follow-up. Int Orthop 1999;23(4):240–3.
42. Pontell D, Gudas CJ. Retrospective analysis of surgical treatment of hallux rigidus/limitus: clinical and radiographic follow-up of hinged, silastic implant arthroplasty and cheilectomy. J Foot Surg 1988;27(6):503–10.
43. Thomas PJ, Smith RW. Proximal phalanx osteotomy for the surgical treatment of hallux rigidus. Foot Ankle Int 1999;20(1):3–12.
44. Mann RA, Coughlin MJ, DuVries HL. Hallux rigidus: a review of the literature and a method of treatment. Clin Orthop Relat Res 1979;(142):57–63.
45. Solan MC, Lemon M, Bendall SP. The surgical anatomy of the dorsomedial cutaneous nerve of the hallux. J Bone Joint Surg Br 2001;83(2):250–2.
46. Wagner E, Ortiz C. The painful neuroma and the use of conduits. Foot Ankle Clin 2011;16(2):295–304.
47. Morton D. The Human foot. New York: Hafner; 1935.
48. Harisboure A, Joveniaux P, Madi K, et al. The Valenti technique in the treatment of hallux rigidus. Orthop Traumatol Surg Res 2009;95(3):202–9.

Deceptions in Hallux Valgus

What to Look for to Limit Failures

Kyung Tai Lee, MD, PhD[a], Young Uk Park, MD, PhD[b],
Hyuk Jegal, MD[a], Thomas H. Lee, MD[c],*

KEYWORDS

- Hallux valgus • Complication • Failures • Prognosis

KEY POINTS

- The treatment of hallux valgus depends on multiple factors, including clinical examination, patient considerations, clinical findings, radiographic assessment, and surgeon preference.
- Appropriate procedure selection and proper technique will usually result in good-to-excellent outcomes. As with any procedure however, there are complications following hallux valgus correction. These commonly include recurrence, transfer metatarsalgia, avascular necrosis, hallux varus, and nonunion and malunion of metatarsal osteotomies.
- In order to decrease the risks of complication, a precise and meticulous physical examination should be conducted preoperatively, and it should assess for the presence of planovalgus deformity, tight heel cord, rigid or correctable hallux valgus, great toe pronation, corns or calluses of the lesser toes, second metatarsaophalangeal joint synovitis, interdigital neuromas, or first tarsometatarsal joint hypermobility.
- A surgeon should select appropriate osteotomies to correct complex hallux valgus deformities.
- As a general principle, the severity of deformity dictates treatment options. A distal chevron osteotomy provides predictable outcomes for mild and select cases of moderate hallux valgus.
- For more severe deformities, multiple proximal first metatarsal procedures, combined with a distal soft tissue procedure, appear to provide satisfactory treatment. These include proximal crescentic, proximal chevron, proximal oblique (Ludloff), proximal closing wedge, scarf osteotomies, and the Lapidus procedure.
- A surgeon should adhere to rigid bone principles to correct complex hallux valgus deformities.

Disclosure Statement: The authors have no disclosures related to this work.
[a] Foot and Ankle Service, KT Lee's Orthopedic Hospital, Seoul, Korea; [b] Division of Foot and Ankle Surgery, Department of Orthopaedic Surgery, Ajou University School of Medicine, 164 World Cup Road, Yeongtong-gu, Suwon, Gyeonggi-do 443-380, Republic of Korea; [c] Orthopedic Foot and Ankle Center, 300 Polaris Parkway, Suite 2000, Westerville, OH 43082, USA
* Corresponding author.
E-mail address: ofacresearch@orthofootankle.com

Foot Ankle Clin N Am 19 (2014) 361–370
http://dx.doi.org/10.1016/j.fcl.2014.06.003
1083-7515/14/$ – see front matter © 2014 Elsevier Inc. All rights reserved.

foot.theclinics.com

OVERVIEW

The correction of hallux valgus deformities is one of the most commonly performed foot and ankle procedures. The goal of operative treatment of hallux valgus is to correct all pathologic elements (hallux valgus, pronation of hallux, metatarsus primus varus, and protruded medial eminence) and yet maintain a biomechanically functional forefoot.[1–3] Successful treatment requires correcting bony alignment, restoring joint congruity, and balancing soft tissues.

Appropriate procedure selection and proper technique will usually result in good-to-excellent outcomes. As with any procedure, however, there are complications following hallux valgus correction, and complications rates from hallux valgus surgery ranges from 10% to 55%.[3] Common complications include recurrence of deformities, transfer metatarsalgia, avascular necrosis, hallux varus, and nonunion and malunion of metatarsal osteotomies. The treatment of hallux valgus depends on multiple factors, including clinical examination, patient considerations, radiographic assessment, and surgeon preference. Patients who have high distal metatarsal articular angle (DMAA), metatarsus adductus, pes planus, or hypermobility are at risk of surgical failure. Hence, treatment must be individualized to address each of these factors, and careful preoperative planning is needed to ensure that the chosen procedure is appropriate for each specific patient. Accurate clinical assessment of hypermobility of the first ray is difficult. Therefore, it should be diagnosed based on clinical or radiographic evidence. The measurement of this DMAA has significant inter- and intraobserver variation, and the valgus orientation of the joint is best assessed intraoperatively under direct vision.

In order to decrease the risks of complication, a precise and meticulous physical examination should be conducted preoperatively, and it should assess for the presence of planovalgus deformity, tight heel cord, rigid or correctable hallux valgus, great toe pronation, corns or calluses of the lesser toes, second metatarsaophalangeal (MTP) joint synovitis, interdigital neuromas, or first tarsometatarsal (TMT) joint hypermobility. A surgeon should select appropriate osteotomies and adhere to rigid bone principles to correct complex hallux valgus deformities.

This article focuses on common complications seen in hallux valgus correction and several points to be considered preoperatively and postoperatively in order to limit failures.

DIFFICULT HALLUX VALGUS

There are conflicting notions about the etiology of hallux valgus. Occupation, shoe wear, genetic predisposition, and pes planus have been implicated as causes of hallux valgus in adults.[4–6] Constricting footwear and high heel shoes are extrinsic factors considered important in the development of hallux valgus.[7,8] Heredity is likely to be a major predisposing factor in some patients, with up to 68% of patients having familial tendency.[9]

The Role of Pes Planus

The role of pes planus is complex. It is unlikely to be the initiating factor in hallux valgus, but progression of hallux valgus is more rapid in the presence of pes planus. This is particularly true in those patients with compromised medial joint capsule in rheumatoid arthritis, collagen deficiency, or a neuromuscular disorder. Scranton reported that 51% of his subjects had pes planus and suggested flatfoot deformity to be a predisposing factor for juvenile hallux valgus.[10] Kalen and Brecher reported that there was 8 to 24 times greater incidence of pes planus in adolescents with hallux valgus.[11] However, Mann and Coughlin found a very low incidence of advanced pes planus in adults with hallux valgus.[12] Some researchers stated that the presence of pes planus does not reduce the success rate of operations for hallux valgus.[4,5]

Hypermobility of the First TMT Joint

Some investigators[13,14] believe that hypermobility of the first TMT joint is a causative component in certain cases of hallux valgus. In these patients, a fusion of the first TMT joint (the Lapidus procedure) should be considered for surgical correction, as opposed to an osteotomy. There is a correlation between hypermobility of the first ray and hallux valgus, and a higher incidence of hypermobility at this site causes a hallux valgus deformity that is painful.[15,16] Accurate clinical assessment of hypermobility of the first ray is difficult. However, a recent cadaver study has shown that correction of hallux valgus deformity by a distal soft tissue procedure and a basal crescentic osteotomy significantly reduces hypermobility of the first ray,[17] implying that hypermobility maybe a secondary phenomenon in a different set of cases.

However, primary hypermobility of the TMT joint does exist. It should be diagnosed based on clinical or radiographic evidence. Clinically, hypermobility is evaluated by determining sagittal motion (the grasping test). Because of its saddle shape, sagittal movement should be dorsolateral and plantar medial. Identifying signs include the presence of a dorsal bunion, intractable plantar keratosis beneath the second metatarsal head, and arthritis of the first and second TMT joint. Radiographically, hypermobility is evaluated by measurements from the modified Coleman block test (for sagittal motion) and the radiographic squeeze test (for transverse motion) and by the identification of signs, such as cortical hypertrophy along the medial border of the second metatarsal shaft, a cuneiform split, a plantar gapping of the first TMT joint, the presence of os intermetatarseum, and the round shape and increased medial slope of the first TMT joint.[14]

Metatarsus Adductus

Metatarsus adductus (MA) has been cited as a cause of hallux valgus, particularly in the juvenile population, and it has been suggested that unrecognized MA deformity is a cause for recurrent HV deformity after surgery.[18,19] MA is described as a structural deformity occurring at the Lisfranc joint (TMT joints),[20] with the metatarsals being deviated medially in reference to the lesser tarsus.

Distal Metatarsal Articular Angle

The DMAA describes the magnitude of the lateral slope of the distal metatarsal articular surface in relation to the long axis of the first metatarsal. The DMAA was measured between the perpendicular and the long axis of the metatarsal and a line uniting the extreme ends (medial and lateral) of the distal metatarsal articular surface. The measurement of this angle has significant inter- and intraobserver variation, and the valgus orientation of the joint should be confirmed intraoperatively.[21] The normal DMAA averages 8°, and higher DMAAs lead to severe deformity of the hallux. On physical examination, it can be suspected when a notable reduction of mobility occurs on the first metatarsophalangeal joint (MTPJ) when the valgus deformity of the toe is manually corrected. Surgical correction of this type of hallux valgus needs special attention. Basal osteotomies have the potential to worsen the valgus orientation of the joint. With distal osteotomies, the typical lateral displacement of the metatarsal head will result in the hallux leaning against the second toe. If one forcefully realigns the hallux when using one of the previous methods, an incongruent joint will be produced.[5,22] In contrast, a double or triple osteotomy can be performed, which is a demanding, extensive and aggressive procedure. Another option is the chevron osteotomy with medial impaction, but this technique is impossible with hard bone and has minimal potential for correction.[23] A chevron osteotomy can also be used with an Akin operation, which aligns the toe, but the joint surface maintains a valgus orientation.[24] A surgical method that can correct the articular angle malposition would be ideal. To correct this angle, medial rotation of the metatarsal head in the horizontal plane must be made.

Theoretically, there is no change in the DMAA in displacement osteotomies like scarf and chevron. These osteotomies can correct only intermediate deformities, however. The scarf osteotomy can be rotated and displaced medially, leading to a limited correction of DMAA. While performing a chevron distal osteotomy of a minor deformity, the distal segment may easily be rotated medially and address the high DMAA.[25] In the presence of an abnormally high DMAA, a soft tissue realignment procedure may place the foot at risk for recurrence. A chevron osteotomy does not significantly realign the DMAA. Many such procedures are associated with significant postoperative recurrence in the presence of an increased DMAA. Correction of a congruous joint with an increased DMAA requires an extra-articular reconstruction. Thus, only an extra-articular correction, such as a double osteotomy, can effectively correct a hallux valgus angle with an increased DMAA.[4]

High DMAA, metatarsus adductus, pes planus, and hypermobility of first metatarsal are also highly associated with juvenile hallux valgus, and surgical intervention for juvenile hallux valgus is noted to have a high failure rate.[26–28] Therefore, patients who have these factors are at an increased risk of surgical failure, and the authors consider these patients to have difficult hallux valgus. Treatment must also be individualized to address each of these factors, and careful preoperative planning is needed to ensure that the chosen procedure is appropriate for each specific patient.

COMPLICATIONS IN HALLUX VALGUS CORRECTION
Recurrence of Deformity

The most apparent complication after a hallux valgus correction is the recurrence of deformity, which is reported to be as high as 16%.[2,23,29–31] Duan and Kadakia[32] reported that recurrence after certain procedures can be caused by factors related to the patient, to the operator, and to components of hallux valgus.

Operator-dependent factors that contribute to recurrent deformities are numerous[3,33,34]:

1. The characteristics of initial deformity must be considered, as well as whether the correct surgical procedure was selected.
2. Poor surgical technique should be avoided.
3. Certain underlying conditions should be evaluated, because conditions associated with a hallux valgus deformity may preclude a satisfactory result.
4. Incomplete reduction of the sesamoids can be a risk factor for the recurrence of hallux valgus.[35]
5. Failure to discuss appropriate postoperative management with the patient may lead to malunion. Patient-dependent factors are poor patient compliance after surgery and poor choice of footwear.[1,36,37] Additionally, smoking is associated with increased rates of nonunion and wound infection in orthopedic surgery.

Certain procedures have specific shortcomings that make recurrence more likely. A simple bunionectomy fails to release the lateral joint contracture and does not reposition the metatarsal head over the sesamoids. Consequently, recurrence is common.[38] For a distal soft tissue procedure to succeed, the soft tissue must be adequately released. The main reason for recurrence after a distal soft tissue procedure is the failure to recognize the presence of significant metatarsus primus varus. A distal soft tissue procedure cannot be used to correct a fixed bone deformity. The Akin procedure consists of a bunionectomy and varus osteotomy of the proximal phalanx. This procedure does not address lateral joint contracture or realign the sesamoids, and has an increased recurrence rate when performed alone. A frequent cause of recurrence after a chevron procedure is that the initial deformity was of greater magnitude than that for which the procedure was designed. Failure to appreciate joint congruency and lateral slope of the distal metatarsal articular surface will prevent full correction in those cases.[1,36] The DMAA should be measured before a chevron procedure, and if the angle is greater than 15°, a medial closing wedge chevron or the addition of Akin procedure should be considered. Recurrent deformity after a crescentic, lateral closing wedge or chevron-shaped proximal metatarsal osteotomy usually results from inadequate bone correction. In a study by Scranton and McDermott,[39] hypermobility was a cause of recurrence. Of the 6 patients with recurrence secondary to hypermobility from that study, a Lapidus procedure was successful in management of the hallux valgus recurrence.

If the recurrent deformity is asymptomatic, the patient is best advised to simply observe the foot, as the likelihood of successful revision is reduced.[37] If the recurrence is symptomatic, however, a revision surgery should be considered. Before the secondary operation, it is imperative to consider the factors that many have contributed to recurrence and to address them properly to minimize the chances of a second recurrence. The same guidelines for correction of a primary hallux valgus deformity apply to the treatment of recurrent hallux valgus. Successful treatment of a recurrence requires special knowledge of the hallux valgus pathomechanics regarding bony alignment, joint congruity, and soft tissue balance. Additionally, bony alignment may require lateral capsule release to correct valgus.

Avascular Necrosis

Avascular necrosis (AVN) of the first metatarsal head is a complication that primarily arises as a result of distal metatarsal osteotomies. Incidence of avascular necrosis is variable and ranges from 0% to 76%.[40–43]

A thorough understanding of vascular anatomy of the first metatarsal head is essential in hallux valgus corrective operations. Careful operative technique permits safe distal osteotomy and lateral soft tissue release. Because the intraosseous blood supply to the metatarsal head is completely disrupted with osteotomy, excessive capsular release and inadvertent injury to the lateral capsular vessels must be avoided. Several investigators have demonstrated a lower incidence of avascular necrosis with the use of a second lateral incision (2%–40%).[42,44] An alternative to the use of a second incision is the release of lateral capsule and adductor tendon through the joint.[45]

Following a distal chevron osteotomy, transient radiographic changes may be seen in the metatarsal head. However, the first metatarsal head has an excellent capacity to accommodate to changes in its blood supply. The radiographic changes following a chevron osteotomy probably represent an adjustment period, as the metatarsal head recovers from vascular compromise, and they rarely progress to symptomatic AVN. Even with slight degree of vascular compromise, the patient may be asymptomatic, and many cases of subclinical radiographic changes probably occur but are most likely never identified. Management of AVN of the first metatarsal head has not been standardized, because symptomatic AVN occurs so infrequently. Anecdotal experience suggests that simple activity and shoe modifications may suffice.

Various procedures have been described to alleviate more pronounced symptoms of metatarsal AVN. For less severe cases, a synovectomy of the first MTP joint is an option, with subchondral drilling as a possible addition. More severe cases of AVN may require either a metatarsophalangeal fusion or a resection arthroplasty, such as a Keller procedure. If arthrodesis is undertaken, it may be necessary to use an interpositional bone graft to maintain the length of the first ray while adequately removing the avascular bone. In the event that a substantial amount of avascular bone must be removed, bone block distraction arthrodesis can be considered to avoid transfer metatarsalgia.

Hallux Varus

Hallux varus is commonly seen as an iatrogenic complication after bunion surgery, resulting from overcorrection of hallux valgus. The incidence is relatively rare and is reported to range between 2% and 15.4% in the literature.[46,47]

Each case of hallux varus must be carefully evaluated to determine the exact etiology. Hallux varus develops due to an imbalance among the osseous, tendon, and capsuloligamentous structures at the first MTP joint, and this imbalance leads to a progressive medial deviation of the great toe. This typically involves a combination of medial contracture and overtightening, with excessive laxity or soft tissue attenuation laterally. In those cases of iatrogenic hallux varus following bunion surgery, there may be loss of medial osseous support due to excessive bone resection or to overcorrected intermetatarsal angle (IMA). Combined with excessive lateral release, such imbalance leads to unopposed tension from the medial muscles, specifically from the abductor hallucis and the medial head of the flexor hallucis brevis. Most patients with hallux varus are asymptomatic. Pain associated with hallux varus can be caused either by subluxation of the MTP joint and subsequent alteration of joint mechanics, or by the use of ill-fitting footwear.

Because of the different factors involved in pathophysiology, surgical decision making concerning hallux varus is a challenging endeavor. In addition to flexibility of varus deformity, it is important to consider interphalangeal (IP) joint contracture, rotational deformity, arthritis, and bony deformity. The first element to consider is the mobility and flexibility of the first MTP joint. In cases of severe stiffness or painful arthritis, an arthrodesis of this joint is the most appropriate solution. If the first MTP joint remains mobile and is painless in the reduced position, the choice of treatment will depend on the IP joint and neighboring rays. Other relevant osseous factors include excessive medial eminence resection, decreased IMA, and malunion of a proximal phalangeal osteotomy. Excessive bone resection at the medial aspect of metatarsal head removes the osseous support of the tibial sesamoid and the proximal phalanx. With good MTP motion in the absence of arthritis, autograft or allograft can be considered for restoration of the osseous buttress. Overcorrection of the IMA following bunion surgery must be recognized. This can be caused by a metatarsal osteotomy with overcorrection or by a soft tissue release of the first web space causing a lateral force vector that obliterates the first interspace. If there is overcorrection of the IMA caused by metatarsal osteotomy, the surgeon must consider revising the osteotomy with release of scar tissue and repair of the lateral ligaments. This soft tissue procedure alone may be sufficient if no metatarsal osteotomy malunion exists. The need for revision osteotomy can be determined by a simulated weight-bearing fluoroscopic image to assess the IMA after the release of scar tissue.

Varus malunion of a proximal phalangeal (Akin) osteotomy can be reversed by a lateral closing wedge osteotomy. For soft tissue deficits such as attenuation or overly aggressive release of the lateral capsule and ligaments, dynamic or static transfers could reconstruct these lateral components of the MTP joint.

Transfer Metatarsalgia Due to Malunion or Shortening

A shortened first metatarsal is generally associated with transfer metatarsalgia. This is usually observed for the second metatarsal, although it has been reported to affect the lateral metatarsal head also. If the first metatarsal shortening is confirmed radiographically, the possibility of a dorsal malunion must also be evaluated.

All metatarsal osteotomies are associated with some degree of shortening. The extent of shortening depends on the type of osteotomy. The distal chevron osteotomy is associated with minimal shortening, and some studies have reported metatarsal shortening of 2.0 to 2.5 mm.[41,42,48] Similarly, proximal metatarsal osteotomies are associated with relatively small amounts of shortening, which are also reported from 2.0 to 2.5 mm.[31,45] The Mitchell osteotomy is associated with the greatest amount of shortening, with reports ranging from 3 to 7 mm.[49,50]

Dorsal malunion of the first metatarsal may be seen with any type of metatarsal osteotomy, but it is most commonly reported with a crescentic osteotomy. This type of malunion arises from a variety of factors. One factor is an improper orientation of the osteotomy. More importantly, improper fixation or fracture at the fixation site may result in dorsal malunion. For this reason, careful protection of the osteotomy should be undertaken until the bone has completely healed. Initial treatment of the transfer lesion should be conservative. This is best addressed with a foot orthosis that includes a metatarsal pad to decrease the pressure being applied to the affected metatarsal heads. If the patient does not respond to conservative treatment, then surgical correction can be undertaken. In the presence of any significant shortening, a lengthening procedure is an option, which may be done either in 1 stage or by distraction osteogenesis using a miniexternal fixator. Lengthening is associated with increased stiffness of the first MTP joint, and it also causes the dorsal skin to become taut on closure. Surgical treatment of dorsal malunion is similar to that used for a shortened metatarsal and includes a corrective osteotomy at the site of dorsal angulation.

SELECTION OF SURGICAL PROCEDURES

There are 3 main categories of surgical hallux valgus correction, which are based on the IMA. Mild valgus deformity has an IMA of less than 15°; intermediate deformity has and IMA of 15° to 20°; and, severe deformity has and IMA of more than 20°. Each category may be subdivided by DMAA. In a mild deformity with normal DMAA, a distal osteotomy can be performed. A mild deformity with high DMAA can be corrected by a distal rotated chevron osteotomy. Intermediate deformities with normal DMAA can be corrected by displacement osteotomies, while an intermediate deformity with high DMAA can be corrected by rotated scarf or double osteotomy, which includes a base osteotomy to correct the IMA and a distal osteotomy to correct the DMAA. Severe deformity can only be corrected by angular osteotomies. These osteotomies inherently increase the DMAA, and can only be performed for deformities with a normal DMAA. Only a base angular osteotomy and distal rotation osteotomy can correct high levels of DMAA and severe deformity.

SURGICAL DECISION MAKING

The goal of operative treatment of hallux valgus is to correct all pathologic elements yet maintain a biomechanically functional forefoot. Successful treatment of a recurrence requires special knowledge of the hallux valgus pathomechanics. It requires correcting bony alignment, restoring joint congruity, and balancing soft tissues. Bony alignment also may require lateral capsule release to correct valgus. Surgical treatment of recurrence should be undertaken using the same guidelines for correction of a primary hallux valgus deformity. A thorough physical examination is critical. Physical examination of a hallux valgus deformity must be performed with the patient sitting and standing.[36,51] The involved foot is examined for pes planus and hindfoot valgus deformities and for contracture of the Achilles tendon, which may affect the choice and success of operation. The metatarsocuneiform joint should be checked for hypermobility, while keeping in mind that there is no absolute amount of motion that is considered to delineate hypermobility. A thorough interview with the patient is important, not only to evaluate the major symptoms associated with hallux valgus deformity, but also to educate the patient with regards to the problem, the alternatives for treatment, and the risks and complications of an indicated operation. The severity of hallux valgus deformity and the magnitude of first–second IMA should be determined with a standing radiographic view. Also, the degree of the DMAA, amount of lateral release, and reduction of sesamoid complex should be assessed. Other deformities and complications of the first operation should be addressed such as limited range of motion in the MTP joint, pronation of hallux, callosities under lesser metatarsal heads, and lesser toe deformities like hammer/claw toes.

REFERENCES

1. Easley ME, Trnka HJ. Current concepts review: hallux valgus part II: operative treatment. Foot Ankle Int 2007;28(6):748–58.
2. Klosok JK, Pring DJ, Jessop JH, et al. Chevron or Wilson metatarsal osteotomy for hallux valgus. A prospective randomised trial. J Bone Joint Surg Br 1993; 75(5):825–9.
3. Thompson FM. Complications of hallux valgus surgery and salvage. Orthopedics 1990;13(9):1059–67.
4. Coughlin MJ. Roger A. Mann Award. Juvenile hallux valgus: etiology and treatment. Foot Ankle Int 1995;16(11):682–97.
5. Coughlin MJ. Hallux valgus in men: effect of the distal metatarsal articular angle on hallux valgus correction. Foot Ankle Int 1997;18(8):463–70.
6. Pouliart N, Haentjens P, Opdecam P. Clinical and radiographic evaluation of Wilson osteotomy for hallux valgus. Foot Ankle Int 1996;17(7):388–94.
7. Kato T, Watanabe S. The etiology of hallux valgus in Japan. Clin Orthop Relat Res 1981;(157):78–81.
8. Sim-Fook L, Hodgson AR. A comparison of foot forms among the non-shoe and shoe-wearing Chinese population. J Bone Joint Surg Am 1958;40A(5): 1058–62.
9. Glynn MK, Dunlop JB, Fitzpatrick D. The Mitchell distal metatarsal osteotomy for hallux valgus. J Bone Joint Surg Br 1980;62B(2):188–91.
10. Scranton PE Jr. Adolescent bunions: diagnosis and management. Pediatr Ann 1982;11(6):518–20.
11. Kalen V, Brecher A. Relationship between adolescent bunions and flatfeet. Foot Ankle 1988;8(6):331–6.

12. Mann RA, Coughlin MJ. Hallux valgus—etiology, anatomy, treatment and surgical considerations. Clin Orthop Relat Res 1981;(157):31–41.
13. Lee KT, Young K. Measurement of first-ray mobility in normal vs. hallux valgus patients. Foot Ankle Int 2001;22(12):960–4.
14. Myerson MS, Badekas A. Hypermobility of the first ray. Foot Ankle Clin 2000; 5(3):469–84.
15. Ito H, Shimizu A, Miyamoto T, et al. Clinical significance of increased mobility in the sagittal plane in patients with hallux valgus. Foot Ankle Int 1999;20(1):29–32.
16. Klaue K, Hansen ST, Masquelet AC. Clinical, quantitative assessment of first tarsometatarsal mobility in the sagittal plane and its relation to hallux valgus deformity. Foot Ankle Int 1994;15(1):9–13.
17. Coughlin MJ, Jones CP, Viladot R, et al. Hallux valgus and first ray mobility: a cadaveric study. Foot Ankle Int 2004;25(8):537–44.
18. Mahan KT, Jacko J. Juvenile hallux valgus with compensated metatarsus adductus. Case report. J Am Podiatr Med Assoc 1991;81(10):525–30.
19. Pontious J, Mahan KT, Carter S. Characteristics of adolescent hallux abducto valgus. A retrospective review. J Am Podiatr Med Assoc 1994;84(5):208–18.
20. Rothbart BA. Metatarsus adductus and its clinical significance. J Am Podiatry Assoc 1972;62(5):187–90.
21. Coughlin MJ, Freund E. Roger A. Mann Award. The reliability of angular measurements in hallux valgus deformities. Foot Ankle Int 2001;22(5):369–79.
22. Hattrup SJ, Johnson KA. Chevron osteotomy: analysis of factors in patients' dissatisfaction. Foot Ankle 1985;5(6):327–32.
23. Austin DW, Leventen EO. A new osteotomy for hallux valgus: a horizontally directed "V" displacement osteotomy of the metatarsal head for hallux valgus and primus varus. Clin Orthop Relat Res 1981;(157):25–30.
24. Mitchell LA, Baxter DE. A Chevron-Akin double osteotomy for correction of hallux valgus. Foot Ankle 1991;12(1):7–14.
25. Barouk LS. Scarf osteotomy for hallux valgus correction. Local anatomy, surgical technique, and combination with other forefoot procedures. Foot Ankle Clin 2000;5(3):525–58.
26. Ball J, Sullivan JA. Treatment of the juvenile bunion by Mitchell osteotomy. Orthopedics 1985;8(10):1249–52.
27. Bonney G, Macnab I. Hallux valgus and hallux rigidus; a critical survey of operative results. J Bone Joint Surg Br 1952;34B(3):366–85.
28. Helal B. Surgery for adolescent hallux valgus. Clin Orthop Relat Res 1981;(157): 50–63.
29. Lehman DE. Salvage of complications of hallux valgus surgery. Foot Ankle Clin 2003;8(1):15–35.
30. Lewis RJ, Feffer HL. Modified chevron osteotomy of the first metatarsal. Clin Orthop Relat Res 1981;(157):105–9.
31. Mann RA, Rudicel S, Graves SC. Repair of hallux valgus with a distal soft-tissue procedure and proximal metatarsal osteotomy. A long-term follow-up. J Bone Joint Surg Am 1992;74(1):124–9.
32. Duan X, Kadakia AR. Salvage of recurrence after failed surgical treatment of hallux valgus. Arch Orthop Trauma Surg 2012;132(4):477–85.
33. Bock P, Lanz U, Kroner A, et al. The Scarf osteotomy: a salvage procedure for recurrent hallux valgus in selected cases. Clin Orthop Relat Res 2010;468(8): 2177–87.
34. Coughlin MJ, Mann RA. Arthrodesis of the first metatarsophalangeal joint as salvage for the failed Keller procedure. J Bone Joint Surg Am 1987;69(1):68–75.

35. Okuda R, Kinoshita M, Yasuda T, et al. Postoperative incomplete reduction of the sesamoids as a risk factor for recurrence of hallux valgus. J Bone Joint Surg Am 2009;91(7):1637–45.
36. Coughlin MJ. Hallux valgus. Instr Course Lect 1997;46:357–91.
37. Kitaoka HB, Patzer GL. Salvage treatment of failed hallux valgus operations with proximal first metatarsal osteotomy and distal soft-tissue reconstruction. Foot Ankle Int 1998;19(3):127–31.
38. Kitaoka HB, Franco MG, Weaver AL, et al. Simple bunionectomy with medial capsulorrhaphy. Foot Ankle 1991;12(2):86–91.
39. Scranton PE Jr, McDermott JE. Prognostic factors in bunion surgery. Foot Ankle Int 1995;16(11):698–704.
40. Horne G, Tanzer T, Ford M. Chevron osteotomy for the treatment of hallux valgus. Clin Orthop Relat Res 1984;(183):32–6.
41. Mann RA, Donatto KC. The chevron osteotomy: a clinical and radiographic analysis. Foot Ankle Int 1997;18(5):255–61.
42. Meier PJ, Kenzora JE. The risks and benefits of distal first metatarsal osteotomies. Foot Ankle 1985;6(1):7–17.
43. Rossi WR, Ferreira JC. Chevron osteotomy for hallux valgus. Foot Ankle 1992; 13(7):378–81.
44. Pochatko DJ, Schlehr FJ, Murphey MD, et al. Distal chevron osteotomy with lateral release for treatment of hallux valgus deformity. Foot Ankle Int 1994; 15(9):457–61.
45. Johnson JE, Clanton TO, Baxter DE, et al. Comparison of Chevron osteotomy and modified McBride bunionectomy for correction of mild to moderate hallux valgus deformity. Foot Ankle 1991;12(2):61–8.
46. Edelman RD. Iatrogenically induced hallux varus. Clin Podiatr Med Surg 1991; 8(2):367–82.
47. Goldman FD, Siegel J, Barton E. Extensor hallucis longus tendon transfer for correction of hallux varus. J Foot Ankle Surg 1993;32(2):126–31.
48. Johnson KA, Cofield RH, Morrey BF. Chevron osteotomy for hallux valgus. Clin Orthop Relat Res 1979;(142):44–7.
49. Karbowski A, Schwitalle M, Eckardt A, et al. Long-term results after Mitchell osteotomy in children and adolescents with hallux valgus. Acta Orthop Belg 1998; 64(3):263–8.
50. Merkel KD, Katoh Y, Johnson EW Jr, et al. Mitchell osteotomy for hallux valgus: long-term follow-up and gait analysis. Foot Ankle 1983;3(4):189–96.
51. Baumhauer JF, DiGiovanni BF. Salvage of first metatarsophalangeal joint arthroplasty complications. Foot Ankle Clin 2003;8(1):37–48, viii.

Iatrogenic Hallux Varus Treatment Algorithm

 CrossMark

Matthew D. Crawford, MD[a], Jaymin Patel, BS[b], Eric Giza, MD[c],*

KEYWORDS

- Iatrogenic hallux varus • Intermetatarsal angle • Corrective surgery
- Hallux valgus complication

KEY POINTS

- Iatrogenic hallux varus is a relatively rare complication of corrective hallux valgus surgery that has multiple pathologic facets.
- It requires a comprehensive assessment that focuses on joint flexibility, joint integrity, soft tissue balance, and bony deformity.
- A step-wise treatment approach is used to address all elements of the deformity.
- The literature on hallux varus treatments consists mainly of retrospective case series, with several proposed procedures addressing various degrees of deformity.
- Comparison of these procedures is a challenging endeavor and each case should be considered on an individual basis.

INTRODUCTION

Iatrogenic hallux varus is a complication of hallux valgus corrective surgery leading to medial deviation of the hallux on the first metatarsal. The deformity may consist of triplane involvement, including phalangeal supination and interphalangeal (IP) joint flexion.[1] A relatively rare occurrence, it was first reported by McBride[2] with an incidence of 5% following his procedure of medial eminence removal, medial capsulorrhaphy, and fibular sesamoid excision. Many investigators have subsequently reported on this complication following various hallux valgus corrective surgeries, with incidences ranging from 2%[3] to 17%.[4,5]

Other causes of hallux varus include trauma, Charcot-Marie-Tooth disease, polio, rheumatoid arthritis, and avascular necrosis of the first metatarsal head.[6] Because

Disclosure: Paid consultant for Arthrex, Inc, Zimmer, Inc, Olympus BioTech, Inc; Research and fellowship funding for Arthrex, Inc (E. Giza).

[a] Department of Orthopaedic Surgery, Duke University Medical Center, Box 3000, Durham, NC 27710, USA; [b] School of Medicine, University of California, Davis, 4610 X Street, Sacramento, CA 95817, USA; [c] Foot & Ankle Surgery, Department of Orthopaedics, University of California, Davis, 4860 Y Street, Suite 3800, Sacramento, CA 95817, USA
* Corresponding author.
E-mail address: eric.giza@ucdmc.ucdavis.edu

this article is dedicated to iatrogenic hallux varus, its pathogenesis arises from excessive surgical correction of the hallux joint itself or an overcorrection of the intermetatarsal angle (IMA). Aggressive surgical correction leads to an imbalance between the soft tissue and bony structures at the first metatarsophalangeal (MTP) joint. The resulting progressive varus deforming force may cause patients to complain of cosmetic deformity, difficulty with footwear, and pain. The goals of treatment are to correct the deformity, relieve pain, and restore the function of the forefoot.

ANATOMY

In a normal foot, the hallux is in similar alignment to the first metatarsal and lateral deviation does not exceed 15°.[7] The intrinsic muscles of the hallux insert on the base of the proximal phalanx and include the flexor hallucis brevis (FHB), extensor hallucis brevis (EHB), adductor hallucis, and abductor hallucis (AbH). These short muscles serve to stabilize the hallux and exert an influence on rotation as well as medial and lateral deviation, particularly when not in balance.[8] The extrinsic muscles of the hallux, flexor hallucis longus (FHL) and extensor hallucis longus (EHL), also provide stability but act more to mobilize the MTP joint into flexion and extension.

The FHB has medial and lateral heads that insert into the proximal phalanx through sesamoid bones. The plantar aspect of the metatarsal head has two longitudinal grooves, separated by a longitudinal ridge, the crista, where the tibial and fibular sesamoids normally glide.

PATHOGENESIS

Two types of iatrogenically induced hallux varus have been described.[7] The static type results from osseous disruption at the MTP joint following overcorrection (aggressive medial eminence resection or overcorrection of the IMA) during osteotomy procedures.[9,10] The dynamic type is a result of disruption of muscle balance at the base of the proximal phalanx.

Although hallux varus can occur due to a combination of intraoperative procedures, it is most commonly reported, and perhaps best explained, after a McBride procedure with fibular sesamoid excision.[11] Fibular sesamoidectomy allows the tibial sesamoid to slide medially, whereas adductor tendon release allows the abductor tendon to operate unopposed, both of which can lead to a varus movement of the proximal phalanx. As the MTP rotates into varus, the EHL, FHL, and EHB become positioned medial to the midline in an axial plane and further contribute to the varus deformity. As the medial head of the FHB slides medially along with the tibial sesamoid, it is no longer able to act as an effective flexor and is overpowered by the extensors of the MTP joint, leading to an extension deformity. MTP joint extension results in a tightened FHL and loosened EHL, which leads to flexion at the IP joint.[5] Additional factors that can contribute to a hallux varus deformity include

- Excessive release of the lateral MTP joint structures: Release of the lateral MTP capsule with release of the adductor hallucis tendon and the lateral head of the FHB in combination[7,11] can lead to MTP imbalance.
- Excessive tightening of the medial MTP joint capsule: Excessive resection and subsequent tight suturing of the medial capsule
- Aggressive postoperative dressing holding the MTP in varus causing medial subluxation
- Excessive resection of the medial eminence: This can lead to loss of the medial bony buttress for the proximal phalanx, allowing for varus rotation of the hallux.

Loss of part of the tibial sesamoid groove will destabilize the tibial sesamoid, allowing medial subluxation and will further contribute to the varus deforming force of the FHB (**Fig. 1**).

- Overcorrection of the IMA (1-2): Although closure of the IMA to neutral or negative is more common with proximal metatarsal osteotomy, it can also occur with a midshaft or distal metatarsal osteotomy. As the IMA decreases, the medial vector pull that helps to correct a hallux valgus deformity now moves in favor of a varus or adducted position.[12]

CLINICAL EVALUATION

The diagnosis of hallux varus is primarily based on clinical observation. There are a range of presentations from the great toe being "too straight" to being medially positioned to occurring in conjunction with deformity at the MTP and IP joints.[1] A patient history should focus on the timing of previous corrective hallux valgus surgery, the procedure type, and the chronicity of symptoms. A patient's chief complaint is more often due to cosmetic deformity or poor shoe fit, rather than pain.[4]

Evaluation should determine if the deformities of the MTP and IP joint are flexible or rigid as this will influence treatment plans (**Fig. 2**). Flexible deformities are passively reducible and should be assessed in a seated and standing position because contractures can change dynamically.[13] Rigid deformities are nonreducible as a result of long-standing contractures.

Clinical findings may include

- Medial displacement of the first MTP joint
- Supination of the hallux
- Extension of the proximal hallux
- Medially bowstrung and taut EHL
- Medially displaced tibial sesamoid that is painful to palpation
- Loss of great toe purchase
- Hammertoe contracture at IP joint with dorsal clavus[1]
- IP joint bursitis
- Long hallux and/or first ray[14]

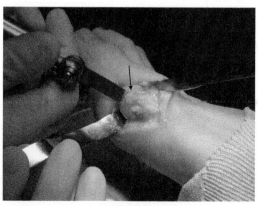

Fig. 1. Example of resection of the medial eminence of the first metatarsal. Aggressive resection or "notching" lateral to the long axis of the metatarsal diaphysis (*arrow*) can lead to hallux varus.

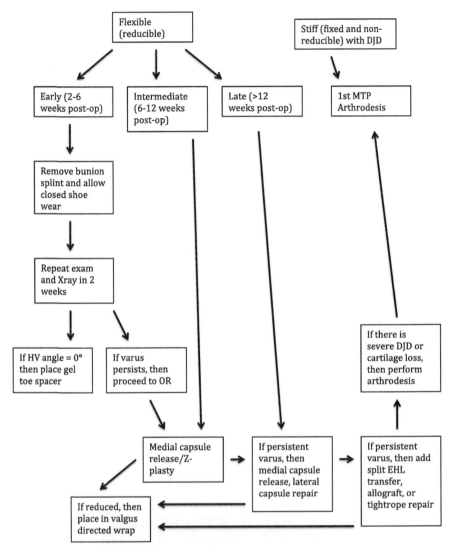

Fig. 2. Iatrogenic hallux varus treatment algorithm. DJD, degenerative joint disease; HV, hallux varus.

- Progressive adductus of the lesser toes[8]
- Compensatory rearfoot supination with lateral metatarsal overload[14] and metatarsalgia as the hallux assists less with the stance phase of the gait cycle.

RADIOGRAPHIC FINDINGS

Radiographic evaluation is necessary in the identification of elements of hallux varus and is considered by some to be the standard for diagnosis.[4] Weight-bearing AP films are most valuable for evaluating the MTP joint deformity; however, oblique or lateral films also help to better understand the deformity in three planes. A sesamoid view can show the position of the sesamoid bones relative to the first metatarsal head.

The hallux varus angle is formed between the longitudinal axis of the first metatarsal and the longitudinal axis of the proximal phalanx. Normal values range from 5° to 15°, whereas it will be 0° or negative in cases of hallux varus. Other findings include

- Excessive medial eminence resection
- Medial subluxation of the tibial sesamoid out of the sesamoid groove
- Absence of a fibular sesamoid
- Decreased IMA, angle between the longitudinal axes of the first and second metatarsals. Normal is 0° to 8°. With hallux varus it will be 0° or negative.
- Longer first metatarsal than second metatarsal
- Phalangeal varus or malunion from previous phalangeal osteotomy
- Cystic or arthritic changes at the MTP and/or IP joint
- Arthritic, deformed or hypertrophied sesamoid bone.

CLASSIFICATION

Due to its multiple pathologic facets, hallux varus is not easily classified. Hawkins[7] categorized the deformity based on its static (supple) or dynamic (fixed) nature. Static deformity does not affect muscle balance and is uniplanar, passively correctible, and usually asymptomatic (**Fig. 3**). Dynamic deformity is multiplanar, fixed, and usually symptomatic as a result of muscle imbalance at the MTP joint.[5] Other classification systems attempt to assess the deformity by categorizing based on the joint involvement (MTP and/or IP) and plane of deformity[15] or by increasing complexity: MTP adduction (+/− arthrosis), MTP adduction and IP joint flexion (+/− arthrosis), complex multiplanar deformity.[14]

Regardless of the method of classification, the important elements that impact treatment include the duration following hallux valgus correction procedure, flexibility

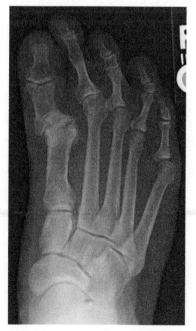

Fig. 3. Radiograph of a 63 year-old woman with an asymptomatic, rigid hallux varus deformity 15 years after a bunion correction.

of the MTP and IP joints, arthritis of the MTP and IP joints, soft tissue balance, and rotational and bony deformity.

EARLY TREATMENT

Early recognition of iatrogenic hallux varus may allow for corrective nonoperative treatment if the deformity is solely a result of soft tissue imbalance. The hallux should be assessed for alignment, range of motion, stability, and any signs of early MTP joint arthritis.

If hallux varus presents within the first 2 to 4 weeks after surgery, treatment can include weekly dressings and tapings of the hallux to 10° to 15° of valgus for 8 to 12 weeks. This can be followed by an additional 3 months of night splinting.[5] Shoe wear modification and antiinflammatories may also provide benefit. Patients should be monitored both clinically and with radiographs to assess for progression. It has been reported that nonoperative treatments are successful in 22% (12/54) of patients[16]; however, this is contingent on severity of deformity and time of presentation.

If nonoperative management fails to correct a flexible deformity or the deformity becomes symptomatic after going unnoticed or untreated for greater than 6 to 8 weeks after surgery, a return to the operating room is warranted (**Fig. 4**). The medial capsule closure can be released or Z-lengthened on the medial aspect of the first MTP joint to help provide correction.

LATE TREATMENT

The treatment algorithm for iatrogenic hallux varus that presents after the window of effective nonoperative measures is determined by joint flexibility, joint integrity, and soft tissue balance of the deformity. Maintaining joint mobility is preferable but is not always possible due to arthritis or rigid contracture. In order for a tendon transfer or tenodesis to correct the deformity, the joint needs to be mobile and reducible. If arthritis exists in either the MTP or IP joint, arthrodesis of that joint is warranted. Similarly if there is a rigid contracture of the MTP or IP joint, then soft tissue correction is unlikely to restore the anatomy. In the rare case that both the MTP and IP joints are

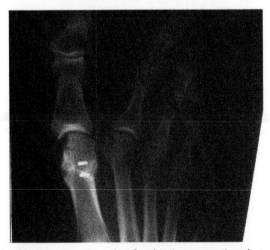

Fig. 4. Radiograph of hallux varus 6 weeks after bunion correction that was treated with a medial capsule release.

deformed due to contracture and/or arthritis, arthrodesis of both joints should not be performed. Instead resection arthroplasty of the MTP joint and IP arthrodesis may be preferable.[13]

The surgical procedures for hallux varus can be divided into procedures that address the soft tissue (tendon transfer or tenodesis, ligamentoplasty, Mini TightRope [Arthrex, Inc, Naples, FL, USA] procedure), the bone (osseous buttress, first metatarsal osteotomy, hallux proximal phalangeal osteotomy), or the joint (arthrodesis of the IP joint and arthrodesis or resection arthroplasty of the MTP joint).[13] Their common goal is to correct deformity, relieve pain, restore function, and produce a first MTP joint that will remain stable and mobile, and not develop degenerative changes. Each procedure proceeds in a step-wise fashion beginning with a wide medial capsular release as described above.

SOFT TISSUE

Current effective soft tissue procedures include the use of autograft (tendon transfer or tenodesis), allograft, or supplement of the lateral ligaments via a Mini TightRope reconstruction for correction. Soft tissue correction is indicated in the case of flexible, nonarthritic deformity. The choice of procedure must be individualized based on the source of deformity (ligament insufficiency, tendon contracture), the patient's unique anatomy, and the patient's goals and expectations for correction. Although many soft tissue procedures exist, there is significant evidence to suggest that static correction with abductor tendon release, conjoined tendon repair, or lateral capsule imbrications are unsuccessful.[7,17]

TENDON TRANSFER OR TENODESIS

Tendon transfers have the potential for dynamic correction of the deformity whereas a tenodesis provides static correction. Advantages of tendon transfer procedures include the preservation of motion and restoration of the dynamic balance of forces about the first MTP joint.[9,17] Contraindications to tendon transfer or tenodesis alone include deformity of the first metatarsal and the presence of arthritis or rigidity of the MTP joint.[13] Plovanich and colleagues[18] conducted a review assessing the sustainability of soft-tissue release with tendon transfer, including eight studies that revealed a 16.6% (11/68) incidence of complications and a 4.4% (3/68) recurrence of hallux valgus (all occurring with Johnson EHL transfers with IP arthrodesis).

ABH TENDON TRANSFER

Hawkins[7] first introduced a technique for a transfer of the AbH tendon. The tendon is released from the base of the proximal phalanx, routed deep to the intermetatarsal ligament, and anchored to the lateral side of the base of the proximal phalanx.[7] This logical procedure takes advantage of medial capsular and AbH tendon release, a requirement for medial joint contracture, by using the AbH tendon for dynamic transfer. Concerns with this method include inadequate length of the harvested tendon and residual supination of the phalanx.[19]

ABH HALLUCIS TENODESIS

Leemrijse and colleagues[20] proposed an anatomic tenodesis using the AbH tendon. One-third of the AbH tendon width is harvested, detached proximally, and completely released from the tibial sesamoid. The tendon is passed through two bone tunnels, from medial to lateral through the proximal phalanx, and then from lateral to medial through the first metatarsal. An advantage of this technique is its physiologic reconstruction in which the tendon largely responsible for deformity is used to anatomically reconstruct the deficient lateral capsular ligament. Reported results of seven cases indicate an American Orthopaedic Foot and Ankle Society (AOFAS) score improving from 61 to 85 and good maintenance of the correction at a mean follow-up of 2 years with the hallux varus angle, IMA, and tibial sesamoid position returning to normal.[20]

FIRST DORSAL INTEROSSEOUS TENDON TRANSFER

Valtin[21] proposed a technique of transferring the first dorsal interosseous tendon to the base of the proximal phalanx. Detachment of the distal insertion from the base of the phalanx of the second toe and transferring it through a bone tunnel in the base of the proximal phalanx of the hallux helps to create a valgus force on the hallux. Concerns include a technically difficult reinsertion due to the small size of the tendon and the unknown long-term effects on the second toe, which is deprived of its interosseous muscle.[6]

EHL TRANSFER

Johnson and Spiegl[22] originally proposed a transfer of the entire EHL tendon to provide dynamic correction. After detachment of the distal insertion, the EHL is redirected beneath the first intermetatarsal ligament, which acts as a pulley, to the plantar-lateral aspect of the proximal phalanx. The procedure intends to transform the EHL deforming force (dorsiflexion of the MTP joint) to assist with lateral pull and plantar flexion of the phalanx. Due to the subsequent unopposed pull of the FHL, IP joint fusion is proposed to avoid a mallet deformity. Advantages include the stoutness and long length of the EHL tendon, which makes it appropriate for transfer. Limitations include reduced extension of the hallux and complete loss of IP motion.[23,24] The results of the 15 feet evaluated indicate uniform improvement in deformity and pain with 14 excellent or good clinical results.

SPLIT EHL TRANSFER

After proposing entire EHL tendon transfer, Johnson[23] described a modified technique using a split transfer. The lateral half of the EHL is transferred in a similar fashion to that described for the complete EHL but half of the EHL insertion is maintained on the proximal phalanx. This makes IP joint fusion unnecessary and hypothetically does not affect the ability to extend the hallux. However, when tension is applied distally to the lateral portion of EHL tendon, it is also transferred to the remaining medial half of EHL tendon, lengthening it and altering its function.[13,24]

MODIFIED SPLIT EHL

Lau and Myerson[24] proposed a modification of Johnson's technique because of concerns about the medial half of the EHL being constrained after tension is applied to the lateral half. Instead of distal release, the lateral half of the EHL is released proximally, run under the intermetatarsal ligament, and attached to the first metatarsal as a tenodesis. The advantage of proximal release is that the tensioning of the tenodesis does not alter the mechanics of the remaining EHL tendon allowing for a more reliable correction.

EHB TENODESIS

Juliano and colleagues[17] proposed using an EHB tenodesis as an alternative to using the EHL because the EHL could have scarred or contracted during previous surgery. In this procedure, the EHB is transected at the musculotendinous junction, then mobilized to its distal insertion, passed plantar to the intermetatarsal ligament, and reattached through a bone tunnel from lateral to medial on the first metatarsal. Care is taken to avoid supination of the proximal phalanx by releasing the dorsal insertion of the EHB if necessary.[9] An advantage compared with EHL techniques is the maintenance of extension of the distal phalanx of the hallux. Results of six corrections indicate excellent correction maintained at a mean follow-up of 28 months and an AOFAS score improvement from 61 to 85.[17]

LIGAMENTOPLASTY

The lateral ligamentous structures can also be reconstructed as an alternative to autologous tendon transfers or tenodeses. These procedures include

- Reconstruction of the lateral collateral ligament using the Saragaglia technique with a Ligapro suture; results of five cases indicate excellent radiographic and clinical outcomes at an average of 4 years[25]
- Reinforcement of the lateral collateral ligament with fascia lata or soft tissue anchors.[26,27]

Disadvantages of these procedures include the cost of artificial or allograft reconstruction, risk of infection with allograft, and poorly studied long-term results.[11]

MINI TIGHTROPE PROCEDURE

The Mini TightRope is an implanted fixation button and suture that was first used for correction of hallux varus by Pappas and Anderson.[28] After medial release, bone tunnels are created in the proximal phalanx and first metatarsal and the Endobutton (Smith & Nephew, Andover, MA, USA) device is passed through each tunnel sequentially, ending with the leading oblong button resting in line with the metatarsal shaft. The trailing round button is tightened and tensioned to the medial side of the proximal phalanx until adequate correction is obtained. Rather than relying on the patient's own soft tissues, the device applies tension to anchor the hallux in proper alignment and can easily be adjusted intraoperatively to ensure appropriate correction (**Fig. 5**). Although there is limited data and no complications have been reported, potential proposed complications include fracture of the base of the proximal phalanx and/or the first metatarsal head if the intraosseous drill holes are made too close to the cortical surfaces of the first MTP joint, overcorrection or undercorrection of the hallux deformity if careful attention is not used when toggling the implanted button and suture device in the corrected position, limitation of first MTP joint range of motion if the hallux deformity is overcorrected, frontal plane deformity of the hallux if the drill holes are not made parallel to the weight-bearing substrate, loss of correction if the FiberWire (Arthrex Inc, Naples, FL, USA) used in the device breaks before sufficient lateral soft tissue scarring has taken place, chronic edema in the first MTP joint, and hematoma formation within the first intermetatarsal space.[29]

BONE

If the iatrogenic hallux varus deformity is a result of overresection of the medial eminence, overcorrection of the IMA, or malunion of a proximal phalangeal (Akin)

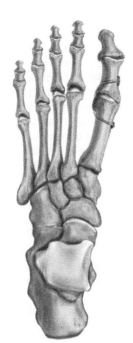

Fig. 5. Illustration of Mini TightRope device placement for correction of hallux varus. (*Courtesy of* Arthrex, Inc, Naples, FL, USA.)

osteotomy, then bony work may be necessary. Excessive bone resection at the medial aspect of the metatarsal head can be restored with an osseous buttress. Overcorrection of the metatarsal with a negative IMA can occur because of proximal or distal metatarsal osteotomy, as well as soft tissue release. Although it has been reported that soft tissue procedures alone can restore normal IMA after overcorrection, this can only occur in the absence of a metatarsal osteotomy malunion. If malunion occurs, osteotomy must be performed to correct metatarsal alignment, sometimes in conjunction with a tendon transfer. Varus malunion of an Akin osteotomy can be reversed with an osteotomy to restore MTP and IP joint line parallelism and equalize the length of the first and second toes.[6]

Numerous reverse osteotomies in conjunction with soft tissue step-wise approaches have been proposed, including reverse Austin osteotomy[30] and revisional osteotomy at the surgical site with metatarsal shaft osteotomy if more IMA correction is required.[31] The following procedures offer effective reconstruction when the hallux varus deformity requires bony correction.

OSSEOUS BUTTRESS

In cases of flexible hallux varus due to excessive resection of the medial metatarsal head, Rochwerger and colleagues[32] proposed the application of bone graft to restore the missing bone following bunionectomy. Restoring the medial bony buttress provides support for the tibial sesamoid to prevent medial subluxation and stabilizes the base of the proximal phalanx. Results of seven cases at an average of 8.6 years indicated no recurrence, good maintenance of range of motion, and six satisfactory results with one subject being dissatisfied due to valgus angulation of 20°.

DISTAL CHEVRON METATARSAL OSTEOTOMY

Choi and colleagues[33] and Lee and colleagues[34] described a method for correction using distal chevron metatarsal osteotomy with medial displacement along with medial capsular release. Choi and colleagues[33] also included a medial closing wedge osteotomy based on the degree of distal metatarsal articular angle. Advantages include mild shortening the first metatarsal, which may relax the first MTP joint and improve range of motion, and the stability of the osteotomy, with no failure of fixation even with immediate weight-bearing. Of the 19 cases reported,[5] the hallux valgus angle improved from −11.6° to 4.7°, the mean first to second IMA improved from −0.3° to 3.3°, the AOFAS scores increased from 77 to 95, and two subjects had recurrence of hallux varus.

REVERSE SCARF AND OPENING WEDGE OSTEOTOMY

Kannegieter and Kilmartin[35] proposed a method of correction for patients who developed hallux varus following combined rotation scarf and Akin osteotomy for hallux valgus. They describe a stepwise approach of soft tissue release and ultimately reverse scarf osteotomy and opening wedge osteotomy of the proximal phalanx. Advantages of this reverse osteotomy in relation to MTP joint fusion include the preservation of the MTP joint, allowing the surgeon flexibility to correct a range of positional abnormalities, and early return to shoe wear and activity without immobilization in a cast. The five cases reviewed at an average follow-up of 38 months indicated an improved hallux valgus angle from −10° to 11°, IMA improved from 5° to 9°, and 100% of subjects felt better off as a result of their revision surgery.

JOINT

Arthrodesis has historically been suggested as the standard treatment of patients who have fixed deformity or degenerative arthritis involving the first MTP joint. It has been shown to reduce pain and maintain a stable medial column for nonreducible, established hallux varus deformities (**Fig. 6**). Known complications include transfer

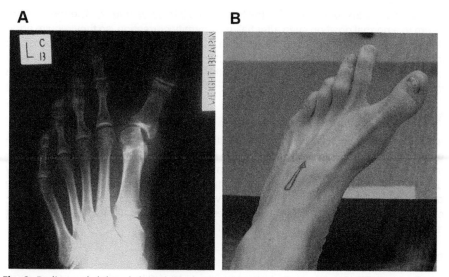

Fig. 6. Radiograph (A) and clinical (B) photograph of a patient with severe hallux varus and degenerative change of the MTP joint requiring first MTP arthrodesis for correction.

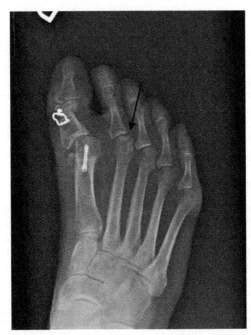

Fig. 7. Iatrogenic hallux varus with secondary second MTP varus (*arrow*).

metatarsalgia, nonunion, IP arthrosis of the hallux, and footwear choice limitations.[35] A treatment guideline for arthrodesis versus resection arthroplasty in patients with degenerative arthritis of the first MTP joint suggests that most patients younger than 65 years should be treated with arthrodesis, whereas most patients older than 65 years should be treated with resection arthroplasty.[11] However, if a contracted or arthritic IP joint presents in conjunction with a fixed or arthritic MTP joint deformity, a resection arthroplasty is necessary.

Over time, hallux varus may pull the lesser toes into varus (**Fig. 7**). The toes will not return to a normal position even after hallux deformity correction, so they require additional realignment. Shortening of the metatarsals, which indirectly lengthens the intrinsic muscles and releases the contracture, provides adequate correction as a standard capsulotomy with release of the medial collateral ligament is often insufficient.

SUMMARY

Iatrogenic hallux varus is a relatively rare complication of corrective hallux valgus surgery. Due to its multiple pathologic facets, hallux varus requires a thorough assessment focusing on joint flexibility, joint integrity, soft tissue balance, and bony deformity. A step-wise treatment approach is used to address all elements of the deformity. Because the literature on hallux varus treatments consists mainly of retrospective case series, comparison of different procedures is a challenging endeavor and each case should be considered on an individual basis.

REFERENCES

1. Edelman RD. Iatrogenically induced hallux varus. Clin Podiatr Med Surg 1991; 8(2):367–82.

2. Mcbride ED. The conservative operation for "bunions" end results and refinements of technic. J Am Med Assoc 1935;105(15):1164–8.
3. Peterson HA, Newman SR. Adolescent bunion deformity treated with double osteotomy and longitudinal pin fixation of the first ray. J Pediatr Orthop 1993; 13(1):80–4.
4. Trnka L, Krejbich F. Tuberculosis in the Czech Republic in 1997. Cas Lek Cesk 1999;138(15):460–4 [in Czech].
5. Richardson EG. Disorders of the hallux. Campbell's operative Orthopaedics. 12th edition. Philadelphia: Mosby; 2013. p. 3878–90.
6. Bevernage BD, Leemrijse T. Hallux varus: classification and treatment. Foot Ankle Clin 2009;14(1):51–65.
7. Hawkins F. Acquired hallux varus: cause, prevention and correction. Clin Orthop Relat Res 1971;76:169–76.
8. Miller JW. Acquired hallux varus: a preventable and correctable disorder. J Bone Joint Surg Am 1975;57(2):183–8.
9. Juliano PJ, Campbell MA. Tendon transfers about the hallux. Foot Ankle Clin 2011;16(3):451–69.
10. Mann RA, Coughlin MJ. Hallux valgus–etiology, anatomy, treatment and surgical considerations. Clin Orthop Relat Res 1981;(157):31–41.
11. Donley BG. Acquired hallux varus. Foot Ankle Int 1997;18(9):586–92.
12. Boike AM, Christein G. Hallux varus and forefoot surgery. London: Churchill Livingstone; 1994. p. 307–12.
13. Myerson MS. Reconstructive foot and ankle surgery: management of complications: Expert Consult. Philadelphia: Elsevier Health Sciences; 2010.
14. Vanore JV, Christensen JC, Kravitz SR, et al. Diagnosis and treatment of first metatarsophalangeal joint disorders. Section 3: Hallux varus. J Foot Ankle Surg 2003;42(3):137–42.
15. Johnson KA, Saltazman CL, Frisca DA. Hallux Varus. In: Gould J, editor. Operative foot surgery. Philadelphia: W.B. Saunders; 1994. p. 28–35.
16. Skalley TC, Myerson MS. The operative treatment of acquired hallux varus. Clin Orthop Relat Res 1994;306:183–91.
17. Juliano PJ, Myerson MS, Cunningham BW. Biomechanical assessment of a new tenodesis for correction of hallux varus. Foot Ankle Int 1996;17(1):17–20.
18. Plovanich EJ, Donnenwerth MP, Abicht BP, et al. Failure after soft-tissue release with tendon transfer for flexible iatrogenic hallux varus: a systematic review. J Foot Ankle Surg 2012;51(2):195–7.
19. Aiyer A, Juliano P. Tendon transfers for hallux varus. Tech Foot Ankle Surg 2013; 12(1):16–24.
20. Leemrijse T, Hoang B, Maldague P, et al. A new surgical procedure for iatrogenic hallux varus: reverse transfer of the abductor hallucis tendon: a report of 7 cases. Acta Orthop Belg 2008;74(2):227–34.
21. Valtin B. First dorsal interosseous muscle transfer in iatrogenic hallux varus surgery. Med Chir Pied 1991;7:9–16.
22. Johnson KA, Spiegl PV. Extensor hallucis longus transfer for hallux varus deformity. J Bone Joint Surg Am 1984;66(5):681–6.
23. Johnson KA. Dissatisfaction following hallux valgus surgery. In: Surgery of the Foot and Ankle. New York: Raven; 1989. p. 35–68.
24. Lau JT, Myerson MS. Modified split extensor hallucis longus tendon transfer for correction of hallux varus. Foot Ankle Int 2002;23(12):1138–40.
25. Tourne Y, Saragaglia D, Picard F, et al. Iatrogenic hallux varus surgical procedure: a study of 14 cases. Foot Ankle Int 1995;16(8):457–63.

26. Labovitz JM, Kaczander BI. Traumatic hallux varus repair utilizing a soft-tissue anchor: a case report. J Foot Ankle Surg 2000;39(2):120–3.

27. Stanifer E, Hodor D, Wertheimer S. Congenital hallux varus: case presentation and review of the literature. J Foot Surg 1991;30(5):509–12.

28. Pappas AJ, Anderson RB. Management of acquired hallux varus with an Endo-button. Tech Foot Ankle Surg 2008;7(2):134–8.

29. Gerbert J, Traynor C, Blue K, et al. Use of the Mini TightRope® for correction of hallux varus deformity. J Foot Ankle Surg 2011;50(2):245–51.

30. Bilotti M, Caprioli R, Testa J, et al. Reverse Austin osteotomy for correction of hallux varus. J Foot Surg 1987;26(1):51.

31. Jenkin WM. Hallux Varus. In: Gerbert J, editor. Textbook of bunion surgery. 3rd edition. Philadelphia: W.B. Saunders; 2001. p. 411–33.

32. Rochwerger A, Curvale G, Groulier P. Application of bone graft to the medial side of the first metatarsal head in the treatment of hallux varus. J Bone Joint Surg Am 1999;81(12):1730–5.

33. Choi KJ, Lee HS, Yoon YS, et al. Distal metatarsal osteotomy for hallux varus following surgery for hallux valgus. J Bone Joint Surg Br 2011;93(8):1079–83.

34. Lee KT, Park YU, Young KW, et al. Reverse distal chevron osteotomy to treat iatrogenic hallux varus after overcorrection of the intermetatarsal 1-2 angle: technique tip. Foot Ankle Int 2011;32(1):89–91.

35. Kannegieter E, Kilmartin TE. The combined reverse scarf and opening wedge osteotomy of the proximal phalanx for the treatment of iatrogenic hallux varus. Foot (Edinb) 2011;21(2):88–91.

Etiology and Management of Lesser Toe Metatarsophalangeal Joint Instability

Jesse F. Doty, MD[a], Michael J. Coughlin, MD[b,c,*],
Lowell Weil Jr, DPM, MBA[d], Caio Nery, MD[e],
From Saint Alphonsus Coughlin Foot and Ankle Clinic, Boise, Idaho, USA

KEYWORDS

- Plantar plate • Lesser MTP joint instability • Crossover toe • Drawer test

KEY POINTS

- A plantar plate tear is associated with instability of the lesser MTP joints and may be associated with collateral ligament tears leading to sagittal and coronal plane malalignment.
- The drawer test is a reliable examination to assess pain and instability of the lesser MTP joint in the presence of plantar plate insufficiency.
- MRI may help to define the presence and magnitude of a plantar plate tear.
- Staging of the clinical examination and grading of the surgical findings are useful in defining the plantar plate tear and formulating the appropriate operative intervention.
- Exposure of the plantar plate is possible through a dorsal approach using a Weil osteotomy.
- Direct repair of the tear is possible allowing anatomic reapproximation and advancement of the plantar plate.

INTRODUCTION

Crossover toe, a term introduced in 1986 as a description of the end result of instability of the metatarsophalangeal (MTP) joint, culminates in sagittal and coronal plane deformity.[1] Deterioration of the collateral ligaments and/or plantar plate is associated with

---

[a] Department of Orthopaedic Surgery, University of Tennessee College of Medicine Chattanooga, 960 East Third Street, Suite 100, Chattanooga, TN 37403, USA; [b] Saint Alphonsus Coughlin Foot and Ankle Clinic, 1075 North Curtis Road, #300, Boise, ID 83706, USA; [c] Department of Orthopaedic Surgery, University of California San Francisco, San Francisco, CA 94143, USA; [d] Weil Foot & Ankle Institute, Des Plaines, IL 60016, USA; [e] Department of Orthopedics and Traumatology, UNIFESP - Federal University of Sao Paulo, Sao Paulo, Brazil
* Corresponding author. Saint Alphonsus Coughlin Foot and Ankle Clinic, 1075 North Curtis Road, #300, Boise, ID 83706.
E-mail address: thefootmd@gmail.com

Foot Ankle Clin N Am 19 (2014) 385–405
http://dx.doi.org/10.1016/j.fcl.2014.06.013
1083-7515/14/$ – see front matter © 2014 Elsevier Inc. All rights reserved.

foot.theclinics.com

instability of the lesser MTP joint and leads to the involved toe crossing over or under the adjacent toes or hallux.[2,3] Multiple reports have described both the progression of the deformity and method of treatment.[4–8] Pain in and around the lesser MTP joints is a common complaint that is difficult to diagnose especially when there is no obvious deformity.[5,9,10] Acute trauma, high-fashion shoe wear, rheumatoid arthritis, and other various inflammatory conditions have all been linked with metatarsalgia and lesser MTP joint deformity.[2,4,7,11,12] The crossover toe deformity has been associated with hallux rigidus, hallux valgus, hammertoes, and interdigital neuromas.[4,6,7] For 25 years, the treatment of lesser MTP joint instability has been characterized by indirect repairs of the deformity using soft tissue releases, balancing procedures, extensor and flexor tendon transfers, and periarticular osteotomies.[1,4–6,8,11,13–24]

A degenerative tear of the plantar plate as a definitive cause of this deformity has now been well documented as the primary pathology.[13–15,21–23,25–27] Classifying the plantar plate tear, based on the location and magnitude of the lesion, helps make it possible to directly repair the plantar plate tear as a means to stabilize the MTP joint.[13–15,21–23,25]

ANATOMY

The lesser MTP joints are stabilized by the dynamic intrinsic and extrinsic muscles of the lesser toes, but also by static stabilizing structures including the plantar plate and collateral ligaments.[20] The plantar plate is the major stabilizing structural force of the lesser MTP joint.[24,28] The plantar plate originates on the proximal neck of the metatarsal metaphysis by a thin synovial attachment. It inserts distally as a firm fibrocartilagenous attachment into the plantar base of the proximal phalanx adjacent to the phalangeal articular cartilage (**Fig. 1**).[26,29] The plantar plate averages 2 cm in length, 1 cm in width, and varies from 2 to 5 mm in thickness. The plate is thicker along the medial and lateral borders but also thickens directly beneath the metatarsal head.[29] The major composition of the plantar plate contains type 1 (75%) and type 2 collagen (21%), which are woven together to create a dense fibrocartilagenous network that lends itself to weight-bearing function.[26,29] The plantar plate serves as a cushion to support compressive forces transferred to the forefoot during weight bearing by functioning similar to the meniscus in the knee, also a structure characterized by type 1 collagen.[26,27,29] Several structures interdigitate with the plantar plate including the plantar fascia, the tendon sheath of the flexor tendons, the transverse intermetatarsal ligament, the collateral ligaments, and the interossei tendons.[26,27,30]

Two distinct collateral ligaments of the MTP joint can be identified, and both ligaments arise from the metatarsal head. The proper collateral ligament attaches to the lateral base of the proximal phalanx, and the accessory collateral ligament attaches directly to the plantar plate (**Fig. 2**).[26] Barg and colleagues found that both collateral ligaments contribute to the stability of the MTP joint, but that the accessory collateral ligament, with its attachment directly to the plantar plate, affords key stability to the joint.[31] With chronic hyperextension forces at the lesser MTP joint, the plantar plate and capsular attachments may become attenuated and insufficient leading to a loss of stability of the MTP joint.[1,4,9,25]

DEMOGRAPHICS OF LESSER MTP JOINT INSTABILITY

Lesser MTP joint instability occurs much more commonly than has been recognized previously.[5] The most frequent presentation of this deformity occurs in older sedentary women.[1,17] However, Coughlin reported this to occur in the younger male athletic population.[5,17] Kaz and Coughlin[17] examined the demographics of a large series of

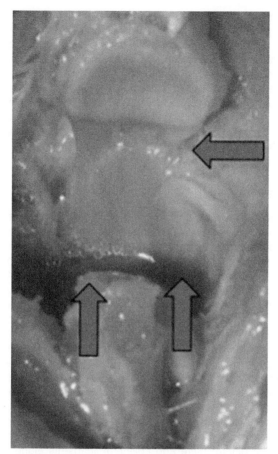

Fig. 1. Operative exposure of the plantar plate with the first metatarsal head displaced proximally. The *horizontal arrow* points to the distal attachment and the two *vertical arrows* point to the proximal origins of the plantar plate. (*Courtesy of* Erin Klein, DPM, Des Plaines, IL.)

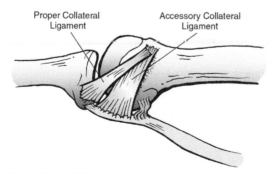

Fig. 2. Diagram of the collateral ligaments of the lesser metatarsophalangeal joint.

patients with the diagnosis of crossover second toe and noted that 86% were women, and the average age at the time of surgery was 59 years. They observed the presence of hallux valgus in nearly 50% of cases, hallux rigidus in 14%, and hallux varus in 7%. Development of a callosity beneath the involved MTP joint was uncommon.[17] Nery and colleagues[21] recently reported on a series of patients with lesser MTP joint instability and observed 71% were female, and the mean age at deformity onset was 58 years. Although many reports on plantar plate insufficiency have indicated it occurs almost universally at the second MTP joint,[1,6,7,17] Nery and colleagues[21] reported in their prospective series of 28 patients (55 MTP joints) that the second MTP joint was affected in 64% of cases, and the third and fourth MTP joints were affected in 32% and 4% of cases, respectively.

PATHOPHYSIOLOGY

On occasion, an acute injury can destabilize the MTP joint,[12,19,31] but more commonly instability develops insidiously with progressive malalignment of the digit. The differential diagnosis of metatarsalgia can include several forefoot conditions **Box 1**. It has been suggested that lesser MTP joint synovitis is an early finding associated with capsular attritional changes.[3] The synovial proliferation associated with rheumatoid arthritis and other inflammatory arthropathies can lead to capsular degeneration and subsequent instability.[2] A long second metatarsal, first ray hypermobility, hallux valgus, hallux rigidus, and pes planus may all contribute to a chronic overload of the lesser MTP joints with resultant instability.[4,7,17,33] Coughlin[4,7] and Nery and colleagues[21] suggested that the high incidence of second MTP joint instability seen in the older female population may be attributed to the long-term use of high-fashion footwear. Chronic hyperextension forces at the lesser MTP joints may lead to elongation or attenuation of the plantar aponeurosis and capsule, eventually leading to plantar plate deterioration and instability.[4,7]

During the gait cycle, the forefoot functions in weight transfer during approximately 40% of stance phase.[6,20] During normal gait, at toe-off, the proximal phalanx is displaced dorsally. The plantar plate and collateral ligaments along with the intrinsic flexors (interossei and lumbricals) resist this force by pulling the proximal phalanx back into a neutral position. With the loss of these stabilizing forces from the plantar plate, collaterals, and intrinsic musculature, the proximal phalanx subluxes in a dorsal or dorsomedial direction with respect to the metatarsal.[13,18,24,25,27,32]

The alignment of the digit is maintained by a balance of static ligamentous and capsular restraints, and the dynamic forces of intrinsic and extrinsic muscles. The

---

Box 1
Differential diagnoses of forefoot pain

- Instability of the lesser MTP joints
- Freiberg infraction
- Degenerative arthritis of lesser MTP joints
- Systemic arthritis with involvement of lesser MTP joints
- MTP joint synovitis
- Metatarsal stress fracture
- Interdigital neuroma
- Synovial cyst formation

extensor digitorum longus tendon has no direct insertion into the proximal phalanx, and thus extension of the lesser MTP joint occurs through the attachment and pull of the extensor digitorum longus through the fibroaponeurotic extensor sling. This extension force is balanced by a flexion force at the MTP joint created mainly by the intrinsic musculature.[1,28] The flexor digitorum longus and brevis tendons flex the proximal interphalangeal and distal interphalangeal joints, but are only weak flexors of the MTP joint.[4] The intrinsic anatomy of the second toe is unique in that there are two dorsal interossei and no plantar interossei.[28] The lumbrical tendon insertion into the medial extensor hood adds an adduction and flexion force on the MTP joint (**Fig. 3**). This may, with the development of a lateral plantar plate or collateral ligament tear, serve as a deforming force in the transverse plane.[5] The tendons of the lumbricals and interossei pass plantar to the MTP joint axis of rotation. With hyperextension of the proximal phalanx, and a shift in the axis of rotation, the interossei become inefficient flexors of the MTP joint.[5,20,28] The tendon of the lumbricals passes beneath the deep transverse metatarsal ligament, and thus remains plantar to the axis of rotation, even with deformity at the joint. However, because of the acute angle of pull, the lumbrical loses its efficiency as a MTP joint flexor, but can still add a medial deforming force to the digit (**Fig. 4**). The remaining constraints on joint stability are the joint capsule, collateral ligaments, and the plantar plate.[7,20,28] Based on cadaveric dissections and surgical findings,[11,13,21,22,25,30] we believe that the primary structure to fail is the plantar plate. This leads to sagittal and transverse plane deformity. Secondarily, the collateral ligaments may also rupture contributing to further malalignment of the toe.[25,30]

HISTORY AND CLINICAL PRESENTATION

Although plantar plate tears can present in acute and chronic settings at any of the lesser MTP joints, the second MTP joint is the most commonly involved.[4,6,7,17,21] Pain localized to the plantar aspect of the forefoot at the base of the second toe is the most common complaint.[7] Patients may describe the feeling of a mass, or "walking on a marble." The pain is accentuated with ambulation and is reduced with rest. Patients may note significant plantar swelling at the base of the involved toe, and in late stages the dorsal base of the proximal phalanx may be palpated when the toe dislocates. In the early stages of plantar plate attenuation, only swelling with no deformity may be present. With time, however, the capsule and ligaments, and the intrinsic musculature lose their capacity to compensate for the torn plantar plate and progressive deformity develops. As the deformity progresses, the second toe may cross either under or, more often, over the hallux, especially in the presence of a hallux valgus deformity.

Plantar plate insufficiency can present a difficult diagnostic dilemma and the diagnosis may sometimes be confused with an interdigital neuroma.[4,5,18] A neuroma is usually associated with numbness and neuritic radicular pain into the toes.

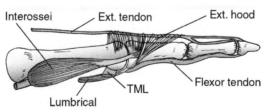

Fig. 3. Diagram of the intrinsic muscles of the lesser metatarsophalangeal joint. The lumbrical tendon is plantar to the transverse metatarsal ligament (TML), whereas the interossei tendon is dorsal to it.

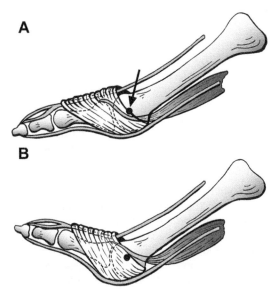

Fig. 4. (*A*) The center of rotation of the metatarsophalangeal joint is the center of the metatarsal head (*arrow*). The lumbrical tendon and the interosseous tendon are plantar to the center of rotation in the neutral position. (*B*) With hyperextension of the joint, the interosseous tendon displaces dorsal to the center of rotation and becomes a deforming extension force. The lumbrical tendon remains tethered plantarly and can become an adduction deforming force.

Reproduction of pain by squeezing the transverse metatarsal arch may result in a "Mulder click."[34,35] This finding is present about 40% of the time with neuromas.[34] Lesser MTP joint instability is not typically associated with radicular pain or numbness unless associated with a concomitant neuroma. Coughlin and colleagues[8] noted that 20% of the cases in which an interdigital neuroma was excised also demonstrated instability of the second MTP joint.

PHYSICAL EXAMINATION

As the plantar plate becomes attenuated or tears, MTP joint instability occurs[13,15,17,19,21,25] with the development of pain initially and then deformity.[4,13,21,25,27] Medial deviation of the digit or the development of a gap between the toes is another clinical sign of instability.[5,7,25] Initially joint swelling without malalignment is typical, but with time progressive dorsal or dorsomedial deviation of the digit develops because of degeneration of the lateral plantar plate and collateral ligament complex. A hammertoe typically develops in later stages of the deformity. On palpation, the location of tenderness depends on the presence of a ligament or capsular tear, and tenderness can be either the medial or lateral aspect of the MTP joint in the presence of a collateral ligament tear, or on the plantar aspect near the base of the proximal phalanx in the presence of a plantar plate tear. Compression of the transverse metatarsal arch typically does not illicit pain radiating into the toes, which is characteristic with interdigital neuroma.[17] However, on occasion an interdigital neuroma can occur in the second intermetatarsal space associated with second toe instability.[8] Distinguishing pain associated with an unstable lesser MTP joint or a neuroma is difficult, and sequential xylocaine injections may help to differentiate the exact location of pain.[7,8,17,34,36] The drawer test is a definitive sign of MTP joint instability (**Fig. 5**).[17,21,25,36,37] The drawer

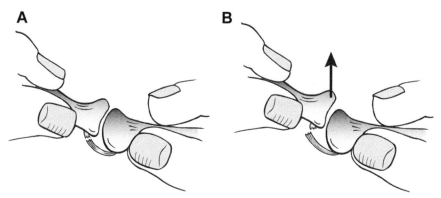

Fig. 5. Drawer test. (*A*) The toe is grasped by the examiner. (*B*) Dorsally directed force causes pain and subluxation at the MTP joint. Arrow denotes dorsal subluxation of the proximal phalanx on the lesser metatarsal head.

test is correctly performed by holding the MTP joint in a neutral position, and then applying vertical stress in a dorsal direction. To assess the position and strength of the digit, the "paper pull-out test" is used to measure the dynamic digital purchase on the ground (**Fig. 6**).[11] A narrow strip of paper is placed beneath the tip of the affected digit. The patient plantar flexes the affected toe to resist the attempt of the examiner to pull the paper out from beneath the digit. When the paper is pulled out without ripping, this is a positive test that confirms the absence of digital purchase. Sung and colleagues[38] reported on a series of 45 patients and noted that the physical examination had a high degree of accuracy. By combining all examination findings, the clinical examination can be highly successful in diagnosing plantar plate tears.

Several reports have proposed grading of second MTP joint instability.[16,18,22,24] A prodromal stage preceding joint subluxation was proposed by Mendicino and colleagues[18] and Yu and colleagues.[24] Haddad and colleagues[16] suggested a clinical description of second MTP instability based on deformity, but did not use the findings of clinical examination. Coughlin[4] proposed a comprehensive clinical staging system based on physical examination that incorporated many of the clinical ratings and attributes of the previous rating systems.[16,18,21,22,24] Based on the findings of the history

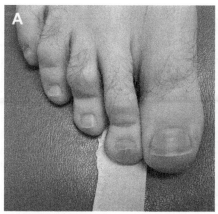
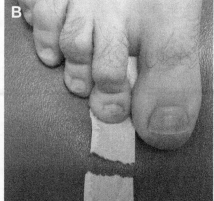

Fig. 6. Paper pull-out test. (*A*) A slip of paper is placed beneath the affected digit. (*B*) With plantar flexion pressure at the digit, tearing of the paper denotes adequate strength.

and physical examination and especially the magnitude of the drawer test, the MTP joint instability is staged based on a 0 to 4 scale (**Table 1**). This staging system defines the severity of the deformity. The preoperative staging is helpful in anticipating surgical findings and predicting the steps necessary for successful surgical treatment. The authors subsequently performed cadaveric dissections of specimens with confirmed plantar plate tears and then developed an anatomic grading scale to match the clinical staging system. These two scales are helpful in the surgical planning and management of plantar plate ruptures. Nery and colleagues[21] reported a high correlation between the clinical staging and surgical findings in a series of 55 plantar plate tears (**Fig. 7, Table 2**).

IMAGING STUDIES

Plain radiographs may give important information regarding lesser MTP joint instability (**Fig. 8**). With progression of a plantar plate tear and capsular degeneration, the orientation of the digit in the transverse plane becomes altered. Standard anteroposterior and lateral radiographs are used in evaluating the magnitude of the angular deformity, assessing joint congruity, evaluating the presence of arthritic changes, and assessing the length of the second metatarsal.[17] The length of the lesser metatarsals can be evaluated on radiographs and may contribute to increased pressure at the MTP joints. A lateral radiograph may define either a hyperextension deformity or dislocation of the joint.[17,24]

Arthrography of a lesser MTP joint can be used to evaluate chronic MTP joint pain. In a cadaveric study, Blitz and colleagues[39] reported the use of arthrography to assess the integrity of the plantar plate. More recently, the use of magnetic resonance imaging (MRI) to evaluate plantar plate integrity has been reported to have high sensitivity and specificity (**Fig. 9**).[38,40] Sung and colleagues[38] reported concordance of 62% between the MRI grade and the surgical grade of the plantar plate tear with greater agreement noted with higher-grade tears. MRI is useful for diagnosing injuries of the plantar plate in cases where the physical examination is equivocal. MRI can also be helpful when attempting to determine the involvement of multiple lesser toes with plantar plate

Table 1		
Clinical staging of examination for second MTP joint instability		
Grade	Alignment	Physical Examination
0	No MTP joint malalignment; prodromal phase with pain but no deformity	MTP joint pain, thickening or swelling of the MTP joint, diminished toe purchase, negative drawer
1	Mild malalignment of MTP joint; widening of the webspace, medial deviation	MTP joint pain, swelling of MTP joint, reduced toe purchase, mildly positive drawer (<50% subluxable)
2	Moderate malalignment; medial, lateral, dorsal, or dorsomedial deformity, hyperextension of the MTP joint	MTP joint pain, reduced swelling, no toe purchase, moderately positive drawer (>50% subluxable)
3	Severe malalignment; dorsal or dorsomedial deformity; the second toe can overlap the hallux; may have flexible hammertoe	Joint and toe pain, little swelling, no toe purchase (dislocatable MTP joint), flexible hammertoe
4	Dorsomedial or dorsal dislocation; severe deformity with dislocation, fixed hammertoe deformity	Joint and toe pain, little if any swelling, no toe purchase, dislocatable MTP joint, fixed hammertoe deformity

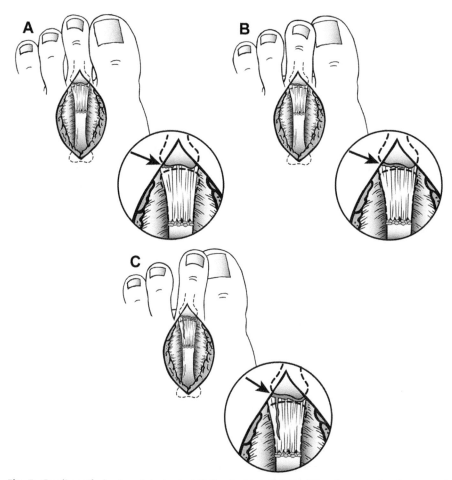

Fig. 7. Grading of plantar plate tears. (*A*) Grade 1 tear (*dotted line* denotes distal extent of metatarsal head, which has been removed to show the plantar plate) with less than 50% tear off of the base of the proximal phalanx. (*B*) Grade 2 tear with greater than 50% tear off of the proximal phalanx base. (*C*) Grade 3 tear with longitudinal component (also includes a horizontal distal tear). (*D 1* and *2*). Grade 4 tear with different patterns of extensive degeneration in the plantar plate. Arrow denotes tear pattern of the plantar plate.

pathology. We have found that a 3-T MRI unit gives excellent imaging capacity without the need for arthrography to make an accurate diagnosis.

CONSERVATIVE TREATMENT

There is often a significant delay between the initial onset of symptoms and the treatment of lesser MTP joint instability. Many patients do not seek out intervention for a mild deformity in the absence of substantial pain. Patients often only seek medical evaluation after the development of a progressive deformity.[7] If recognized in its early stages, the initiation of conservative measures may not only relieve pain but may slow the progression of the deformity. Nonsurgical measures may be initiated by changing footwear to a low-heeled shoe with a roomy toe box. A rocker-bottom sole may

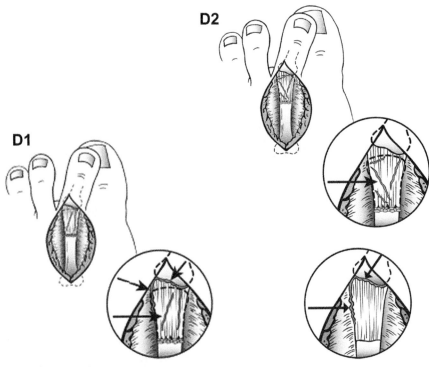

Fig. 7. (*continued*)

diminish pain and relieve dorsiflexion stress to the forefoot.[36] Adding a cushioned insole or a metatarsal pad[6,25] may reduce plantar pressure (**Fig. 10**). A graphite foot-plate can stiffen the toe box and reduce dorsiflexion stress across the MTP joint.[25] Padding over a symptomatic hammertoe may decrease discomfort and prevent rapid progression of deformity. Although nonsurgical treatment of an unstable second MTP joint deformity may temporarily relieve pain, it cannot be expected to permanently correct the malalignment.[1,6,7] In a report on the conservative treatment of patients with a crossover toe deformity, Coughlin observed that digital taping slowed progression of the deformity but the patients continued to have pain.[7] The purpose of taping is to

Table 2	
Surgical grading of plantar plate tears	
Grade	**Patterns of Tears**
0	Plantar plate or capsular attenuation, and/or discoloration.
1	Transverse distal tear adjacent to insertion into proximal phalanx (<50%; medial/lateral/central area) and/or midsubstance tear (<50%).
2	Transverse distal tear (>50%); medial/lateral/central area and/or midsubstance tear (<50%).
3	Transverse and/or longitudinal extensive tear (may involve collateral ligaments). Frequently also a distal transverse tear present.
4	Extensive tear with button hole (dislocation); a combination of transverse and longitudinal tears, with an extensive tear, little plantar plate to repair.

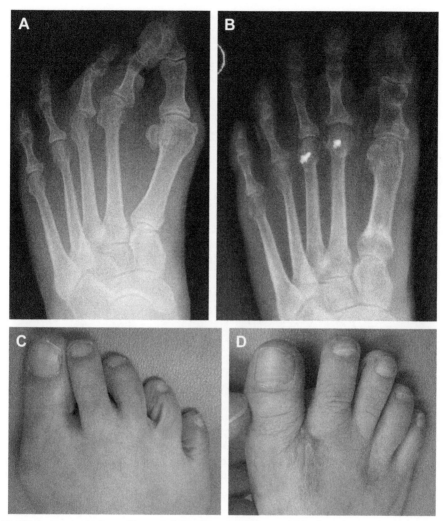

Fig. 8. Anteroposterior radiograph (*A*) before treatment and (*B*) after plantar plate repair of the second and third MTP joints. Clinical photograph (*C*) before and (*D*) after surgical realignment.

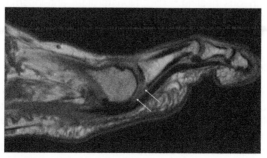

Fig. 9. MRI demonstrating a complete plantar plate rupture (*arrows*).

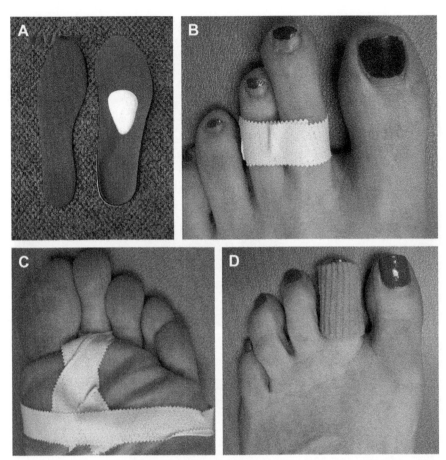

Fig. 10. Conservative treatment. (*A*) Graphite insole on the left and a soft insole with a metatarsal pad on the right. (*B*) Dorsal and (*C*) plantar view of taping technique. (*D*) Padding of a hammertoe deformity.

stabilize the toe in a neutral position with the development of scarring or healing of the capsular deformity. Taping, however, is not effective with capsular disruption or dislocation.[7] Because the plantar plate and knee meniscus are similarly composed of primarily type 1 collagen, some believe that a plantar plate tear has a minimal chance of undergoing spontaneous healing.[22,26,29] Nonsteroidal anti-inflammatory drugs and intra-articular corticosteroid injections have been reported to have temporary efficacy; however, injections should be used judiciously and not on a repetitive basis.[25,36]

SURGICAL TECHNIQUE

The patient is positioned supine with a bump under the ipsilateral hip and a tourniquet on the calf. The authors prefer an alcohol followed by chlorhexidine surgical preparation. The surgical technique uses a dorsal approach to expose the plantar plate. A 3- to 4-cm dorsal webspace incision allows access to the dorsal MTP joint and then dissection is continued deeper between the two extensor tendons. The distal capsular attachments to the base of the proximal phalanx are released medially and laterally. A

McGlamry elevator is used plantarly to release the proximal plantar plate from the metatarsal while carefully preserving the collateral ligament origins on the metatarsal head. A Weil metatarsal osteotomy is performed and the metatarsal head is temporarily translated proximally 5 to 10 mm and held in position with a vertical Kirschner wire (**Figs. 11** and **12**). A separate Kirschner wire is placed centrally in the metaphysis of the proximal phalanx and the MTP joint is distracted. Longitudinal tears of the plantar plate are visualized and repaired using a mini-Scorpion (mechanical suture-passer; Arthrex, Inc, Naples, FL) or a Micro-Suture-Lasso (curved suture-passer or a viper suture-passer; Arthrex, Inc, Naples, FL). A distally based partial plantar plate tear is converted to a complete tear and detached from the base of the proximal phalanx (**Fig. 12**). Following placement of Fiberwire (Arthrex) sutures in the plantar plate, the distractor is removed and a Kirschner wire is used to drill a medial and lateral hole in the base of the proximal phalanx through which the sutures are passed from plantar to dorsal. The Weil osteotomy is reduced and fixed in a more anatomically appropriate position with typical shortening of 2 to 3 mm. Lastly, the sutures from the plantar plate are tied dorsally over a bone bridge of the proximal phalanx with the toe MTP joint held in a corrected position. The soft tissue and skin are approximated in a routine fashion (**Fig. 13**). Postoperatively, a gauze and tape compression dressing is used to protect the toe. Ten days following surgery, passive and active exercises are commenced to rehabilitate the digit. The patient is allowed to weight bear flat-footed in a postoperative shoe immediately after surgery and can begin walking with a normal gait in athletic footwear 6 weeks postsurgery.

COMPLICATIONS AND MANAGEMENT

With any procedure it is imperative to appropriately identify and address complications. The most common complications of plantar plate repair are misdiagnosis, residual plantar forefoot pain, transfer metatarsalgia, MTP joint stiffness, intrinsic muscle weakness, dorsal contracture, and recurrence of the deformity. Many patients have been treated with lengthy conservative care or indirect repair, and their surgical correction may be more difficult based on prolonged neglect or previous reconstructive procedures.

Misdiagnosis

Often plantar plate tears are misdiagnosed as an adjacent interdigital neuroma. Following neurectomy, these patients may experience continued pain and progressive transverse plane deformity resulting from a missed plantar plate tear or intraoperative injury to the collateral ligament, joint capsule, interosseus tendon, or lumbrical tendon. Frequently, these patients are successfully managed with reoperation and direct plantar plate repair. A prior neuroma excision does not preclude reconstruction.

Residual Plantar Forefoot Pain

A vertically performed Weil osteotomy may contribute to residual forefoot pain. If the Weil osteotomy is performed too vertical, surgical shortening also displaces the metatarsal head plantarly and leads to increased plantar pressure. It is paramount to start the osteotomy in the dorsal cartilaginous surface of the metatarsal head and maintain the osteotomy closely parallel to the plantar aspect of the foot. This usually equates to a 15-degree angle with the metatarsal shaft. Maintaining this angle and limiting shortening to 1 to 3 mm can help prevent the metatarsal head fragment from becoming prominent plantarly.

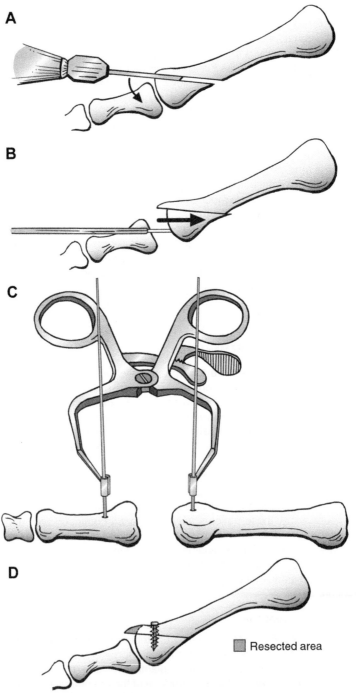

Fig. 11. Diagram of surgical treatment. (*A*) Weil osteotomy. (*B*) Capital fragment is pushed proximally and (*C*) secured with a vertical Kirschner wire. A second Kirschner wire is placed in the proximal phalanx and a distractor exposes the plantar plate. (*D*) Sutures securing the plantar plate through drill holes in the proximal phalanx.

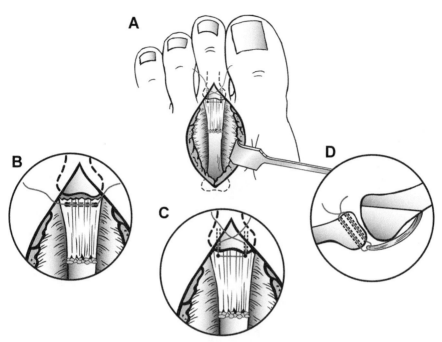

Fig. 12. (*A*) Placement of a horizontal mattress suture in the plantar plate. (*B*) Close up of the suture technique. (*C*) Sutures pulled through holes in the proximal phalanx. (*D*) Lateral view of sutures through the proximal phalanx.

Transfer Metatarsalgia

This can result from the surgically corrected metatarsal being overshortened. It is critical to maintain an appropriate metatarsal arc with the length of metatarsals progressively shortening from medial to lateral. Often shortening of 1 to 3 mm is adequate. To avoid postoperative length issues, shortening the adjacent metatarsal during the index procedure may be beneficial.

Joint Stiffness

Development of postoperative stiffness can occur for multiple reasons. A significant amount of surgical dissection is done in a confined area and the resulting inflammation, swelling, and immobilization can contribute to soft tissue contracture. Aggressive joint mobilization and an early return to flexible footwear is advised. Joint stiffness often improves with time, which may take up to a year postoperatively. If stiffness does not spontaneously resolve, manipulation under sedation or surgical release may be beneficial.

Flexion Weakness

It is often difficult for the flexor intrinsic musculature to overcome the dorsal extensor moment and there may be residual hyperextension and plantar flexion weakness as a result. One of the most common causes of flexor weakness is excessive shortening of the metatarsal. Excessive shortening can cause laxity in the flexor musculature that may be difficult to overcome postoperatively. Plantar translation of the axis of rotation when performing the Weil osteotomy may also alter the force vector of the intrinsic

400

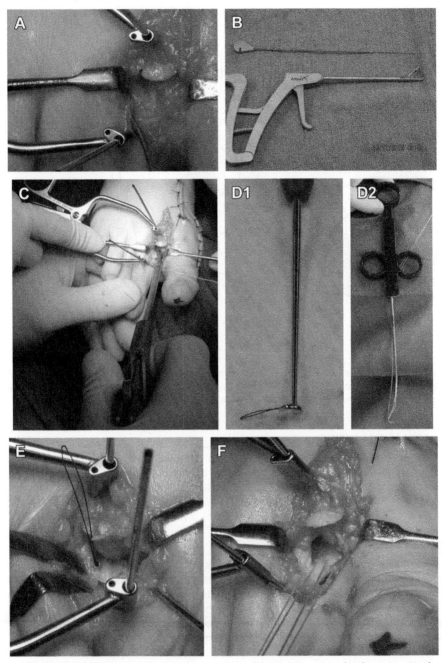

Fig. 13. (*A*) Distraction reveals the plantar plate. (*B*) Mini-Scorpion (Arthrex Inc, Naples, FL) is used to deliver the sutures. (*C*) Placement of the sutures in the plantar plate. (*D1*) Suture lasso with internal loop to transfer the suture. (*D2*) Viper (Arthex Inc, Naples, FL) is a suture passer that can be used without performing a Weil osteotomy. (*E*) The suture-lasso can be used in a constricted joint to pass the sutures. (*F*) Suture pattern with two horizontal mattress sutures of Fiberwire (Arthrex). (*G*) Drilling the vertical bone tunnels (medial and lateral) in proximal phalanx. (*H*) Sutures in plantar plate are passed through the proximal phalanx drill hole with a wire loop retriever. (*I*) The Weil osteotomy is secured with a clamp and fixed with a screw.

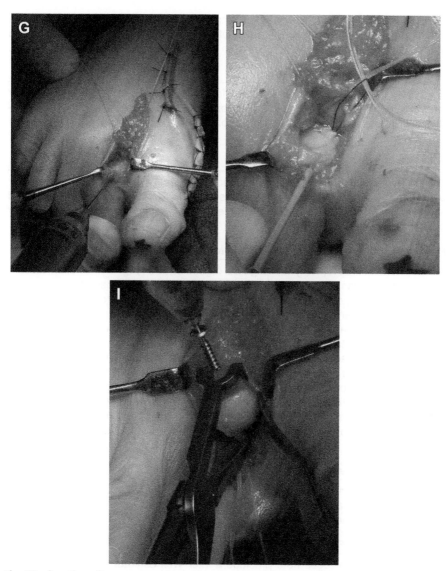

Fig. 13. (*continued*)

tendons. Limiting the amount of metatarsal shortening and plantar translation and early aggressive range of motion exercises may mitigate this complication.

Dorsal Contracture

During the recovery process, the flexor musculature may not have enough power to overcome the dorsal extensors. This coupled with dorsal adhesions from bone and capsular healing may result in a dorsal contractures. This is different from the "floating toe" associated with a Weil osteotomy. The dorsally contracted toe still maintains vertical stability indicating successful plantar plate repair but the dorsal contracture prevents desired alignment and function. Night splinting the toe in plantarflexion for 4 weeks postoperatively may help prevent the development of dorsal contractures.

Early and aggressive physiotherapy to strengthen the flexors and maintain joint mobility is crucial. Percutaneous capsulotomy and manipulation between 4 and 9 months postoperatively has been used to successfully correct dorsal contractures.

Deformity Recurrence

This is rare in our experience. In severe deformities, it may be necessary to consider more aggressive procedures, such as a flexor tendon transfer or metatarsal arthroplasty. We believe these yield less favorable results but they may be necessary for salvage procedures.

Prior Soft Tissue Release, Capsular Reefing

Soft tissue release and realignment does not preclude a Weil osteotomy and plantar plate repair. Usually old scar tissue and soft tissue contractures can be released and the Weil osteotomy adequately mobilized to allow for joint distraction and plantar plate visualization.

Prior Phalangeal Osteotomy or Weil Osteotomy

A prior phalangeal osteotomy to realign the digit rarely is a long-term solution. Reconstruction with a plantar plate repair is still possible if phalangeal osteotomy has been previously performed. A prior Weil osteotomy without plantar plate repair remains an area of concern. Performing a subsequent Weil osteotomy may present an increased risk for avascular necrosis (AVN) of the metatarsal head. Also, mature scar tissue in and around the metatarsal head may preclude adequate metatarsal head displacement and joint distraction and therefore make a plantar plate repair difficult. However, if the metatarsal has been appropriately aligned previously, creating a new osteotomy for exposure and repair of the plantar plate is reasonable and realigning the metatarsal to its previous position is advocated. This is similar to the use of a medial malleolar osteotomy to access an osteochondral defect on the talus. One may choose to release the collateral ligament, distract the joint, and repair the plantar plate without an osteotomy.

Prior Metatarsal Head Condylectomy

This was an early form of treatment to stabilize the MTP joint. A Weil osteotomy can be performed, and a careful proximal plantar plate release using a McGlamry elevator aids in mobilizing the plantar plate sufficiently to allow a repair.

Prior Extensor and Flexor Tendon Transfer

Prior tendon transfer does note preclude a later Weil osteotomy and plantar plate repair. With more extensive tear patterns (Grade 4), a flexor tendon transfer may be necessary because there is insufficient plantar plate to repair. Preoperative MRI is helpful in determining the extent and magnitude of the tear for surgical planning.

SURGICAL OUTCOMES

In the past, the operative intervention of a lesser MTP joint instability has consisted of an indirect repair of the MTP joint subluxation. Commonly reported treatments consist of MTP joint synovectomy,[3] capsular soft tissue release,[1,5,6,16,17,19,20] extensor and flexor tendon transfers,[1,5,8,11,16–18,20,24] and periarticular osteotomies.[4,18,23,24] The introduction of the Weil osteotomy led to improved outcomes with decompression and realignment of the involved joint.[4,6,18,24] However, all of these methods neglect the treatment of the plantar plate tear. New surgical techniques to directly repair the plantar plate have used a plantar and dorsal surgical exposure.[11,14,15,21,22,25,29] Powless and Elze[22] and Bouche and Heit[11] reported on a total of 78 plantar plate repairs done using a plantar approach. An anatomic study of the surgical exposure of the lesser MTP joints demonstrated that a dorsal approach could also be used to allow adequate exposure of the plantar plate.[9] In a series of 35 plantar plate repairs in 23 patients performed through the dorsal surgical approach, Gregg and colleagues[15] reported substantial correction of deformity and marked reduction of pain. Weil and colleagues[23] reported that they performed 15 plantar plate repairs using a dorsal approach with a Weil osteotomy and had acceptable results. In the first prospective evaluation of direct plantar plate repair and capsular reefing, Nery and colleagues[21] and Coughlin[7] evaluated 22 patients (40 MTP joints). They reported marked improvement in pain scores and improved joint stability as measured by the drawer test. Two-thirds of the patients regained marked toe strength as measured with the paper pull-out test (see **Fig. 8**).

SUMMARY

The development of lesser MTP joint instability has been recognized for more than two decades. Until recently, there has been a lack of understanding of the true pathoanatomy responsible for the deformity. A clear understanding of plantar plate degeneration and collateral ligament dysfunction has led to the development of direct plantar plate repair techniques. A dorsal surgical exposure allows extensive visualization that can include inspection of the common underlying anatomic causes of the deformity including metatarsal position and plantar plate insufficiency. The results of direct repair of the plantar plate are very encouraging, although long-term follow-up is necessary. The addition of a direct plantar plate repair does not preclude any of the prior treatment options including soft tissue release, capsular reefing, and metatarsal shortening osteotomy.

REFERENCES

1. Coughlin MJ. Crossover second toe deformity. Foot Ankle 1987;8:29–39.
2. Mann RA, Coughlin MJ. The rheumatoid foot: review of literature and method of treatment. Orthop Rev 1979;8:105–12.
3. Mann RA, Mizel MS. Monarticular nontraumatic synovitis of the metatarsophalangeal joint: a new diagnosis? Foot Ankle 1985;6:18–21.
4. Coughlin MJ. Lesser toe deformities, surgery of the foot and ankle. In: Coughlin MJ, Mann CL, Saltzman CL, editors. Surgery of the foot and ankle. 9th edition. Philadelphia: Mosby Elsevier Inc; 2007. p. 366–400.
5. Coughlin MJ. Second metatarsophalangeal joint instability in the athlete. Foot Ankle 1993;14:309–19.
6. Coughlin MJ. Subluxation and dislocation of the second metatarsophalangeal joint. Orthop Clin North Am 1989;20:535–51.
7. Coughlin MJ. When to suspect crossover second toe deformity. J Muscoskel Med 1987;39–48.
8. Coughlin MJ, Schenck RC Jr, Shurnas PS, et al. Concurrent interdigital neuroma and MTP joint instability: long-term results of treatment. Foot Ankle Int 2002;23:1018–25.
9. Cooper MT, Coughlin MJ. Sequential dissection for exposure of the second metatarsophalangeal joint. Foot Ankle Int 2011;32:294–9. http://dx.doi.org/10.3113/fai.2011.0294.
10. DuVries HL. Dislocation of the toe. JAMA 1956;160:728.

11. Bouche RT, Heit EJ. Combined plantar plate and hammertoe repair with flexor digitorum longus tendon transfer for chronic, severe sagittal plane instability of the lesser metatarsophalangeal joints: preliminary observations. J Foot Ankle Surg 2008;47:125–137. http://dx.doi.org/10.1053/j.jfas.2007.12.008.

12. Brunet JA, Tubin S. Traumatic dislocations of the lesser toes. Foot Ankle Int 1997; 18:406–11.

13. Coughlin MJ, Schutt SA, Hirose CB, et al. Metatarsophalangeal joint pathology in crossover second toe deformity: a cadaveric study. Foot Ankle Int 2012;33: 133–40. http://dx.doi.org/10.3113/fai.2012.0133.

14. Ford LA, Collins KB, Christensen JC. Stabilization of the subluxed second metatarsophalangeal joint: flexor tendon transfer versus primary repair of the plantar plate. J Foot Ankle Surg 1998;37:217–22.

15. Gregg J, Silberstein M, Clark C, et al. Plantar plate repair and Weil osteotomy for metatarsophalangeal joint instability. Foot Ankle Surg 2007;13:116–21.

16. Haddad SL, Sabbagh RC, Resch S, et al. Results of flexor-to-extensor and extensor brevis tendon transfer for correction of the crossover second toe deformity. Foot Ankle Int 1999;20:781–8.

17. Kaz AJ, Coughlin MJ. Crossover second toe: demographics, etiology, and radiographic assessment. Foot Ankle Int 2007;28:1223–37. http://dx.doi.org/10.3113/fai.2007.1223.

18. Mendicino RW, Statler TK, Saltrick KR, et al. Predislocation syndrome: a review and retrospective analysis of eight patients. J Foot Ankle Surg 2001;40:214–24.

19. Murphy JL. Isolated dorsal dislocation of the second metatarsophalangeal joint. Foot Ankle 1980;1:30–2.

20. Myerson MS, Jung HG. The role of toe flexor-to-extensor transfer in correcting metatarsophalangeal joint instability of the second toe. Foot Ankle Int 2005;26: 675–9.

21. Nery C, Coughlin MJ, Baumfeld D, et al. Lesser metatarsophalangeal joint instability: prospective evaluation and repair of plantar plate and capsular insufficiency. Foot Ankle Int 2012;33:301–11. http://dx.doi.org/10.3113/fai.2012.0301.

22. Powless SH, Elze ME. Metatarsophalangeal joint capsule tears: an analysis by arthrography, a new classification system and surgical management. J Foot Ankle Surg 2001;40:374–89.

23. Weil L Jr, Sung W, Weil LS Sr, et al. Anatomic plantar plate repair using the Weil metatarsal osteotomy approach. Foot Ankle Spec 2011;4:145–50. http://dx.doi.org/10.1177/1938640010397342.

24. Yu GV, Judge MS, Hudson JR, et al. Predislocation syndrome. Progressive subluxation/dislocation of the lesser metatarsophalangeal joint. J Am Podiatr Med Assoc 2002;92:182–99.

25. Coughlin MJ, Baumfeld DS, Nery C. Second MTP joint instability: grading of the deformity and description of surgical repair of capsular insufficiency. Phys Sportsmed 2011;39:132–41. http://dx.doi.org/10.3810/psm.2011.09.1929.

26. Deland JT, Lee KT, Sobel M, et al. Anatomy of the plantar plate and its attachments in the lesser metatarsal phalangeal joint. Foot Ankle Int 1995;16: 480–6.

27. Deland JT, Sung IH. The medial crosssover toe: a cadaveric dissection. Foot Ankle Int 2000;21:375–8.

28. Sarrafian SK, Topouzian LK. Anatomy and physiology of the extensor apparatus of the toes. J Bone Joint Surg Am 1969;51:669–79.

29. Johnston RB 3rd, Smith J, Daniels T. The plantar plate of the lesser toes: an anatomical study in human cadavers. Foot Ankle Int 1994;15:276–82.

30. Barg A, Courville XF, Nickisch F, et al. Role of collateral ligaments in metatarsophalangeal stability: a cadaver study. Foot Ankle Int 2012;33:877–82. http://dx.doi.org/10.3113/fai.2012.0877.

31. Rao JP, Banzon MT. Irreducible dislocation of the metatarsophalangeal joints of the foot. Clin Orthop Relat Res 1979;(145):224–6.

32. Gallentine JW, DeOrio JK. Removal of the second toe for severe hammertoe deformity in elderly patients. Foot Ankle Int 2005;26:353–8.

33. Morton DJ. Metatarsus atavicus:the identification of a distinctive type of foot disorder. J Bone Joint Surg 1927;9:531–44.

34. Coughlin MJ, Pinsonneault T. Operative treatment of interdigital neuroma. A long-term follow-up study. J Bone Joint Surg Am 2001;83-A:1321–8.

35. Mulder JD. The causative mechanism in Morton's metatarsalgia. J Bone Joint Surg Br 1951;33-B:94–5.

36. Trepman E, Yeo SJ. Nonoperative treatment of metatarsophalangeal joint synovitis. Foot Ankle Int 1995;16:771–7.

37. Thompson FM, Hamilton WG. Problems of the second metatarsophalangeal joint. Orthopedics 1987;10:83–9.

38. Sung W, Weil L Jr, Weil LS Sr, et al. Diagnosis of plantar plate injury by magnetic resonance imaging with reference to intraoperative findings. J Foot Ankle Surg 2012;51:570–4. http://dx.doi.org/10.1053/j.jfas.2012.05.009.

39. Blitz NM, Ford LA, Christensen JC. Second metatarsophalangeal joint arthrography: a cadaveric correlation study. J Foot Ankle Surg 2004;43:231–40. http://dx.doi.org/10.1053/j.jfas.2004.05.009.

40. Yao L, Cracchiolo A, Farahani K, et al. Magnetic resonance imaging of plantar plate rupture. Foot Ankle Int 1996;17:33–6.

Recurrent Metatarsalgia

Pierre Barouk, MD

KEYWORDS

- Recurrent metatarsalgia • Hallux valgus surgery • Lateral ray surgery
- First metatarsal

KEY POINTS

- In hallux valgus surgery, recurrent metatarsalgia can be a problem of the position of the first metatarsal after an inappropriate or poorly done first metatarsal osteotomy and/or a problem of gastrocnemius tightness not previously recognized.
- The best treatment is to restore the normal anatomy but it is not always possible, and surgery on affected rays could be the solution.
- Recurrent metatarsalgia after lateral ray surgery depends on the technique (remove a second layer–double oblique osteotomy to shorten and elevate) and indications (respect the parabola) of the Weil osteotomy, which is the most used technique for lateral rays.
- Conservative realignment osteotomies can be done most of the time. Percutaneous osteotomy of lateral rays seems interesting but needs to be evaluated.
- Barouk, Rippstein, Toullec (BRT) osteotomy provides solutions in cases of excess of metatarsal slope/plantarflexion.

INTRODUCTION

Recurrent metatarsalgia can be considered a failure of a first surgery. This article looks at 2 scenarios: (1) recurrent metatarsalgia after surgery of the first ray for hallux valgus and (2) metatarsalgia that did not disappear after a lateral ray surgery. Whatever the type, it can be a problem of indication or achievement. This article tries to understand the reasons for this failure and ways to prevent and treat it.

RECURRENT METATARSALGIA AND HALLUX VALGUS

One of the unanswered questions for every foot surgeon is, When is it necessary to do lesser metatarsal osteotomies when patients present with hallux valgus and metatarsalgia? In other words, When is the first ray correction sufficient to treat the metatarsalgia? There is no consensus around this question. Only a randomized double-blind study can provide a solution.

Understanding the mechanism of the metatarsalgia associated with hallux valgus might help reduce the number of failures of treatment and also help determine the correct surgical approach.

Disclosures: None.
Foot and Ankle Surgery Center, Sport's Clinic, 33700 Bordeaux-Mérignac, France
E-mail address: pierre.barouk@wanadoo.fr

Foot Ankle Clin N Am 19 (2014) 407–424
http://dx.doi.org/10.1016/j.fcl.2014.06.005
foot.theclinics.com

Etiology of Metatarsalgia Associated with Hallux Valgus

Several reasons:

a. First ray insufficiency is most common. It can be due to
  - Short first metatarsal
    - Congenital
    - Functional shortening due to metatarsus primus varus
    - Surgical shortening
  - Cuneometatarsal hypermobility[1–3]

This first ray insufficiency leads to a lesser head overload, especially because the metatarsus varus disturbs the windlass mechanism.[4–6]

b. Gastrocnemius tightness

A frequent cause of metatarsalgia associated with hallux valgus, but sometimes difficult to quantify, is gastrocnemius tightness. This is the most common explanation of lesser metatarsalgia in cases of a fairly normal first ray and mild hallux valgus.

An illustration of the association hallux valgus–metatarsalgia–gastrocnemius tightness is the case in **Figs. 1** and **2** that shows a patient with bilateral callus and metatarsalgia under the second, third, and fourth metatarsal head. Pain is more significant on the left side. Looking only at the right side, it is theoretically possible that the metatarsalgia is the result of the hallux valgus. Looking at the left forefoot overload, however, in particular, examining the patient, this metatarsalgia is seen due to the gastrocnemius tightness (Silfverskiold test: equinus when the knee is extended, reduced when the knee is flexed). This tightness has certainly worsened or even created the right hallux valgus.

The association between hallux valgus and gastrocnemius tightness has been highlighted by several investigators.[7–10] They all explained the correlation of forefoot overload due to the equinus and the close relationship of the gastrocnemius to the plantar aponeurosis, especially at the medial part.[6,10]

The metatarsalgia-gastrocnemius tightness association was highlighted in a biomechanical study by Cazeau and colleagues,[11] that shows that overpressure under the metatarsal heads is at maximum when the gastrocnemius are contracted. It was also highlighted by Maceira[12] as the metatarsalgia of the end of the secundo rocker (**Fig. 3**).

This metatarsalgia-gastrocnemius tightness association was also highlighted in a clinical study by Colombier[13] with the term, *metatarsalgia sine materia*. He noted the

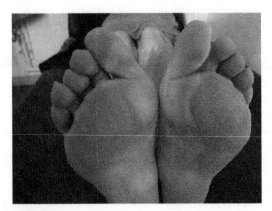

Fig. 1. Bilateral metatarsalgia.

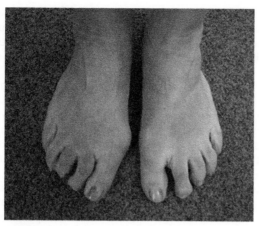

Fig. 2. Right hallux valgus.

efficiency of the proximal medial gastrocnemius lengthening in reducing the pressure under the metatarsals.

The hallux valgus–metatarsalgia–gastrocnemius tightness association was emphasized by Barouk and Barouk.[10] In a series of 106 cases of hallux valgus with gastrocnemius tightness, 61% had associated metatarsalgia, which is quite high.

This phenomenon of gastrocnemius tightness has to be taken into account when analyzing a metatarsalgia associated (or not) with a hallux valgus.

Metatarsalgia After Hallux Valgus Surgery

Metatarsalgia and plantar callosities disappear between 48% and 93% of cases after hallux valgus surgery due to the correction of the medial ray function and normalization of the windlass mechanism.[14–17]

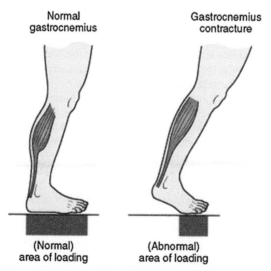

Fig. 3. Gastrocnemius contraction and forefoot overload. (*From* Bannerjee R, Nickisch F, Easley ME, et al. Foot injuries. In: Browner BD, Jupiter JB, Levine AM, et al, editors. Skeletal trauma. 4th edition. Philadelphia: Elsevier; 2009; with permission.)

The stress is redistributed to the first ray: cortical thickness of second metatarsal decreases[18] and contact pressure under second and third metatarsal decrease.[19]

In cases of a shortening first metatarsal osteotomy, however, like the Mitchell, the rate of plantar callosity recovery is low (48% for Yamamoto and colleagues[16] and 35% for Dermon and colleagues[20] and Toth and colleagues[21,22]). The metatarsal pressure reduces if the procedure is combined with lesser metatarsal shortening osteotomies.[16]

For a well-done distal osteotomy, like the chevron, the recovery rate is higher: in 80%, plantar callosity and metatarsalgia disappear. In 93%, metatarsalgia disappear but 13% have persistence of asymptomatic callosities. There are studies that report a 50% recurrence rate after chevron osteotomy.[23] This is especially true if the first metatarsal was shortened at the time of the osteotomy.

Mann and colleagues,[15] with a proximal crescentic osteotomy, reported a slightly lower recovery rate of plantar callosities and metatarsalgia, perhaps because of the possible elevation of the first metatarsal produced with this type of osteotomy.

A proximal basilar closing wedge osteotomy results in approximately 10% of postoperative metatarsalgia (8.5% of recurrent metatarsalgia and 1.5% of appearance of metatarsalgia),[24] possibly because of the shortening this kind of osteotomy induces. In contrast, an opening wedge osteotomy that effectively lengthens the first metatarsal seldom leads to metatarsalgia.[25] In a study by García-Bordes and colleagues,[26] a basilar opening wedge associated with a Keller procedure for severe deformity and MTPJ1 arthrosis had no recurrence of metatarsalgia.

At the level of diaphysal osteotomy, the scarf osteotomy seems more effective than the Ludloff osteotomy,[27] possibly because of the ease of plantarization of the metatarsal with the scarf osteotomy.

Nevertheless, no study, except the one by Barouk and Barouk,[10] took into account the gastrocnemius tightness. On 56 hallux valgus associated with metatarsalgia treated by scarf osteotomy and proximal medial gastrocnemius lengthening, they obtained a recurrence rate of only 5% (89% cured and 6% improved). It was evident that the gastrocnemius lengthening played a critical role in the treatment of metatarsalgia.

Prevention

Overall, the recurrence rate is 20% after correction of the first ray alone. Knowing that, a case can be made never to do lesser metatarsal osteotomies at the time of surgery and reserve them for recurrent metatarsalgias that do not respond to medical treatment. A better approach might be to try to identify the factors responsible for recurrence of metatarsalgia and either prevent them or add additional procedures.

A review of the literature does not show any studies looking at the factors that could decrease this recurrence rate of metatarsalgia. This article tries to identify them. Looking at the published studies, recurrent metatarsalgia in hallux valgus depends on the final position of the first metatarsal: too elevated or too short leads to the recurrence or appearance of metatarsalgia.

The choice of the first metatarsal osteotomy is important in preoperative analysis of cases. In cases of a short M1, a shortening osteotomy preferably should not be done (Mitchell, Wilson, or proximal closing wedge). Having said that, in some cases shortening of the first metatarsal might be critical for the correction. With a high M1M2 angle or arthrosis and/or stiffness of the first metatarsophalangeal joint (MTPJ), shortening of the metatarsal is beneficial to the correction and to unload the first MTPJ. The presence in these cases of preoperative metatarsalgia should prompt surgeons to do lesser metatarsal shortening osteotomies at the same time.

In cases where shortening of the first metatarsal is not mandatory, the author prefers nonshortening osteotomies to correct the hallux valgus (chevron, scarf, or opening wedge).

Lowering first metatarsal osteotomies is useful in situations where there is a metatarsus elevatus or even in cases of relative hypermobility of the first tarsometatarsal joint. In these cases, a lowering scarf osteotomy or Lapidus is preferable.

It is always an interesting conversation to have with a patient when metatarsalgia is the main complaint and when the mechanical issues around the first metatarsal are the reason for lesser metatarsal overload. It might be difficult to convince a patient that correcting the first ray will solve the metatarsalgia.

It is important

- To be sure to resolve what for the patient came for
- That if metatarsalgia is the main symptom, longstanding, and in an advanced stage, there is less of a chance to resolve it with the first ray surgery alone and lesser metatarsal osteotomies should be considered as well

Finally, gastrocnemius tightness has to be taken into account. It is critical to evaluate the association between hallux valgus and metatarsalgia. If there is an obvious contracture, a proximal medial gastrocnemius lengthening could give satisfactory resolution of symptoms.[10]

Treatment of Recurrent Metatarsalgia After Hallux Valgus Correction

Nonsurgical treatment should always be attempted first to try and resolve or accommodate the metatarsalgia. The options are orthotics, shoe wear changes, and stretching of the triceps surae. If these attempts fail, surgical treatment is often required.

Case of a well-reduced hallux valgus and good position of M1 (not too short, not too elevated)

If there is gastrocnemius tightness, lengthening of the gastrocnemius is a more logical and less-invasive alternative than lesser metatarsal osteotomies. The author's experience is to cut the tendinous fibers of the medial gastrocnemius close to their insertion on the femur. Moreover, this technique not only is effective in terms of equinus reduction but also has advantages of not interrupting the muscle continuity (respect of the red fibers), being minimally invasive (cosmetically and for the postoperative recovery), having a low complication rate, and not requiring immobilization. It could be done bilaterally at the same time.

The author also has observed that this procedure has a positive effect on other symptoms of gastrocnemius tightness, including a reduction of cramps, tension of the calf, lower limb instability, difficulty walking without a heel, and lumbar pain.[28] It also still leaves the option open to do metatarsal osteotomies if metatarsalgia persists.

If there is no gastrocnemius tightness or if lengthening does not resolve the metatarsalgia, it seems that lesser metatarsal osteotomies are required. There are 3 commonly used osteotomies:

1. Distal percutaneous for small/minimal shortening
2. Open Weil osteotomy for shortening more than 5 mm
3. BRT osteotomy: It is a basal dorsal closing wedge that mainly elevates and slightly shortens the metatarsals. This is the simplest way to maintain the normal parabola of the metatarsals.[29]

In cases like the one described previously (normal length and so forth), a small shortening of the lesser metatarsal is most often indicated, and the author prefers a percutaneous osteotomy.

Case of well-reduced hallux valgus but abnormality of M1 position

M1 too short Lengthening of the first metatarsal is possible either with a scarf osteotomy (first description by Burutaran[30] and clinical study by Singh[31]) or by external fixator.[32] These techniques are effective in reducing metatarsalgia and they have the advantage of restoring a normal anatomy. Joint stiffness might be an issue, however.

On the other hand, if lengthening is not possible due to skin problems, arthritic MTPJ, or other soft tissue compromises, shortening of lesser metatarsals is indicated. A Weil osteotomy is most appropriate to achieve the required shortening (**Figs. 4** and **5**).

M1 elevated Pure lowering of M1 is not easy. The standard Weil osteotomy shortens but also lowers the lesser metatarsal (MT), so is not indicated in case of metatarsalgia.

A proximal osteotomy can also be done: opening dorsal wedge or plantar closing wedge of the first MT (**Figs. 6** and **7**).

Elevation of the lesser metatarsal is another option, with BRT osteotomy (**Fig. 8**) or distal percutaneous (**Figs. 9** and **10**).

Case of recurrent hallux valgus Correction of the recurrent hallux valgus is essential. In these cases, the shortening of the first metatarsal is often needed as well as shortening of the lesser rays, especially when metatarsalgia is associated with a metatarsophalangeal dislocation (**Figs. 11** and **12**).

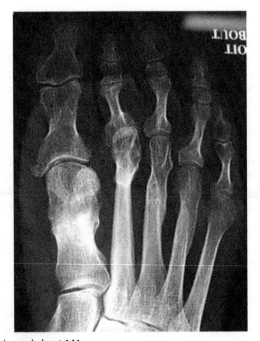

Fig. 4. Metatarsalgia and short M1.

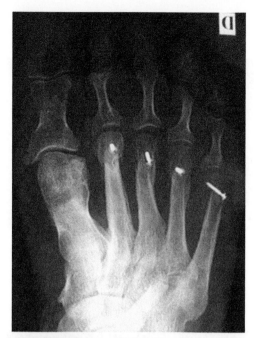

Fig. 5. Shortening with Weil osteotomies of MT 2–5.

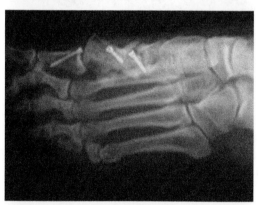

Fig. 6. Iatrogenic elevation of M1. (*Courtesy of* Toullec E, MD, Bordeaux, France.)

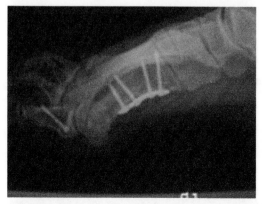

Fig. 7. M1 lowering by plantar closing wedge. This could be done is the first metatarsal has adequate length. The alternative is to do a dorsal open wedge osteotomy to plantarflex the first ray. (*Courtesy of* Toullec E, MD, Bordeaux, France.)

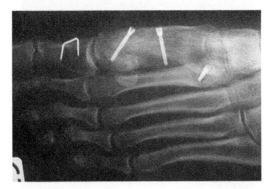

Fig. 8. BRT of M2.

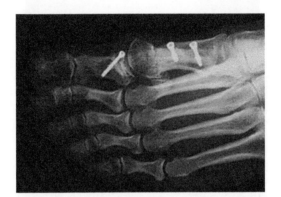

Fig. 9. M1 elevated.

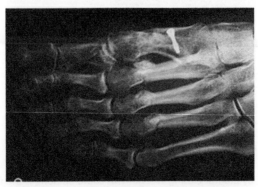

Fig. 10. Elevation of M2M3M4 by distal percutaneous osteotomy.

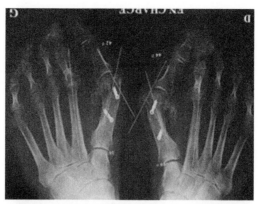

Fig. 11. Recurrent HV and MTPJ2 dislocation.

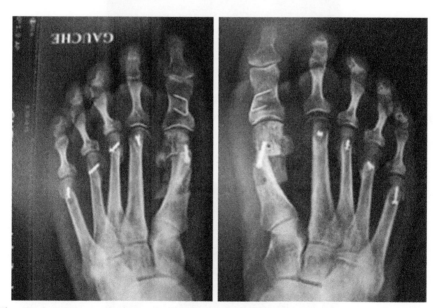

Fig. 12. Correction with shortening by scarf and Weil osteotomy.

RECURRENT METATARSALGIA AFTER LATERAL RAY SURGERY

Metatarsalgia can occur at the same level or recur at the adjacent metatarsal (transfer metatarsalgia).

1. Recurrent metatarsalgia on the operated ray

The most studied and most likely used osteotomy is the Weil osteotomy. It is the most popular because it is the safest way to shorten a metatarsal, and metatarsal shortening is required in many indications: severe disorders, hammer toes due to metatarsal over length, MTPJ dislocation, and metatarsalgia.

The most reported complication is recurrent metatarsalgia (**Figs. 13** and **14**). An analysis of 17 articles of Weil osteotomy (1131 osteotomies) showed a 15% recurrence rate of metatarsalgia.[33,34]

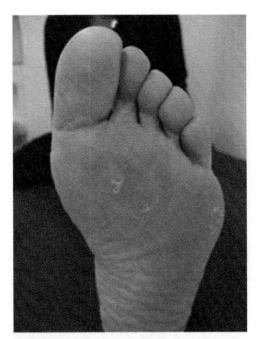

Fig. 13. Recurrent metatarsalgia and Weil osteotomy.

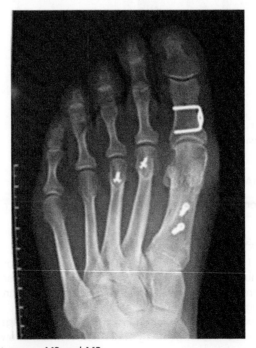

Fig. 14. Weil osteotomy on M2 and M3.

The most advocated reason for that is the lowering of the head induced by a single oblique cut.[35,36] This lowering induces more pressure under the head and increases the slope of the metatarsal. It has been demonstrated that postoperative plantar prominence of the head is related to recurrent metatarsalgia.[37] Lowering or plantar flexion of the metatarsal with a single-cut Weil osteotomy could also be responsible for stiffness in plantar flexion. This is caused by malpositioning of the intrinsic muscles and lowering of the center of rotation of the head.[36] Stiffness and recurrent metatarsalgia are related. Does the stiffness that creates a vertical force on the metatarsal head give the metatarsalgia, or does the excessive slope of the metatarsal create the stiffness? It is difficult to answer.

To resolve this problem, the most proposed modification is elevating the metatarsal by removing a second layer,[29,35,36,38–43] which improves the results by reducing pressure and also positioning the intrinsic muscle more anatomic.[37] This is for prevention. But to treat the problem, an elevation of the metatarsal is required:

- Distally, by a new Weil osteotomy with second layer or by a dorsal closing wedge (called in France the *Gauthier osteotomy*, used in Freiberg disease) or by the distal metatarsal minimally invasive osteotomy (DMMO).[29]
- Proximally by the BRT osteotomy.[29]

If there is stiffness, an arthrolysis must be done to remove the intra-articular fibrosis.

Specific indications
- Arthrolysis alone: dorsal soft tissue contracture is more apparent than the position of the metatarsal (**Figs. 15** and **16**).
- Gauthier osteotomy (see **Fig. 20**): to reorientate the articular surface when the cartilage is more plantar than dorsal. It also elevates the MT a few degrees.
2. Metatarsal overlength, despite a previous Weil osteotomy. It is possible to do a Weil osteotomy on a previous Weil osteotomy. In this case, it is preferable to do Weil osteotomy on M2345. The other option is DMMO if there is no need for an open arthrolysis (**Figs. 17** and **18**).
3. Frontal parabola disturbed (excess of metatarsal slope) (**Fig. 19**): BRT osteotomy (**Fig. 20**).

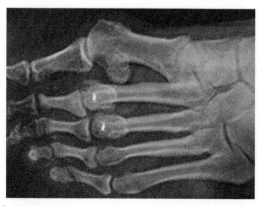

Fig. 15. Dorsal impingement.

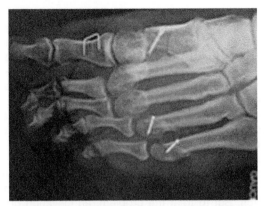

Fig. 16. Screw removal and arthrolysis on M2 M3.

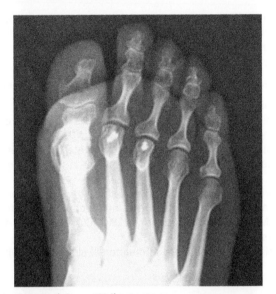

Fig. 17. Recurrent metatarsalgia on Weil osteotomy.

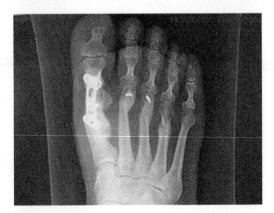

Fig. 18. DMMO on Weil osteotomy.

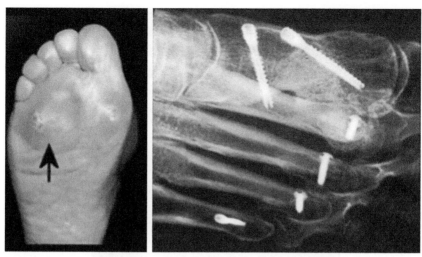

Fig. 19. Recurrent metatarsalgia on M3 M4. (*From* Barouk LS. Forefoot reconstruction. Paris: Springer-Verlag; 2003; with permission.)

4. Cases of MTPJ arthrosis: there are 2 options. The first is if it is thought that the MTPJ could be preserved. In that case, a Gauthier osteotomy is preferred (see **Fig. 23**). The second is when the joint cannot be preserved due to degenerative changes. In that situation, either an excision arthroplasty or a form of interposition arthroplasty can be done (**Figs. 21** and **22**).[29]

Transfer Metatarsalgia

Transfer metatarsalgia is most often due to nonrespect of the metatarsal parabola in the frontal plane (criteria of Maestro)[44] or in the sagittal plane.

As for Weil osteotomy, performing a single metatarsal osteotomy has been recognized as increasing the problems of recurrence, transfer, or stiffness.[29] The removal of

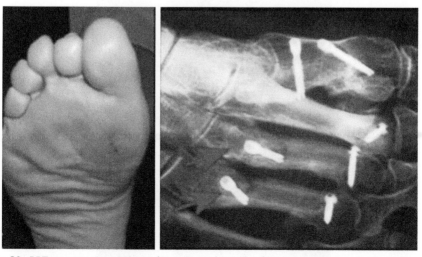

Fig. 20. BRT osteotomy on M3 M4. (*From* Barouk LS. Forefoot reconstruction. Paris: Springer-Verlag; 2003; with permission.)

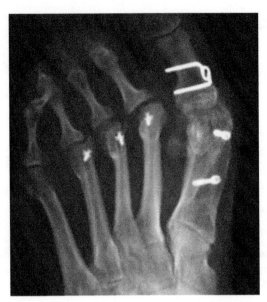

Fig. 21. MTPJ2 artrosis.

a second layer does not protect of transfer metatarsalgia, when a single osteotomy is done; it may even exacerbate it. There is a high rate of complications when the shortening is small and focused on a single metatarsal.[42] Restoring good alignment in all planes is the best way to solve the problem. In these cases, the complete parabola should be restored by doing mutliple osteotomies (**Figs. 23** and **24**).

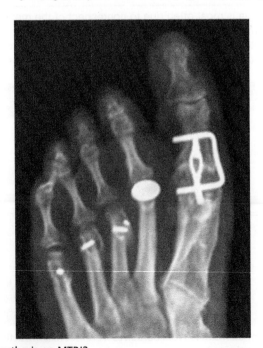

Fig. 22. Button prosthesis on MTPJ2.

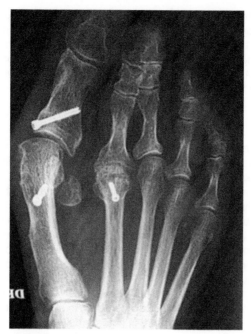

Fig. 23. Recurrent and transfer metatarsalgia.

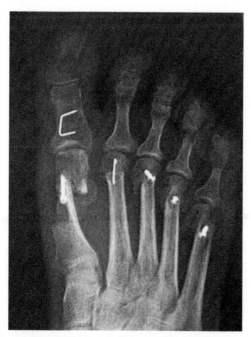

Fig. 24. Gauthier osteotomy on M2 (dorsal closing wedge) and parabola restored with Weil osteotomy on M345 and short scarf osteotomy on M1.

The risk of transfer exist also for the BRT osteotomy on a single metatarsal if the removed edge is too large. It is a base osteotomy, so it is powerful. One millimeter removed dorsally at the base elevates the head 3 mm. The author does not recommend routinely doing BRTs on several metatarsals. If it is used, close attention should be paid to get the MT head at the same level. BRTs are valuable when used for cavus foot surgery due to the power of correction.

SUMMARY

Recurrent metatarsalgia has a multifactorial etiology. The analysis of the cause is critical in planning the appropriate treatment. Understanding the etiology helps understand the mechanism of prevention, which is the best treatment. Like many failures in orthopedic surgery, recurrent metatarsalgia is often due to either poor technique or poor understanding of the underlying problem.

In hallux valgus surgery, recurrent metatarsalgia can be a problem of the position of the first metatarsal after an inappropriate or poorly done first metatarsal osteotomy and/or a problem of gastrocnemius tightness not previously recognized. The best treatment is to restore the normal anatomy but that is not always possible, and surgery on affected rays could be the solution.

Recurrent metatarsalgia after lateral ray surgery depends on the technique (remove a second layer–double oblique osteotomy to shorten and elevate) and indications (respect the parabola) of the Weil osteotomy, which is the most used technique for lateral rays. Conservative realignment osteotomies can be done most of the time. Percutaneous osteotomy of lateral rays seems interesting but needs to be evaluated. BRT osteotomy provides solutions in cases of excess of metatarsal slope/plantarflexion.

REFERENCES

1. Greisberg J, Sperber L, Prince DE. Mobility of the first ray in various foot disorders. Foot Ankle Int 2012;33(1):44–9.
2. Greisberg J, Prince D, Sperberg L. First ray mobility increase in patients with metatarsalgia. Foot Ankle Int 2010;31(11):P954–8.
3. Van Beek C, Greisberg J. Mobility of the first ray: review article. Foot Ankle Int 2011;32(9):917–22.
4. Huerta JP. Brièveté des gastrocnémiens et son effet sur l'aponévrose plantaire et le comportement sagittal. Brièveté des gastrocnémiens. Sauramps; 2012. p. 119–41.
5. Hicks JH. The foot as a support. Acta Anat (Basel) 1995;25(1):34–45.
6. Kirby KA. Foot and lower extremity biomechanics III: Precision Intrincast Newsletters, 2002–2008. Payson (AZ): Precision Intrincast Inc; 2009. p. 88.
7. DiGiovanni CW, Kuo R, Tejwani N, et al. Isolated gastrocnemius tightness. J Bone Joint Surg Am 2002;84:962–70.
8. Kowalski C. La retraction du tríceps sural et ses conséquences biomécaniques et pathologiques. La rétraction du triceps sural. Conséquences podologiques. Montpellier (France): Sauramps; 2006. p. 33–47.
9. Barouk LS, Diebold P, et al. Hallux valgus congénital. Symposium Journées de printemps SFMCP. Med Chir Pied 1990;7(2–3):65–112.
10. Barouk LS, Barouk P. Hallux valgus et gastrocnémiens courts: étude de deux séries cliniques. In: Sauramps, editor. Brièveté des gastrocnémiens. Montpellier, France: Sauramps; 2012. p. 265–80.

11. Cazeau C, Stiglitz Y. Analyse des conséquences biomécaniques de la brièveté du gastrocnémien sur l'avant-pied. In: Sauramps, editor. Brièveté des gastrocnémiens. Montpellier, France: Sauramps; 2012. p. 79–90.

12. Espinosa N, Maceira E, Myerson MS. Current concept review: metatarsalgia. Foot Ankle Int 2008;29(8):871–9.

13. Colombier JA. Brièveté des gastrocnémiens dans les métatarsalgies. In: Sauramps, editor. Brièveté des gastrocnémiens. Montpellier, France: Sauramps; 2012. p. 285–94.

14. Okuda R, Kinishita M, Morikawa j, et al. Surgical treatment for hallux valgus with painfull plantar callosities. Foot Ankle Int 2001;22:203–8.

15. Mann RA, Rudicel S, Graves SC. Repair of hallux valgus with a distal soft tissue procedure and proximal metatarsal osteotomy. A long term follow up. J Bone Joint Surg Am 1992;74:124–9.

16. Yamamoto K, Imakiire A, Katori Y, et al. Clinical results of modified Mitchell's osteotomy for hallux valgus augmented with oblique lesser metatarsal osteotomy. J Orthop Surg 2005;13:245–52.

17. Lee KB, Park JK, Park YH, et al. Prognosis of painfull plantar callosity after hallux valgus correction without lesser metatarsal osteotomy. Foot Ankle Int 2009; 30(11):1048–52.

18. Opsomer G, Deleu PA, Bevernage BD, et al. Cortical thickness of the second metatarsal after correction of hallux valgus. Foot Ankle Int 2010;31(9):770–6.

19. Lorei TJ, Kinast C, Klärner H, et al. Pedographic, clinical, and functional outcome after scarf osteotomy. Clin Orthop Relat Res 2006;451:161–6.

20. Dermon A, Tilkeridis C, Lyras D, et al. Long-term results of Mitchell's procedure for hallux valgus deformity: a 5- to 20-year followup in 204 cases. Foot Ankle Int 2009;30(1):16–20.

21. Toth K, Huszanyik I, Kellermann P, et al. The effect of first ray shortening in the development of metatarsalgia in the second through fourth rays after metatarsal osteotomy. Foot Ankle Int 2007;28(1):61–3.

22. Toth K, Huszanyik I, Boda K, et al. The influence of the length of the first metatarsal on transfer metatarsalgia after Wu's osteotomy. Foot Ankle Int 2008;29(4): 396–9.

23. Potenza V, Caterini R, Farsetti P, et al. Chevron osteotomy with lateral release and adductor tenotomy for hallux valgus. Foot Ankle Int 2009;30(6):512–6.

24. Day T, Charlton TP, Thordarson DB. First metatarsal length change after basilar closing wedge osteotomy for hallux valgus. Foot Ankle Int 2011;32(5):S513–8. http://dx.doi.org/10.3113/FAI.2011.0513.

25. Shurnas PS, Watson TS, Crislip TW. Proximal first metatarsal opening wedge osteotomy with a low profile plate. Foot Ankle Int 2009;30(9):865–72.

26. García-Bordes L, Jiménez-Potrero M, Vega-García J, et al. Opening first metatarsal osteotomy and resection arthroplasty of the first MPJ in the treatment of first ray insufficiency associated with degenerative hallux valgus. Foot Ankle Surg 2010;16(3):132–6.

27. Robinson AH, Bhatia M, Eaton C, et al. Prospective comparative study of the scarf and Ludloff osteotomies in the treatment of hallux valgus. Foot Ankle Int 2009;30(10):955–63. http://dx.doi.org/10.3113/FAI.2009.0955.

28. Barouk P. Technique, indications, résultats de l'allongement proximal du gastrocnémien médial. In: Sauramps, editor. Brièveté des gastrocnémiens. Montpellier, France: Sauramps; 2012. p. 331–44.

29. Barouk LS. Forefoot reconstruction. Paris: Springer; 2003. p. 117, 109–48, 168–72.

30. Burutaran JM. Hallux valgus y cortedad anatomica del primer metatarsano (correction quirugica). Actual Med Chir Pied 1976;XIII:261–6.
31. Singh D, Dudkiewicz I. Lengthening of the shortened first metatarsal after Wilson's osteotomy for hallux valgus. J Bone Joint Surg [Br] 2009;91(12):1583–6.
32. Hurst JM, Nunley JA 2nd. Distraction osteogenesis for the shortened metatarsal after hallux valgus surgery. Foot Ankle Int 2007;28(2):194–8.
33. Highlander P, VonHerbulis E, Gonzalez A, et al. Complications of the Weil osteotomy. Foot Ankle Spec 2011;4(3):165–70.
34. Melamed EA, Schon LC, Myerson MS, et al. Two modifications of the Weil osteotomy: analysis on sawbone models. Foot Ankle Int 2002;23(5):400–5.
35. Trnka HJ, Nyska M, Parks BG, et al. Dorsiflexion contracture after the Weil osteotomy: results of cadaver study and three-dimensional analysis. Foot Ankle Int 2001;22(1):47–50.
36. Khurana A, Kadamabande S, James S, et al. Weil osteotomy: assessment of medium term results and predictive factors in recurrent metatarsalgia. Foot Ankle Surg 2011;17(3):150–7.
37. Pérez-Muñoz I, Escobar-Antón D, Sanz-Gómez TA. The role of Weil and triple Weil osteotomies in the treatment of propulsive metatarsalgia. Foot Ankle Int 2012;33(6):501–6.
38. Espinosa N, Brodsky JW, Maceira E. Metatarsalgia. J Am Acad Orthop Surg 2010;18(8):474–85.
39. Maceira E, Farinas F, Tena J, et al. Analysis of metatarsophalangeal stiffness following Weil osteotomies. Rev Med Chir Pie 1998;12:35–40.
40. Barouk LS, Barouk P. Reconstruction de l'Avant Pied. Paris: Springer; 2005. p. 123.
41. Garg R, Thordarson DB, Schrumpf M, et al. Sliding oblique versus segmental resection osteotomies for lesser metatarsophalangeal joint pathology. Foot Ankle Int 2008;29(10):1009–14.
42. Schuh R, Trnka HJ. Metatarsalgia: distal metatarsal osteotomies. Foot Ankle Clin 2011;16(4):583–95.
43. Henry J, Besse JL, Fessy MH, AFCP. Distal osteotomy of the lateral metatarsals: a series of 72 cases comparing the Weil osteotomy and the DMMO percutaneous osteotomy. Orthop Traumatol Surg Res 2011;97(Suppl 6):S57–65.
44. Maestro M, Besse JL, Ragusa M, et al. Forefoot morphotype study and planning method for forefoot osteotomy. Foot Ankle Clin 2003;8:695–710.

Problems Associated with the Excision of the Hallux Sesamoids

Clare F. Taylor, BM, MRCS, Michael Butler, MA, MB BS, FRCS (Tr&Orth),
Stephen W. Parsons, MA, BS, FRCS, FRCS (Ed)*

KEYWORDS

- Sesamoid • Sesamoidectomy • Indications for sesamoidectomy • Sesamoiditis
- Sesamoid fracture • Complications post sesamoidectomy

KEY POINTS

- Sesamoids have a complex function within the forefoot.
- A careful history, examination, and appropriate investigations are required to diagnose patients with sesamoid abnormality.
- Other underlying abnormalities can give symptoms that arise from the region of the sesamoids, and will not respond to sesamoidectomy.
- Any pathologic deformity should be addressed before sesamoidectomy.
- Sesamoidectomy must only be considered following failure of conservative treatment.

INTRODUCTION

Anatomy

A sesamoid bone is embedded within a tendon, usually found at locations where these tendons run over a joint. There are 2 sesamoids associated with the first metatarsophalangeal joint (MTPJ) of the hallux, the medial (tibial) sesamoid and lateral (fibular) sesamoid. The hallux sesamoids ossify around the eighth year in girls and the twelfth year in boys, with congenital absence being extremely rare.[1] Bipartite sesamoids are present in around 19% to 31% of the population.[2] The literature reports that approximately 80% are in the medial sesamoid[3] and that up to 90% of people with bipartite sesamoids have them bilaterally.[4]

The hallux sesamoids are located within the medial and lateral slips of the flexor hallucis brevis (FHB) tendon, which insert into the base of the proximal phalanx,

Funding Sources: None.
Conflicts of Interest: None.
Department of Trauma and Orthopaedics, Royal Cornwall Hospital, 5 Penventinnie Lane, Truro, Cornwall TR1 3LJ, UK
* Corresponding author.
E-mail address: Stephen.Parsons@rcht.cornwall.nhs.uk

forming part of the plantar plate. The 2 sesamoids are connected by a strong interse-samoid ligament with the flexor hallucis longus (FHL) tendon running in the groove be-tween them. The dorsal facets of the sesamoids are covered by articular cartilage and articulate with the plantar aspect of the first metatarsal (MT) head.[1] Abductor hallucis and adductor hallucis tendons have fibrous insertions into the medial and lateral ses-amoids, respectively, as do the medial and lateral FHB tendons. The lateral sesamoid has an attachment to the deep transverse ligament. These attachments, together with the medial and lateral sagittal hoods, transverse metatarsal ligament, and importantly the plantar fascia create the sesamoid complex.[1]

The medial sesamoid receives a greater weight-bearing load, is larger than the lateral sesamoid, and is more commonly injured.

Function

In general, the presence of a sesamoid bone within a tendon acts to hold the tendon further from a joint's center of rotation, thereby increasing its moment arm. The hallux sesamoids increase the mechanical advantage of FHB, thereby increasing MTPJ flexion power. These sesamoids act as a platform to the floor as the metatarsal head roles and glides over the plantar plate and as the weight-bearing load moves for-ward through the medial column. Friction is reduced at the metatarsal head, and the FHL tendon is protected as it glides between the 2 sesamoids.[5,6]

Windlass Mechanism

As part of the plantar plate and its attachments to the plantar fascia, the hallux sesa-moids play an important role in the windlass mechanism of the foot. In 1954 Hicks[7] discussed the mechanics of the foot, focusing on the relationship of the plantar aponeurosis to the arch. He believed that functionally there were 2 structures of impor-tance, the plantar plates of the MTPJs and the plantar aponeurosis, which is attached to them through 5 digital processes.

Hicks[7] observed that each plantar plate with its attached process of plantar aponeu-rosis was seen to constitute a continuous strong band forming a direct connection be-tween the proximal phalanx and the calcaneus, like a tie or bow-string. When the toes are extended the ties pull the plantar plates forward around the heads of the metatar-sals, akin to a cable being wound on to a windlass. The longitudinal arch of the foot is induced to rise because the distance between the MT heads and the calcaneus is shortened. Thus when the toes are in the extended position toward the end of the stance phase of gait, the arch rises by this ligamentous mechanism, namely the wind-lass mechanism.[7] This effect is greatest in the hallux and gradually reduces in the sec-ond, third, and fourth rays. It is almost completely absent in the fifth ray, which may be related to the size of the MT head acting as the pulley and the length of the toe as the lever.[8]

The reversed windlass mechanism occurs at the foot-flat stage phase of gait. It can be observed when standing with toes over the edge of a surface. When weight bearing on the MT heads, the toes flex down and the proximal phalanges resist being pushed up into dorsiflexion. The interphalangeal joints remain mobile, indicating that the long flexor and extensor tendons are not responsible, and that flexion of the proximal pha-langes is due to the tight plantar fascia tethering the plantar plates.[7] Therefore in this phase of gait, the reverse windlass mechanism passively holds the great and lesser toes in line with the MT heads and in contact with the ground.

It therefore follows that pathologic disorder or surgery that disrupts the plantar plate of the first ray will interfere with both active and passive functions of the first MTPJ and the foot more proximally. Deformities such as hallux valgus, varus, or clawing thus can be exacerbated.

AIMS

This article focuses on the importance of appropriate assessment and correct diagnosis of pain under the MT head. It is clearly crucial to distinguish whether symptoms are due to sesamoid abnormality or other causes of pain. The excision of sesamoids, the complications that can arise, and the management of these consequent problems are discussed, alongside a review of the current literature.

SESAMOID ABNORMALITY

Sesamoid abnormality includes acute fracture, acute separation of bipartite sesamoids, sesamoiditis caused by repetitive trauma or infection, chondromalacia, osteochondritis dissecans, and osteoarthritis. Damage to the plantar plate/sesamoid complex arises from forced dorsiflexion of the first MTPJ, resulting in degrees of avulsion of the plantar plate from the base of the phalanx. Proximal migration of the sesamoids can occur. Chronic injuries can be caused by repetitive trauma, as seen in dancers and runners.

Painful symptoms are observed beneath the first MT head arising from mechanical overload associated with overpronation, hallux valgus, and the pathologic plantar-flexed first ray, for example in pes cavus. Diseases of the joint such as primary osteoarthritis and seronegative and positive inflammatory arthropathies may give rise to plantar pain rather than global joint symptoms. Plantar soft tissue may be a source of pain from traumatic neuromas, bursitis, and tumors, or referred pain from more proximal neurologic abnormality such as nerve entrapment or even S1 nerve-root compression.

In particular, bilateral symptomatic sesamoiditis raises the suspicion of an underlying disease to be identified or excluded.[9]

HISTORY AND EXAMINATION

Careful history, precise examination, and targeted investigations of pain under the hallux MTPJ are needed to establish the correct pathologic nature, or in some cases combinations of pathologic features. In the case of the latter, all abnormalities may need to be addressed to offer patients the best outcome. Patients may present with generalized hallux pain, but also report symptoms being worse in the terminal part of the stance phase of gait. Imaging includes standing anterior-posterior and lateral radiographs of the foot, and a medial oblique/sesamoid view. Proximal migration of the sesamoids may be seen. The preferably weight-bearing sesamoid view assesses sesamoid subluxation. Multiplanar and more complex imaging including bone scans and single-photon omission computed tomography scans may help establish the diagnosis and position of the abnormality. The use of targeted image-guided injections can further establish the sesamoid articulation as the source of pain.

TREATMENT

Treatment is clearly directed at the identified abnormality. Classic teaching states that the initial approach for sesamoid disorder is conservative, but once these measures have been exhausted surgical procedures can be considered, including sesamoid-preserving surgery such as sesamoid shaving, fixation of fractures, or sesamoidectomy itself. However, inappropriate or inept removal can further compromise the finely balanced mechanism, which emphasizes the need to establish the correct diagnosis.

Conservative methods work to reduce the weight transmitted through the first MT head. These methods include:

- Limitation of activities/weight bearing and activity modification
- Orthoses to offload/accommodate the first MTPJ
- Avoidance of high heels
- A rocker-sole shoe designed to reduce the movement at the first MTPJ and especially at the sesamoid-MT articulation
- Physiotherapy
- Immobilization for acute fractures

In addition to these measures, nonsteroidal anti-inflammatories can work synergistically to relieve symptoms.[9]

Surgical options should be carefully considered and should only be used if the clearly defined indications are met. Plantar prominence of one or both sesamoids can cause localized pain that may be due to pes cavus, a plantarflexed first ray, gastrocnemius tightening, or fixed equinus of the ankle. A pronated forefoot can also overload the medial sesamoid. Primary surgical treatment, which should treat the underlying condition, can involve tendo-Achilles or gastrocnemius lengthening, dorsiflexion osteotomy at the base of the first MT, or corrective osteotomies or fusions for the fixed pes cavus foot.

INDICATIONS FOR SESAMOIDECTOMY

- When the correct conservative management (for at least 6–12 months) fails and the patient has ongoing debilitating symptoms
- Normal alignment of first ray: no excessive metatarsal plantarflexion
- Absence of clawing

CONTRAINDICATIONS TO SESAMOIDECTOMY

- Inadequate diagnosis
- Previous excision of a sesamoid/absence of a sesamoid on the same foot

Relative contraindications are similar for all foot and ankle surgery, and include peripheral vascular disease, soft-tissue and wound-healing problems, diabetes mellitus, and smoking.

SESAMOIDECTOMY

Sesamoidectomy can be used after failure of conservative management for various disorders including fractures (acute and nonunion), osteonecrosis, and chondromalacia, and at times may be indicated in inflammatory disorders.

Both partial and complete sesamoidectomy can be used. The surgical approach depends on which sesamoid is to be removed, and should take into account skin tension lines to minimize postoperative scar formation and to provide adequate visualization of the flexor tendons and sesamoids. The approaches used are medial, plantar, and dorsal, each with advantages and disadvantages.

The approach commonly used to the medial sesamoid is medial plantar,[1,10,11] whereby the medial plantar nerve of the hallux is displaced with the plantar flap, but this still carries the risk of injury to a branch of the nerve, creating a neuroma and ongoing pain. The approach to the lateral sesamoid is usually a longitudinal plantar incision directly over the sesamoid. There is a risk of damage and neuropraxia to a branch of the lateral plantar nerve of the hallux or first common branch to the first web space, and caution is mandatory during dissection.[1]

COMPLICATIONS OF SESAMOIDECTOMY

A significant group of complications has been observed and described throughout the last century of orthopedic surgery, including the development of hallux valgus (medial sesamoid) or hallux varus (lateral sesamoid). The practice of lateral sesamoidectomy in association with correction of hallux valgus has fallen into disrepute for this very reason. Claw deformity can develop following removal of both sesamoids if the integrity of the plantar plate attachments is compromised and the FHB tendons are weakened. A meticulous repair and adequate time to heal is necessary after such excision. By contrast, stiffness has also been reported. Additional soft-tissue complications include painful scar, wound dehiscence or infection, and nerve injury. To compound the problem, transfer metatarsalgia of the lesser toes can also occur.[10,12–14]

NEW TECHNIQUE: ARTHROSCOPIC SESAMOIDECTOMY

Chan and Lui[15] described a case of arthroscopic sesamoidectomy in the management of lateral sesamoid osteomyelitis in a 55-year-old patient. First MTPJ arthroscopy is a well-described technique. In this report an arthroscopic synovectomy was performed, and the fibular sesamoid was approached through medial and plantar-medial portals. The arthroscopic approach results in good intra-articular visualization and minimal soft-tissue dissection, leaving the ligamentous attachments intact with excellent cosmetic and functional results. The patient was followed up for 49 months with no reports of morbidity, no deformity, range of movement comparable with that of the other side, and good functional recovery, returning to work as a driver 2 months postoperatively. However, there are no large series of such surgery and "one swallow doth not a summer make" (Aristotle, Greek Philosopher 384–322 BC).

BIOMECHANICAL STUDIES

Aper and colleagues[6,16] studied the biochemical effects of sesamoid excision on the function of the hallux in cadaver studies. In their 1994 study[6] they concluded that removal of the distal part of either sesamoid or the whole tibial sesamoid has little effect on the FHB moment arm, but resection of both bones reduced the moment arm by one-third in dorsiflexion.

Their 1996 study[16] looked at the effects of selective sesamoid resections on the effective tendon moment arm of the FHL tendon. Statistical analysis showed that significant decreases in the effective tendon moment arms occurred with full medial sesamoid resection, full lateral sesamoid resection, and resection of both.

REVIEW OF THE EVIDENCE ON SESAMOIDECTOMY

The identified literature is summarized in **Table 1**. The outcomes documented in these articles are better than those reported historically. Previously the levels of discomfort following sesamoidectomy have been recorded at 41% to 50%[17,18] and development of deformity at 5% to 42%,[18,19] with difficulty with range of movement reported as 33% to 59.5%.[17,18]

Bichara and colleagues[12] looked at the return to activities of a cohort of 24 athletic patients with a hallux sesamoid fracture who were treated with sesamoidectomy. The mean age was 32.2 years (range 17–54) and the mean follow-up 35 months (range

Table 1
Summary of case series of sesamoidectomy

Authors,[Ref.] Year	Study Design and Numbers	Outcomes	Surgical Approach	Deformity	Return to Sports/Work	Nerve Damage	Complications
Lee et al,[10] 2005	Retrospective review of case notes and radiographs between 1989 and 2002 32 patients: 24 F/8 M Mean age: 37.2 (18–65) y Follow-up mean: 4 (3–5) mo 12 could not be contacted 14 of 20 (70%) returned for examination and radiographs	Documented hallux alignment and functional outcome after medial sesamoidectomy, for medial sesamoiditis from any cause 20 patients completed the passive ROMs SF-36, FFI, VAS for pain and a questionnaire on activity levels Preoperatively no significant hallux valgus	Medial sesamoidectomy through longitudinal medial skin incision	14 available for radiographs Mean: (9–105) mo postoperatively No statistically significant differences in pre- and postoperative angles HV IM DMAA Wilcoxon signed rank test Computerized dynamic pedographic measurements for 12 patients did not reveal altered plantar pressures in region of hallux MTPJ	18/20 (90%) returned to preoperative levels of activity Mean time to maximal improvement 10.7 (6–40) wk Postoperative outcome measures for 20 patients: VAS score for pain mean 18.5 (0–77) The score of 77 was for the patient with transfer metatarsalgia FFI mean 18.4 SF-36 compared with group representing USA norm = equivalent scores	1 plantar cutaneous neuritis	2 (14.3%) developed transfer metatarsalgia, only symptomatic in 1 patient. 30% had extreme difficulty/inability to stand on tiptoe but no impact on daily function or athletic activity

| Biedert & Hintermann,[11] 2003 | 5 patients 6 symptomatic stress fractures 4 gymnasts, 1 long jumper 5 F/0 M Mean age: 16.8 (13–22) y Final follow-up at a mean 50.6 (20–110) mo | Aimed to discover whether partial sesamoidectomy successfully treats symptomatic stress fractures All patients had failed conservative treatment and had surgical excision of the proximal fragment of the medial sesamoid Documented clinical and radiographic examination findings with a questionnaire AOFAS scale Mean postoperative score: 95.3 (75–100) points | Medial incision from base of first MT toward the first MTPJ with great toe held in neutral, allowing identification of medial plantar nerve The proximal fragment was removed leaving the distal fragment in place, and a meticulous repair of FHB tendon was performed to restore continuity | All pain free; 4 returned to full sporting activity, 1 returned to sporting activity with a mild limitation, all within 6 (2.5–6) mo At final follow-up all clinical results were graded as good/excellent 1 patient had mild restriction of sporting activities | No complications reported following surgery 1 had plantar fasciitis diagnosed on MRI but no functional restrictions |
| Birchara et al,[12] 2012 | Retrospective case series 24 patients: 24 sesamoid fractures (5 elite athletes, 19 athletically active) Mean age: 32.2 (17–54) y Follow-up mean: 35 (8–70) mo | Reported outcomes in sesamoid fractures treated with sesamoidectomy after failed nonoperative treatment Mean preoperative VAS: 6.2 ± 1.4 Mean postoperative VAS: 0.7 ± 1 | Medial sesamoid through medial approach Lateral sesamoid through dorsal approach | 92% RTA at mean time 11.6 (8–24) wk 1 hallux valgus after medial sesamoidectomy | 2 did not RTA 1 hallux valgus 1 metatarsalgia with flexor hallucis tenosynovitis |

(continued on next page)

Table 1
(continued)

Authors,[Ref.] Year	Study Design and Numbers	Outcomes	Surgical Approach	Deformity	Return to Sports/Work	Nerve Damage	Complications
Saxena & Krisda-kumtorn,[13] 2003	Retrospective 24 patients: 26 sesamoidectomies (11 athletes, 13 sporting individuals) 21 F/3 M Mean age: 35.4 (16–68) y Follow-up mean: 86.4 (33–135) mo	Reported outcomes of sesamoidectomy in sesamoiditis, displaced fractures, and nonunions Documented approach, return to activity and complications	Medial sesamoid through midline medial (4) or dorsomedial (12) approach Lateral sesamoid through dorsolateral (7) or plantar lateral (3) approach	Hallux varus following dorsolateral approach 1 mild preoperative hallux valgus had increased deformity post dorsomedial approach	20/24 reached desired level of activity 11 athletes Mean RTA: 7.5 (4–10) wk 13 sporting individuals Mean RTA: 12 (8–26) wk Significant difference: P<.02	2 neuromas post dorsolateral approach	1 lost to follow-up 1 hallux valgus required bunionectomy 1 developed loss of hallux flexion and went on to arthrodesis 2 neuromas, symptoms resolved post steroid injection
Tagoe et al,[14] 2009	Retrospective case study 33 patients 36 procedures 25 F/8 M Mean age: 54 (38–66) y Clinical assessment of 31 patients, 34 cases (excluded 2 who required joint replacements) Follow-up between 2 and 4 y	Results following total sesamoidectomy for painful hallux rigidus/limitus AOFAS measured pre- and postoperatively Clinical assessment 94.4% happy they proceeded with surgery 81.6% would recommend the procedure to others	Initial incision placed dorsally (29) over first MTPJ, repositioned medially (5) for better access to sesamoids	No significant malalignment found	No significant functional impairment found. Statistically significant improvement in AOFAS scores (P<.001) Mean ROM at first MTPJ of 34 cases 35.7° (10°–70°)		In 27 feet (79.4%) no complications reported 1 case of continued pain 2 superficial infections 1 case of delayed healing 3 patients required further surgery 2 joint replacements 1 MUA

Abbreviations: AOFAS, American Orthopaedic Foot and Ankle Society; DMAA, distal metatarsal articular angle; F, female; FFI, Foot-Function Index; FHB, flexor hallucis brevis; HV, hallux valgus; IM, intermetatarsal; M, male; MRI, magnetic resonance imaging; MT, metatarsal; MTPJ, metatarsophalangeal joint; MUA, manipulation under anesthetic; ROM, range of movement; RTA, return to activity; SF-36, Short Form-36 Questionnaire; VAS, visual analog scale.

8–70). Ninety-one percent returned to activity at a mean time of 11.6 weeks (range 8–24). Patients reported excellent pain relief postoperatively recorded on the visual analog scale for pain. One patient (4.2%), who suffered symptomatic hallux valgus, did not return to sporting activities postoperatively.

Saxena and Krisdakumtorn[13] reviewed 26 sesamoidectomies in 24 athletes or active individuals for chronic sesamoiditis, symptomatic displaced fractures, or nonunion. The mean age was 35.4 years (range 16–68) and the mean follow-up 86.4 months (range 33–135). Eleven athletes had an average return to activity of 7.5 weeks (range 4–10). Thirteen active patients had an average return to activity of 12 weeks (range 8–26). The difference in return to activity of the 2 groups was statistically significant (P<.02). Eighty-three percent were able to return to their desired level of activity, and none developed injury to the adjacent sesamoid. Three patients (12.5%) reported deformity or progression of deformity. One patient (4.2%) developed a hallux varus deformity following lateral sesamoidectomy through the dorsolateral approach. One patient undergoing bilateral medial sesamoidectomies through the dorsomedial approach had progression of mild preoperative bilateral hallux valgus deformity. Two of 7 patients who had undergone a dorsolateral approach to the lateral sesamoid developed nerve symptoms postoperatively, both of which resolved with steroid injections.

Lee and colleagues[10] reviewed 20 patients following isolated medial sesamoidectomy for sesamoiditis. Eighteen patients (90%) were able to return to preoperative levels of activity. The mean time to maximal improvement was 10.7 weeks (range 6–40). Fourteen patients were available for clinical review, which identified 2 patients (14.3%) with transfer metatarsalgia; however, only 1 of the 2 was symptomatic, presenting 2 years after the initial procedure. Clinical examination did not elicit any postoperative hallux valgus deformity or tenderness under the medial sesamoid region. Preoperative and postoperative radiographs were reviewed in 14 patients at a mean of 58.5 months (range 9–105) after surgery. There was no statistically significant difference in hallux valgus angle, intermetatarsal angle, or distal metatarsal articular angle (Wilcoxon signed rank test). Computerized dynamic pedographic measurements for 12 patients did not reveal any altered plantar pressures in the region of the hallux MTPJ. There was no significant difference in range of motion between the affected and unaffected sides. In 12 (85.7%) patients there was less than a 10° difference in arc of motion. One patient had a 25° loss of dorsiflexion, whereas another had a 35° increase in dorsiflexion when compared with the other side. One patient (7%) had evidence of plantar cutaneous neuritis without functional impairment. Surgery was performed through a medial slightly plantar incision. Six patients (30%) reported extreme difficulty or inability to stand on tiptoe.

Biedert and Hintermann[11] reviewed 5 athletes who had excision for symptomatic sesamoid stress fractures, with bilateral fractures present in 1 patient. The mean age was 16.8 years (range 13–22). The fractures all involved the medial sesamoid. Follow-up of all 5 patients was complete at a mean time of 50.6 months (range 20–110). All patients returned to sporting activities within 6 months (range 2.5–6). One patient reported mild limitation in sporting activities but no limitations in daily life.

Tagoe and colleagues[14] retrospectively reviewed 33 (36 operations) patients out of a potential 52 identified for review at 2 to 4 years who had undergone total (medial and lateral) sesamoidectomy, with removal of osteophytes, for hallux rigidus/limitus. A dorsal approach was used initially (29 procedures) but was later changed to a medial approach (5 procedures). Gripping the ground using the hallux postoperatively was said to be possible in 88.9%. Two patients went on to have joint replacements. No significant functional impairment or malalignment was seen in the cases reviewed. One patient required postoperative manipulation under anesthetic.

DEALING WITH COMPLICATIONS OF SESAMOIDECTOMY

As with all operative complications, avoidance is preferred to attempts at correction. Correct diagnosis and indication are mandatory. If one is not convinced, surgery should not be initiated.

If surgery is undertaken, correct, meticulous technique is required. Injury to the plantar digital nerves leading to neuromas can be minimized by identification, careful retraction, and protection. The choice of approach is important, which is more commonly seen with lateral sesamoidectomy. The incidence of neuroma/neuritis is reported at 7% to 8%[10,13]; one article in particular reports the incidence as 29% with the dorsolateral approach.[13] Neuromas can settle with conservative management including avoidance of high heels and shoes with constricting toe boxes, or the addition of a metatarsal pad. It may be necessary to make a referral to an orthotist for a metatarsal dome orthotic. If patients remain symptomatic after failure of conservative management for at least 6 months then in experienced hands an ultrasound guided injection of corticosteroid and local anaesthetic can be inserted into the relevant web space placed on the plantar side of the deep transverse inter-metatarsal ligament. Surgery to perform a neurectomy is the most common surgical treatment although should be a last resort as results are not guaranteed and can be variable.[20]

The integrity of the FHB tendons and capsular structures should be maintained or restored to avoid weakness and instability at the first MTPJ. If the integrity of these structures is compromised during the surgery patients can develop symptoms of instability, pain, and deformity. If conservative measures fail including orthoses or a targeted injection then a fusion should be considered in an anatomical position. In the authors experience this is a definitive solution for this problem- although movement at the joint is lost, the pain relief is often very marked and the patients tolerate this procedure well. If patients develop iatrogenic hallux valgus and varus treatment is based on symptoms and degree of deformity. Conservative measures with orthotics will be successful in some at controlling symptoms. For patients that develop painful deformity that limits function significantly there is the option of surgical intervention but only following the appropriate discussion with patient regarding risks and expectations. As discussed previously prevention is better than cure. If the MTPJ surface is preserved then there are a variety of first metatarsal corrective osteotomies and soft tissue releases that can be used such as a scarf for Hallux valgus. Patients should be warned that corrective osteotomies may not offer a total solution to their symptoms whereas a first MTPJ fusion is generally very successful for the relief of pain and could be preceded with a targeted injection. If there is any degree of arthrosis within the MTPJ then a corrective fusion is the only sensible option. If the deformity is particularly large and the fusion does not fully correct the deformity and the foot remains wide at the time of surgery then a combined proximal metatarsal osteotomy and fusion should be considered.

Any preexisting deformity has potential for progression postoperatively. Deformity and weakness require osteotomies and balance of soft tissues. Extreme coronal deformity would require first MTPJ arthrodesis, and claw deformity first interphalangeal joint arthrodesis.

Aper and colleagues[6,16] concluded that isolated removal of the medial sesamoid was unlikely to compromise the mechanical advantage of FHB but that removal of the lateral sesamoid would significantly decrease the moment arm of FHL. Lee and colleagues[10] reported 30% of patients having extreme difficulty standing on tiptoe after sesamoidectomy, but this was said to not affect their daily activities, and no further treatment was required.

Stiffness and a reduced range of movement can occur after any operation. Manipulation under anesthesia and/or a steroid injection can be performed, but arthrodesis may be indicated for pain.

SUMMARY

The hallux sesamoids have a complex role in foot function in transferring load to the medial forefoot, giving mechanical advantage to the FHB and protecting the FHL tendon, and form an important part of the plantar plate and, thus, the windlass mechanism. The hallux sesamoids are vulnerable to injury from shear and loading forces, and pain from the sesamoids can be incapacitating. The diagnosis of abnormality can be challenging and involves careful history (paying particular attention to work, athletic activities, and hobbies), thorough examination, and appropriate targeted investigations. Although conservative management is the mainstay of treatment, surgery including partial or complete sesamoidectomy may be an option when this fails and if other disorders have been excluded or corrected. However, when excising a sesamoid bone it is extremely important to maintain the function of the plantar plate, and excision of both sesamoids should be avoided if possible.

Recent literature reports high percentages of good pain relief and return to activities in sesamoids removed for fracture, especially in high-level athletes. However, inability to stand on tiptoes has been noted, which is consistent with the findings of Aper and colleagues[6,16] and reiterates the importance of reinforcing the repair of the FHB. Hallux deformity resulting in functional loss can be reduced by careful surgical technique and careful repair of the soft tissues. Although Saxena and Krisdakumtorn[13] evaluated only a small number of patients, they reported less deformity with plantar approaches and a faster return to activity when the lateral sesamoid was removed.

One must conclude that despite these series the literature is limited, retrospective, and weak. This surgery cannot be said to be strongly evidence-based or protocol-driven. Here, as with most foot and ankle surgery, in avoiding problems nothing surpasses careful assessment, time, judicious planning, and well-executed surgical technique. Although several procedures are available to aid in rectifying the problems arising from this surgery, one only has to encounter a small number of patients who have endured multiple operations from well-meaning surgeons and still suffer from intractable pain to remember the Irish proverb, "The best thing is not to start from here."

REFERENCES

1. Leventen E. Sesamoid disorders and treatment: an update. Clin Orthop Relat Res 1991;269:236–40.
2. Coughlin MJ. Sesamoids and accessory bones of the foot and ankle. In: Coughlin MJ, Mann RA, editors. Surgery of the foot and ankle. 7th edition. St Louis (MO): Mosby; 1999. p. 437–99.
3. Dobas DC, Silvers MD. The frequency of the partite sesamoids of the first metatarsophalangeal joint. J Am Podiatry Assoc 1977;67:880–2.
4. Rowe MM. Osteomyelitis of metatarsal sesamoids. BMJ 1963;2:1071–2.
5. Coughlin MJ. Sesamoid pain: causes and surgical treatment. Instr Course Lect 1990;39:23–35.

6. Aper RL, Saltzman CL, Brown TD. The effect of hallux sesamoid resection on the effective moment of the flexor hallucis brevis. Foot Ankle Int 1994;15(9):462–70.
7. Hicks JH. The mechanics of the foot. II. The plantar aponeurosis and the arch. J Anat 1954;88:25–30.
8. Stainsby GD. Pathological anatomy and dynamic effect of the displaced plantar plate and the importance of the integrity of the plantar plate-deep transverse metatarsal ligament tie-bar. Ann R Coll Surg Engl 1997;79:58–68.
9. Grace DL. Sesamoid problems. Foot Ankle Clin 2000;5(3):609–27.
10. Lee S, James WC, Cohen BE, et al. Evaluation of hallux alignment and functional outcome after isolated tibial sesamoidectomy. Foot Ankle Int 2005;26(10):803–9.
11. Biedert R, Hintermann B. Stress fractures of the medial great toe sesamoids in athletes. Foot Ankle Int 2003;24(2):137–41.
12. Bichara DA, Henn FR, Theodore GH. Sesamoidectomy for hallux sesamoid fractures. Foot Ankle Int 2012;33(9):704–6.
13. Saxena A, Krisdakumtorn T. Return to activity after sesamoidectomy in athletically active individuals. Foot Ankle Int 2003;24(5):415–9.
14. Tagoe M, Brown HA, Rees SM. Total sesamoidectomy for painful hallux rigidus: a medium-term outcome study. Foot Ankle Int 2009;30(7):640–6.
15. Chan PK, Lui TH. Arthroscopic fibular sesamoidectomy in the management of the sesamoid osteomyelitis. Knee Surg Sports Traumatol Arthrosc 2006;14:664–7.
16. Aper RL, Saltzman CL, Brown TD. The effect of hallux sesamoid excision on the flexor hallucis longus moment arm. Clin Orthop Relat Res 1996;325:209–17.
17. Inge GAL, Ferguson AB. Surgery of the sesamoid bones of the great toe: an anatomic and clinical study, with a report of forty-one cases. Arch Surg 1933; 27:466–89.
18. Mann RA, Coughlin MJ, Baxter D. Sesamoidectomy of the great toe. In: Mann RA, Coughlin MJ, editors. Surgery of the Foot. St. Louis CV: Mosby; 1993. p. 498.
19. Nayfa TM, Sorto LA. The incidence of hallux abductus following tibial sesamoidectomy. J Am Podiatry Assoc 1982;72:617–20.
20. National Institute for Health and Care Excellence. Clinical knowledge summaries: mortons neroma. London: National Institute for Health and Care Excellence; 2010. Available at: http://cks.nice.org.uk/mortons-neuroma. Accessed September 11, 2013.

The Recurrent Morton Neuroma: What Now?

David R. Richardson, MD[a],*, Erin M. Dean, MD[b]

KEYWORDS

- Interdigital neuroma • Recurrence • Surgical treatment • Surgical exposures
- Nerve transposition

KEY POINTS

- Symptoms may recur because of an incorrect initial diagnosis, inadequate resection, or adherence of or pressure on a nerve stump neuroma. Double crush phenomena or more proximal nerve compression should be suspected in patients with recurrent symptoms or multiple interspaces involved.
- When revision surgery is planned, the recurrent interdigital neuroma can be approached through a dorsal, plantar longitudinal, or plantar transverse incision. The plantar longitudinal incision provides optimal exposure along the proximal extent of the common digital nerve.
- Transposition of the proximal nerve stump into bone or muscle should be considered to avoid traction or pressure on the nerve ending that can result in a painful stump neuroma.
- A thorough preoperative discussion with the patient will help ensure a full understanding of the limitations of neuroma surgery, including the possibility of continued pain and difficulty with shoe wear.

INTRODUCTION

Interdigital neuromas are a common cause of forefoot pain. Initial treatment generally is nonoperative, but approximately 80% of patients eventually require surgical resection of the neuroma because of continued symptoms and intolerance of shoe wear modifications.[1] Reported outcomes of surgical treatment of interdigital neuromas are variable, but overall, 50% to 85% of patients obtain significant improvement after surgery.[1-8] Our experience with primary neuroma resections is somewhat less encouraging. A retrospective review of 120 patients treated at our institution found only 50% good or excellent results at an average follow-up of 67 months.[8] Although our study may have more heavily weighted postoperative numbness in the outcomes scoring than previous studies, it does suggest that patient outcomes may not be as good as reported.

---

[a] Department of Orthopaedic Surgery & Biomedical Engineering, University of Tennessee-Campbell Clinic, 1211 Union Avenue, Suite 510, Memphis, TN 38104, USA; [b] Crystal Clinic Orthopaedic Center, 1310 Corporate Drive, Hudson, OH 44236, USA
* Corresponding author.
E-mail address: drrichardson@campbellclinic.com

Foot Ankle Clin N Am 19 (2014) 437–449
http://dx.doi.org/10.1016/j.fcl.2014.06.006
1083-7515/14/$ – see front matter © 2014 Elsevier Inc. All rights reserved.

foot.theclinics.com

Accurate diagnosis and recognition of concomitant diagnoses are essential to planning for neuroma surgery. At the time of surgery, care must be taken to adequately identify and resect the neuroma proximally enough to allow retraction of the nerve end. Even with accurate diagnosis and surgical resection, recurrent symptoms may develop.

BIOLOGY OF NEUROMA FORMATION

A true neuroma forms at the transected end of a nerve and generally shows proliferative histologic changes. Histology shows dense fibrous tissue formation with irregular nervous tissue proliferation.[9] This is in contrast to the findings in a primary interdigital neuroma, which, in fact, is not a true neuroma (**Figs. 1–3**). What is commonly referred to as a primary interdigital neuroma usually histologically shows signs of nerve degeneration, including degeneration of myelinated fibers, thickening of the epineurium and perineurium, thickening and hyalinization of the walls of the neural vessels, and concentric edema within the nerve.[5,9] Therefore, a primary interdigital neuroma is not a true neuroma. A recurrent neuroma, however, often is a true neuroma that has formed at the cut end of the common digital nerve.

Neuromas tend to form at the transected end of nerves, and proliferation is directed toward the skin or distal portion of the transected nerve.[10,11] This process generally is termed a stump neuroma and often is the cause of recurrent symptoms after primary interdigital neuroma resection.

PRESENTATION OF RECURRENT NEUROMAS

Primary interdigital neuromas frequently cause pain localized in the metatarsal head. Pain is aggravated by ambulation and shoe wear but is relieved by rest.[1,12–14] The most common complaints tend to be pain in the front part of the foot, improvement in pain with shoe removal, pain between the toes, and inability to wear fashionable shoes.[14] Patients with recurrent neuromas report symptoms similar to their original

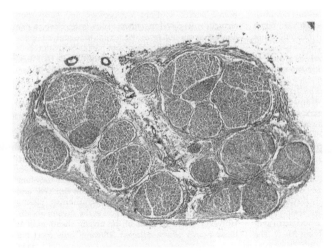

Fig. 1. Normal nerve in cross section (hematoxylin-eosin, original magnification ×40). The entire nerve is surrounded by epineurium, and smaller nerve fascicles are encompassed by perineurium. (*From* Weiss SW, Goldblum JR. Enzinger and Weiss's soft tissue tumors. 4th edition. St Louis (MO): Mosby; 2001. p. 1112–21.)

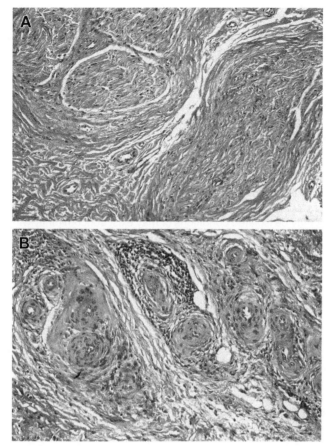

Fig. 2. Morton neuroma (hematoxylin-eosin, original magnification ×200). Dense perineural (*A*) and perivascular (*B*) fibrosis characterize the lesion. (*From* Weiss SW, Goldblum JR. Enzinger and Weiss's soft tissue tumors. 4th edition. St Louis (MO): Mosby; 2001. p. 1112–21.)

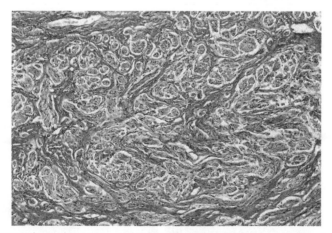

Fig. 3. Traumatic (stump) neuroma composed of small proliferating fascicles of nerve enveloped in collagen (hematoxylin-eosin, original magnification ×100). (*From* Weiss SW, Goldblum JR. Enzinger and Weiss's soft tissue tumors. 4th edition. St Louis (MO): Mosby; 2001. p. 1112–21.)

neuroma symptoms.[1,12] Most also describe a fullness or a lumplike sensation in the symptomatic area of the forefoot.[1,12]

MAKING THE CORRECT DIAGNOSIS

Correct diagnosis is mandatory for successful treatment of the patient with a suspected recurrent neuroma. A thorough history and physical examination are imperative. If the examining physician is not the surgeon who performed the original resection, clinical records, especially the operative report, should be obtained and reviewed. Physical examination should include placing the patient prone and identifying the point of maximal tenderness. Although a Mulder's click may not be present, palpation and axial compression often exacerbate the symptoms (**Fig. 4**).

Other causes of forefoot pain must be ruled out radiographically and clinically (**Box 1**). These may be isolated conditions or may exist concomitantly with a recurrent neuroma.[2,12,13,15]

Other areas of nerve compression, including a double-crush phenomenon, should be considered in all patients with suspected recurrent neuromas.[13,15,16] Tarsal tunnel or more proximal compression of the tibial nerve may cause diffuse distal nerve irritability or tenderness in multiple web spaces that mimics multiple adjacent web-space neuromas.[13,15,16] Electromyography and nerve conduction testing allow evaluation of more proximal areas of compression.[13,16]

Wolfort and Dellon[16] reported that 7 of 13 patients presenting with recurrent neuromas also had proximal compression of the tibial nerve. They suggested that multiple coexisting neuromas or neuromas of the first or fourth web space are rare and may actually represent misdiagnosed tarsal tunnel syndrome. Electrodiagnostic testing can help delineate these findings.

When the diagnosis remains in question despite thorough radiographic and physical examinations, sequential diagnostic injections of local anesthetics may be helpful.[3,7,12,15]

IF THE DIAGNOSIS IS CORRECT, WHY DO SYMPTOMS RECUR AFTER SURGERY?
Anatomy of the Interdigital Nerve

Cadaver dissections to evaluate the anatomy and branching patterns of the common digital nerves found plantarly directed nerve branches consistently present along the course of the second and third common digital nerves.[17] These plantarly directed

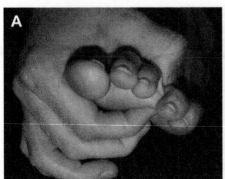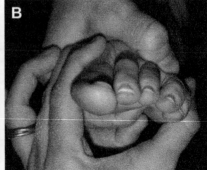

Fig. 4. Diagnosis of interdigital neuroma. Palpation (*A*) and axial compression (*B*) often exacerbate symptoms.

Box 1
Conditions that must be ruled out in diagnosing interdigital neuroma or that may coexist with interdigital neuroma

- Metatarsophalangeal joint derangement

    Arthritis

    Synovitis

    Instability
- Osteonecrosis of the metatarsal head
- Transfer metatarsalgia from adjacent toe deformity
- Space-occupying lesions

    Bursa in the plantar or web spaces

    Synovial or ganglion cysts

    Lipoma
- Plantar fat pad atrophy
- Plantar warts
- Painful surgical incisions
- Iatrogenic superficial neuromas

---

branches were more highly concentrated along the distal few centimeters of the nerve. To avoid tethering of the nerve stump, the common digital nerve should be resected at least 3 cm proximal to the proximal edge of the transverse metatarsal ligament.[17] This is thought to allow better proximal retraction of the nerve stump off the weight-bearing surface of the foot by severing the tethering plantar branches. These branches also are postulated to form painful postoperative traumatic neuromas when the nerve is not excised more proximally.[17] Similarly, when a neuroma is resected and the proximal end of the resected nerve is left in an area of movement, tension, or pressure, a stump neuroma may develop.[16]

Failure to Fully Resect

Johnson and colleagues[9] analyzed 37 histologic specimens resected during reoperations for recurrent neuromas and noted that 21% showed features of a primary interdigital neuroma, indicating residual unresected neuroma; 21% showed features of a stump neuroma, indicating failure to resect proximal enough or continued pressure on or tethering of the nerve; and 46% showed features of both primary neuroma and stump neuroma, indicating incomplete resection at the index procedure. Interestingly, 12% showed no neuromatous tissue and instead had features of fibrofatty tissue or foreign body–reactive tissue. These patients actually were the most satisfied after reoperation.

Adherence to Surrounding Structures

Distal nerve stumps also can adhere to surrounding tissues such as the adjacent metatarsal, plantar fascia, tendons, muscle, or other surrounding structures. In the experience of the senior author, the neuroma is most commonly adhered to the third metatarsal. Some authors have recommended burying the nerve ending into a known tissue to avoid adherence to a structure with excursion or extrinsic pressure. Tension or pressure on the nerve in this setting can irritate the nerve ending, leading to painful stump neuroma formation.[16,18]

Nelms and colleagues[18] described a technique for recurrent neuroma excision that includes transfer of the nerve stump into a drill hole in the metatarsal shaft. They reported 89% good or excellent results with this technique. Histologic evaluation found that a nerve ending buried in a bone canal will form a neuroma with a more regular structure but similar appearance to a nerve ending left outside of the bone canal.[19] Therefore, although a neuroma will likely still form, it is protected from mechanical stimulation and the generation of pain with this technique.

Wolfort and Dellon[16] reported 80% excellent and 20% good results with implantation of the nerve stump into plantar intrinsic muscle belly. Because selected muscles should have little excursion, the interosseous musculature is well suited for this purpose. The idea of placing a nerve end into an innervated muscle has proven successful in the upper extremity and appears to work well in the foot as well.[16] Histologic evaluation found that a nerve stump buried in muscle will form little or no neuroma and remains completely contained within the muscle.[19,20]

Colgrove and colleagues[10] used a technique with a similar goal of burying the nerve stump within the intrinsic muscles of the foot. Their technique involves transposing the interdigital nerve between the transverse head of the adductor hallucis muscle and the interossei muscles. The distal nerve stump is anchored in place with a suture that is passed through the plantar foot and is removed 3 to 4 weeks after surgery. They compared the results of transposition with those of standard resection and found that although early results at 1-month and 6-month follow-up showed lower pain scores for the resection group, at 1-year and 3- to 4-year follow-up, the transposition group had significantly lower pain scores. At final follow-up, 96% of the transposition group was completely pain free, whereas only 68% of the resection group was pain free. The authors hypothesized that the excellent results obtained with transposition of the nerve may be related to the formation of a smaller transaction neuroma that is removed from the weight-bearing surface of the foot and cushioned by muscle. These reports suggest that improved outcomes are possible with transposition techniques, but more studies are needed to fully delineate the techniques that produce the best long-term outcomes.

APPROACH FOR REVISION SURGERY: PLANTAR OR DORSAL

Several surgical approaches to the neuroma exist. Those most commonly used include longitudinal dorsal, longitudinal plantar, and transverse plantar.[9,12,15,18,21]

Although the dorsal approach usually is used for primary neuroma resection, its use in recurrent resections can be more difficult because of scar tissue and limited access to the more proximal extent of the nerve.[12] The dorsal incision allows better exposure of the distal extent of the nerve for excision of primary neuromas and bursal tissue. The plantar incision offers better exposure proximally along the common digital nerve where stump neuromas tend to form. The dorsal incision has been used successfully, however, for excision of recurrent neuromas. Stamatis and Myerson[15] used a dorsal approach in 47 of 49 patients with recurrent neuromas with only 22% of patients dissatisfied with their results.

Plantar incisions are more commonly used for reoperation of the web space. One concern with use of a plantar incision is hypertrophic or sensitive scar formation along the weight-bearing surface of the foot. Faraj and Hosur[21] compared outcomes in patients who had excision of interdigital neuromas through dorsal and plantar approaches. They found that the plantar approach was associated with a significant increase in postoperative wound infection, hematoma, and scar problems. Full weight bearing and return to work and recreational activities were earlier in those with a dorsal incision. Several reports, however, show few or no issues with scar sensitivity or other complications with plantar approaches.[9,12,15,18] Johnson and colleagues[9] used a longitudinal plantar incision in 33 of 37 patients and achieved cosmetic and functionally satisfactory incisional scars in all but 1 patient in whom mild thickening and callus of the proximal extent of the incision developed. This patient's original resection was also through a plantar approach.

Beskin and Baxter[12] used a dorsal incision in 12 patients and a transverse plantar incision in 18 patients for recurrent neuroma resection and found no difference in outcomes between the 2 approaches. No patients complained of painful scars. In fact, most patients reported that their plantar scar healed faster and less painfully than their original dorsal incision. Caution is advised in the use of the plantar incision, however, in patients who are known to form keloid scars and in those with thick callosities because their risk of scar sensitivity is higher.[12]

The largest series of plantar incisions is that of Richardson and colleagues[22] who reported outcomes of 150 plantar incisions for various forefoot procedures. They found a 96% satisfaction rate; only 9 (6%) of 150 feet had an incisional keratosis, of which 3 were symptomatic enough to require excision of the keratosis, and 4 patients had delayed wound healing. Overall, outcomes were good or excellent in 84% of patients with plantar incisions.

AUTHORS' PREFERRED APPROACH FOR TREATMENT OF RECURRENT INTERDIGITAL NEUROMA

Nonoperative options are discussed at length with the patient. Shoe modifications are recommended, including properly sized shoes with a wide toe box. A metatarsal pad is positioned just proximal to the metatarsal heads of the involved interspace to offload the inflamed nerve (**Fig. 5**). If satisfactory symptom relief is not achieved with these modifications, an injection of 1 mL of Bupivacaine and 1 mL of corticosteroid (**Fig. 6**) into the involved interspace is recommended. We do not recommend injection of an alcohol solution. In our experience, this has been associated with poor results and at times resulted in worsening pain. If the diagnosis is in question, serial injections of lidocaine are used instead to delineate the location of pathology. If temporary relief is achieved with injection into the interspace, surgical resection is considered.

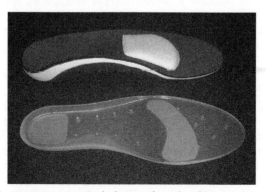

Fig. 5. Nonoperative treatment may include use of a gel cushion insert or metatarsal pad to offload the inflamed nerve.

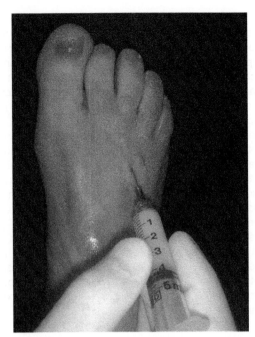

Fig. 6. Injection of corticosteroid into affected web space may relieve symptoms, but relief may be temporary.

Generally, we prefer a dorsal incision for primary neuroma resections and a plantar longitudinal incision for recurrent neuromas. In our experience, recurrent symptoms often are related to adherence of the nerve stump to adjacent structures, such as the plantar fascia or metatarsal head, or to stump neuroma formation with scar or bursal tissue at the site of previous resection. Adherence to the plantar fascia should be suspected if a Tinel sign is positive plantarly along the course of the common digital nerve.

The plantar longitudinal incision provides better exposure of the more proximal aspect of the common digital nerve, allowing a more proximal resection or excursion length for transposition into intrinsic muscle. A plantar transverse incision can be used, especially in the rare situation in which multiple interspaces are to be explored. Although it does not provide the same proximal exposure of the common digital nerve as the longitudinal incision, the incision and subsequent scar are kept off the weight-bearing aspect of the forefoot. The dorsal approach can be used for revision surgery if an inadequate primary resection is suspected.

Plantar Surgical Approach

Before anesthesia, the patient is reexamined and the point of maximal tenderness is marked (**Fig. 7**A). With the patient supine, intravenous anesthesia is administered, and a forefoot block is placed with a combination of lidocaine and Marcaine without epinephrine. An ankle Esmarch tourniquet is placed. A plantar longitudinal incision is made centered over the involved interspace, with care to ensure that the incision is not placed directly over the metatarsal head (**Fig. 7**B). Blunt dissection is carried down through the subcutaneous tissues. The plantar fascia is incised longitudinally in line with the incision, and the common digital nerve is identified (**Fig. 7**C). The nerve

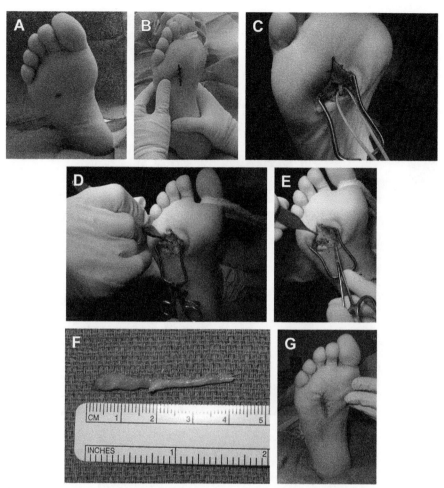

Fig. 7. Surgical technique, plantar approach. (*A*) Before induction of anesthesia, point of maximal tenderness is marked. (*B*) Plantar longitudinal incision. (*C*) Common digital nerve is identified through longitudinal incision in plantar fascia. (*D*) Nerve is inspected for stump neuroma, accessory branches, or adherence to surrounding structures, (*E*) dissected as far proximally as possible, and (*F*) resected or transposed. (*G*) Plantar incision is closed carefully to avoid excessive inversion or eversion of skin edges.

is inspected for stump neuroma, accessory branches, or adherence to surrounding structures (**Fig. 7**D) and then is dissected as far proximally as possible (**Fig. 7**E) and is resected or transposed into muscle as needed (**Fig. 7**F). The skin is closed with 3–0 nonabsorbable suture with care taken to avoid excessive inversion or eversion of the skin edges (**Fig. 7**G). Non–weight bearing is suggested until the incision is healed, usually at 2 weeks. Then full weight bearing is allowed in a stiff soled postoperative shoe for 2 more weeks.

Dorsal Surgical Approach

Patient preparation and anesthesia are as described for the plantar approach. A dorsal longitudinal approach is centered over the involved interspace (**Fig. 8**A). Blunt

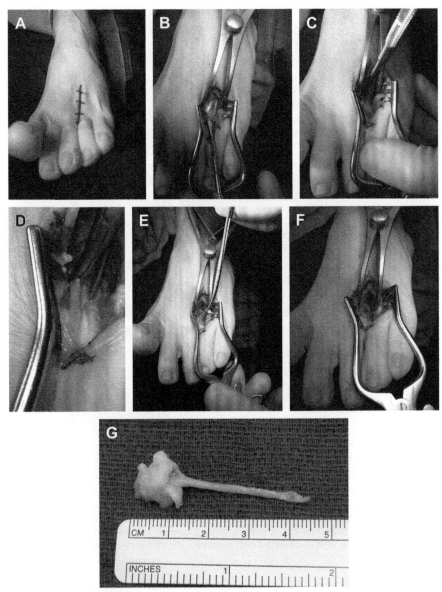

Fig. 8. Surgical technique, dorsal approach. (*A*) Dorsal longitudinal incision. (*B*) Reformed transverse metatarsal ligament after previous dorsal approach. (*C*) Normal interdigital nerve is identified proximal to the stump neuroma. (*D*) Hemostat is placed as far proximally on the nerve as possible to apply gentle traction before (*E*) transection of the nerve. (*F, G*) The neuroma and surrounding bursa are dissected free from the interspace.

dissection is carried down through the subcutaneous layer, and a lamina spreader is placed between the metatarsal necks allowing distraction through the interspace for improved exposure. The transverse metatarsal ligament usually has reformed after surgery through a previous dorsal approach to the interdigital neuroma (**Fig. 8**B). A

Freer elevator is placed just deep to the transverse metatarsal ligament, and the ligament is incised longitudinally. The stump neuroma and occasional associated bursa are visible directly below the incised ligament. The stump neuroma usually is found on the tibial (medial) side of the interspace and often is adherent to the lumbrical muscle or flexor tendon in this area. Proximally in the interspace the normal interdigital nerve is identified proximal to the stump neuroma (**Fig. 8C**). A hemostat is placed on the nerve as far proximally as possible (**Fig. 8D**). Gentle traction is placed on the nerve, and it is transected as far proximally as possible (**Fig. 8E**). Alternatively, the nerve can be transected slightly more distally and the nerve end transposed into muscle as needed. The neuroma and surrounding bursa are then dissected free from the interspace, with care to transect any plantarly directed branches or communicating branches to surrounding interspaces (**Fig. 8F, G**). The skin is closed with 5–0 nonabsorbable suture, and a lightly compressive forefoot bandage is applied. The patient will not bear weight until the incision is healed, usually at 2 weeks. Then full weight bearing is allowed in a stiff-soled postoperative shoe for 2 more weeks.

OUTCOMES AFTER REOPERATION FOR RECURRENT INTERDIGITAL NEUROMA

Most patients with reoperation for recurrent neuromas have improvement in symptoms. Mann and Reynolds[1] reported that 9 of 11 patients who had excision of a recurrent neuroma had at least 50% improvement in their symptoms. Beskin and Baxter[12] reported that 86% of 30 patients (39 neuromas) had at least 50% improvement in symptoms, although fewer than half of patients were completely symptom free. Twenty-four (80%) reported no limitations in postoperative activities, whereas 6 had mild restrictions, mostly relating to shoe wear and long distance ambulation.

Johnson and colleagues[9] reported that 23 (70%) of 33 patients were satisfied after reoperation for recurrent neuroma, and 75% would have the surgery again; 11 (31%) of 36 feet were pain free, 17 (47%) had only mild residual pain, and 8 (22%) had no improvement or were made worse by the surgery. Stamatis and Myerson[15] reported similar findings in 49 patients, with approximately 31% completely satisfied, 27% satisfied with minor reservations, 20% satisfied with major reservations, and 22% dissatisfied.

Shoe wear restriction is a common complaint after reoperation for recurrent neuromas, with only about 15% of patients able to wear any type of shoe.[9,12,15] Discomfort is most commonly related to high-heeled shoes.[12]

Effect of Multiple Interdigital Neuromas on Outcome

The best treatment for patients with suspected multiple interdigital neuromas in adjacent web spaces remains a matter of controversy. Because of the low frequency of adjacent interspace neuromas, reported to be 2% to 3%, more proximal nerve compression or other diagnoses must be ruled out before treatment of suspected adjacent interspace neuromas.[4,23] Thompson and Deland[23] suggested that it is exceedingly rare to find 2 neuromas present simultaneously in the same foot that are symptomatic enough to warrant surgical resection of both. In fact, they cautioned against operating in 2 adjacent web spaces at the same setting because of the risk of damage to the vascular supply of the toe. They recommended selective xylocaine injection testing to find the more symptomatic web space followed by surgical excision of the more symptomatic interdigital neuroma. Friscia and colleagues[4] reported a dissatisfaction rate of 42% after resection of both adjacent neuromas, a significant increase over the dissatisfaction rate of 8% to 11% after single interspace surgery.

Other authors, however, have reported no difference in outcomes when 1 or 2 adjacent web spaces were explored. Benedetti and colleagues[13] reported their experience with primary neuroma resection in simultaneous adjacent web spaces and found results similar to those after excision of a single interdigital neuroma: 10 (53%) of 19 feet had complete relief of symptoms, 6 (31%) had mild residual discomfort, and 3 (16%) had continued severe pain. Recurrent neuromas were suspected in patients with continued pain. All patients had dense sensory loss along the plantar third toe, with variable loss along the plantar second and fourth toes; however, only 9 of the 15 patients reported subjective residual numbness when asked. Stamatis and Myerson[15] reported similar findings after excision of recurrent neuromas; no significant difference in outcomes were found after exploration of an isolated or 2 adjacent interspaces at a single surgical setting.

Effect of Concomitant Forefoot Surgeries on Outcome

Reports in the literature suggest that the addition of other forefoot procedures does not adversely affect the outcome of neuroma excision.[3,8,15]

PATIENT EXPECTATIONS AND PREOPERATIVE COUNSELING

Although good or excellent results are expected after excision of a recurrent neuroma, this result should not be promised or assumed. The patient must be fully counseled on the limits of the procedure. Noting that despite an 80% satisfaction rate almost two-thirds of patients experience some tenderness over the cut end of the common digital nerve, Mann and Reynolds[1] emphasized the importance of preoperative counseling. Shoe wear restrictions also are a common complaint after primary or recurrent interdigital neuroma surgery, and patients should be informed that up to 85% of patients have restrictions in shoe wear. A full disclosure of expected outcomes will allow a better educated patient decision on whether to proceed and a more satisfied patient after surgery when patient expectations are better aligned with the potential outcomes.

REFERENCES

1. Mann RA, Reynolds JC. Interdigital neuroma—a critical clinical analysis. Foot Ankle 1983;3(4):328–43.
2. Bradley N, Miller WA, Devans JP. Plantar neuroma: an analysis and results following surgical excision of 145 patients. South Med J 1976;69:853–4.
3. Coughlin MJ, Pinsonneault T. Operative treatment of interdigital neuroma. A long-term follow-up study. J Bone Joint Surg Am 2001;83(9):1321–8.
4. Friscia DA, Strom DE, Parr JW, et al. Surgical treatment for primary interdigital neuroma. Orthopedics 1991;14(6):669–72.
5. Giannini S, Bacchini P, Ceccarelli F, et al. Interdigital neuroma: clinical examination and histopathologic results in 63 cases treated with excision. Foot Ankle Int 2004;25(2):79–84.
6. Lee KT, Kim JB, Young KW, et al. Long-term results of neurectomy in the treatment of Morton's neuroma: more than 10 years' follow-up. Foot Ankle Spec 2011;4(6):349–53.
7. Pace A, Scammell B, Dhar S. The outcomes of Morton's neurectomy in the treatment of metatarsalgia. Int Orthop 2010;34(4):511–5.
8. Womack JW, Richardson DR, Murphy GA, et al. Long-term evaluation of interdigital neuroma treated by surgical excision. Foot Ankle Int 2008;29(6):574–7.
9. Johnson JE, Johnson KA, Unni KK. Persistent pain after excision of an interdigital neuroma. Results of reoperation. J Bone Joint Surg Am 1988;70(5):651–7.

10. Colgrove RC, Huang EY, Barth AH, et al. Interdigital neuroma: intermuscular neuroma transposition compared with resection. Foot Ankle Int 2000;21(3):206–11.
11. Dellon AL. Treatment of recurrent metatarsalgia by neuroma resection and muscle implantation: case report and proposed algorithm of management for Morton's "neuroma". Microsurgery 1989;10(3):256–9.
12. Beskin JL, Baxter DE. Recurrent pain following interdigital neurectomy—a plantar approach. Foot Ankle 1988;9(1):34–9.
13. Benedetti RS, Baxter DE, Davis PF. Clinical results of simultaneous adjacent interdigital neurectomy in the foot. Foot Ankle Int 1996;17(5):264–8.
14. Bennett GL, Graham CE, Mauldin DM. Morton's interdigital neuroma: a comprehensive treatment protocol. Foot Ankle Int 1995;16(12):760–3.
15. Stamatis ED, Myerson MS. Treatment of recurrence of symptoms after excision of an interdigital neuroma. A retrospective review. J Bone Joint Surg Br 2004;86(1): 48–53.
16. Wolfort SF, Dellon AL. Treatment of recurrent neuroma of the interdigital nerve by implantation of the proximal nerve into muscle in the arch of the foot. J Foot Ankle Surg 2001;40(6):404–10.
17. Amis JA, Siverhus SW, Liwnicz BH. An anatomic basis for recurrence after Morton's neuroma excision. Foot Ankle 1992;13(3):153–6.
18. Nelms BA, Bishop JO, Tullos HS. Surgical treatment of recurrent Morton's neuroma. Orthopedics 1984;7:1708–11.
19. Petropoulos PC, Stefanko S. Experimental observations on the prevention of neuroma formation. Preliminary report. J Surg Res 1961;1:241–8.
20. Mackinnon SE, Dellon AL, Hudson AR, et al. Alteration of neuroma formation by manipulation of its microenvironment. Plast Reconstr Surg 1985;76:345–53.
21. Faraj AA, Hosur A. The outcome after using two different approaches for excision of Morton's neuroma. Chin Med J (Engl) 2010;123(16):2195–8.
22. Richardson EG, Brotzman SB, Graves SC. The plantar incision for procedures involving the forefoot. An evaluation of one hundred and fifty incisions in one hundred and fifteen patients. J Bone Joint Surg Am 1993;75(5):726–31.
23. Thompson FM, Deland JT. Occurrence of two interdigital neuromas in one foot. Foot Ankle 1993;15:15–7.

Recurrent Tarsal Tunnel Syndrome

John S. Gould, MD

KEYWORDS

- Tarsal tunnel syndrome • Chronic heel pain • Tibial nerve • Traction neuritis
- Medial plantar nerve • Lateral plantar nerve • Calcaneal nerves • Barrier materials

KEY POINTS

- Detailed knowledge of the tarsal tunnel anatomy is essential.
- A complete tarsal tunnel release decompresses the tibial nerve and all its branches.
- The extensile tarsal tunnel release after failure of the initial release begins more proximally where the nerve is normal, divides the abductor hallucis, plantar fascia, and flexor digitorum brevis, with complete exposure of the nerves after ligation of crossing vessels.
- Magnetic resonance imaging, ultrasonography, and electrodiagnostic studies may be helpful to establish the precise diagnosis.
- Careful hemostasis is essential during surgical decompression to avoid extensive scarring and resultant traction neuritis.
- Nerve wrapping with autogenous vein or collagen barrier material is an option to aid neurolysis; and collagen or vein conduits may be a useful adjunct in the management of neuromas.
- Chronic hypersensitivity of a nerve may be treated with wrapping, peripheral nerve and dorsal column stimulators, and systemic medications.
- A multidisciplinary approach is often required for the chronic nerve pain patient.

INTRODUCTION

The tarsal tunnel syndrome has been a poorly understood entity and consequently the outcomes of a variety of surgical interventions are highly variable. The diagnosis for plantar heel pain, which includes variations of the tarsal tunnel syndrome, also is murky and non-neurogenic factors may be present (Gould JS. Plantar heel pain. OKU Foot and Ankle 2013; 5. Chapter 18; accepted for publication). For the purposes of this presentation, the author is defining "recurrent tarsal tunnel syndrome" as the *failure of a tarsal tunnel release*, which has been reported to be as high as 40% to 60%[1,2] and as low as 5%.[3,4]

Disclosure: Neither the author nor his family have received anything of value related to the contents of this article. There is no conflict of interest related to this material.
Division of Orthopaedic Surgery, Section of Foot and Ankle, University of Alabama at Birmingham (UAB), 1313 13th Street South, Birmingham, AL 35243, USA
E-mail addresses: Gouldjs@aol.com; jgould@uabmc.edu

It is therefore essential to make a proper initial diagnosis of the tarsal tunnel syndrome, understand the detailed anatomy of the tunnel with its potential variations, possible variations of the nerves, potential pathology, and then to carry out a proper release.

The failed release is due to the following factors[5]:

- An inaccurate diagnosis or multifactorial confounding pathology, including neuropathy and radiculopathy
- An inadequate release due to a lack of understanding of the tarsal tunnel anatomy and variations in the neuroanatomy
- A failure to properly perform the procedure
- Inadequate hemostasis during the release, leading to scarring and subsequent traction neuritis
- Persistent hypersensitivity of the nerve
- Damage to the nerve or its branches during the release
- Intrinsic damage to the nerve that occurred before the surgical release

ANATOMY OF THE TARSAL TUNNEL

The classic or *proximal* tarsal tunnel syndrome is an entrapment of the entire tibial nerve behind the medial malleolus and under the laciniate ligament or flexor retinaculum, formed by the deep and superficial fasciae of the leg and closely attached to the flexor sheaths of the posterior tibial, flexor digitorum, and flexor hallucis tendons. The syndrome was described by Kopell and Thompson[6] and later named by Keck[7] and Lam.[8] The *distal* tarsal tunnel, described by Heimkes and colleagues,[9] is under the abductor hallucis muscle and fascia, the confluence of the deep fascia of the abductor, and the medial edge of the plantar fascia and over the fascia and muscle of the quadratus plantae. Williams and colleagues[10] have described an even more proximal tibial nerve compression site at the "soleal sling."

ANATOMY OF THE TIBIAL NERVE AND BRANCHES

The *tibial nerve* and the accompanying posterior tibial artery and venous comitans, pass under the laciniate ligament about midway between the posterior edge of the medial malleolus and the medial edge of the tendo Achilles. The nerve lies deep to and somewhat more posterior than the vessels. In most instances, the nerve divides into the medial and lateral plantar branches just above the superior border of the abductor hallucis. The *lateral plantar nerve* continues in the same direction as the tibial and enters the foot under the confluence of distal edge of the abductor hallucis deep and superficial fasciae and medial border of the plantar fascia, where there is a distinct "soft spot" along the medial border of the heel (**Fig. 1**). The lateral plantar passes over the fibrous fascial bands of the quadratus plantae at this point, where it make a 45° angle and passes under the flexor digitorum brevis muscle extending distally toward the intermetatarsal nerves to 4/5 and 3/4 (**Fig. 2**).

The *first branch of the lateral plantar* emerges from the lateral plantar just under the superior border of the abductor hallucis, but it may exit the tibial nerve itself just proximal to the abductor. It passes distally in the tunnel posteriorly to the lateral plantar, continues under the fascial confluence noted previously and over the quadratus, sending motor branches to the short flexors, sensory to the periosteum at the medial tubercle of the calcaneus,[9] a sensory branch to the central heel pad, and a motor branch to the abductor digiti quinti on the lateral border of the heel. Baxter and Thigpen[11] popularized the awareness of the branch as the cause of "central heel pad" syndrome in runners.

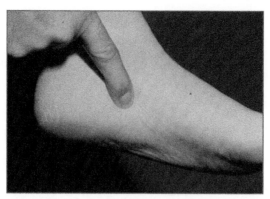

Fig. 1. The "soft spot" on the posteromedial heel where the neurovascular bundle (lateral plantar nerve, first branch of the nerve, and lateral plantar artery with its venous comitans) enters the foot. (*Courtesy of* John S. Gould, MD, Birmingham, AL.)

The *medial plantar nerve* divides from the tibial with the lateral plantar and passes distally under the abductor hallucis muscle and fascia along with the medial plantar artery and veins. The nerve is deep to the artery. As it passes under the muscle, it runs in its own potentially constricting channel or tunnel. It innervates the abductor hallucis and medial intrinsics and forms the intermetatarsal nerves to 1/2, 2/3, and contributes to 3/4. At the Master Knot of Henry, it is medial and adjacent to the flexor digitorum and flexor hallucis tendons. When these tendons develop tenosynovitis, they can irritate the nerve with referred pain into the heel (Jogger's Foot).[12]

The *medial calcaneal nerve(s)* emerges from the tibial nerve above the abductor hallucis and passes posteriorly into the subcutaneous tissue and skin. On occasion, the nerve may emerge under the superior edge of the abductor and then pierce the muscle to enter the subcutaneous and skin tissue. It is important to remember that the first branch of the lateral plantar passes under the abductor and continues to the foot, whereas the calcaneal typically passes superficial to the muscle and goes to the subcutaneous, as both of these small nerves may leave the tibial fairly close to each other.

ETIOLOGIES OF THE "ENTRAPMENT" SYNDROMES

The proximal tarsal tunnel symptomatology is typically caused by a "space-occupying lesion," such as a ganglion, lipoma,[13] neurolemmoma,[14] or bony fragments from a calcaneal fracture. Accessory muscles (flexor digitorum accessorius) and venous varicosities[15] also have been implicated, along with the "soleal sling."

The distal tarsal tunnel syndrome is a traction neuritis[16] commonly associated with the attenuation of the plantar fascia in chronic plantar fasciitis,[17] facial rupture, and, on occasion, with posterior tibial tendon dysfunction.[18]

INDICATIONS FOR PRIMARY TARSAL TUNNEL SURGERY

In *plantar fasciitis*, the patient experiences pain in the heel with the first step in the morning and on arising during the day after a period of sitting or lying down. After a few steps, it remits. In *tarsal tunnel* syndrome, the pain is also in the heel, may be in the posteromedial ankle or in the longitudinal arch, and is brought on by walking and more slowly remits with rest than it does in plantar fasciitis. The pain may occur at rest or at night in bed. The "afterburn,"[13] which continues after the initiation of rest, may be relatively brief or lengthy. The typical neurologic complaints may be either

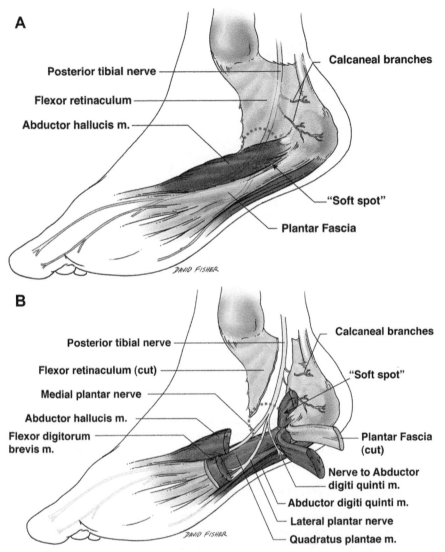

Fig. 2. Artist's rendition of the tibial nerve and its branches. (*A*) With superficial structures intact. (*B*) With the abductor hallucis and flexor digitorum brevis cut away. (*Courtesy of John S. Gould, MD, Birmingham, AL.*)

subtle or severe. In *chronic plantar fasciitis with neuritic symptoms*, the patient may have a combination of pain with the first step *and* with further activity. It is important to know that there are 3 distinct history scenarios.

By physical examination, in plantar fasciitis, the tenderness is at the origin of the plantar fascia on the medial tubercle of the calcaneus and nowhere else (**Fig. 3**). If there has been a rupture of the plantar fascia, the medial definition of the plantar fascia cannot be palpated with the ankle and great toe dorsiflexed. There also may be a palpable defect in the continuity of the plantar fascia. In tarsal tunnel syndromes, there is often tenderness over the course of the nerve posteromedially and in the arch, and a Tinel sign may be present. In distal tarsal tunnel, there is usually significant tenderness

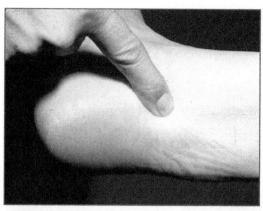

Fig. 3. Location of tenderness over the medial tubercle of the calcaneus in plantar fasciitis. (*Courtesy of* John S. Gould, MD, Birmingham, AL.)

over the "soft spot" noted previously, where the nerve enters the foot. Neurologic findings (sensory, autonomic, and motor) are present only in very severe dysfunction of the nerve(s).

Electrodiagnostic tests are frequently not positive; particularly nerve conduction, but electromyographic (EMG) testing of the intrinsics, particularly the abductor hallucis and abductor digiti quinti may show changes.[19]

With a clear-cut history and physical findings compatible with tarsal tunnel involvement, most patients are given a trial of treatment with a total contact insert with a nerve relief channel (**Fig. 4**).[20]

If the patient is compliant and fails to respond to the conservative approach after 6 weeks, surgery is considered. If the patient is somewhat improved, the nonoperative approach is continued. If the patient reaches a plateau of improvement that is satisfactory or is well, surgery is not needed. If this state is not reached by 3 months, surgery is recommended.

THE COMPLETE RELEASE OF THE TARSAL TUNNEL AND PLANTAR FASCIA

In cases of recalcitrant plantar fasciitis with neurogenic symptoms, a complete release of both the proximal and distal tarsal tunnels and the entire plantar fascia is performed (Gould JS. Plantar heel pain. OKU Foot and Ankle 2013; 5. Chapter 18; accepted for publication.).[3–5,13,17] When there is a discrete space-occupying lesion of the proximal tunnel, only the laciniate ligament is incised and the lesion removed.

In the *complete release*, with the patient in the supine position, under general or spinal anesthesia, with a thigh tourniquet in place, the leg is exsanguinated and the tourniquet inflated. It is important to have absolute hemostasis, so that if the thigh is particularly large, 2 well-padded wide tourniquets are put in place and used simultaneously. Visibility is essential, so the author uses ×4.5 loupes and excellent lighting (×3.5 loupes are probably adequate for most surgeons). The leg is externally rotated, and if hip motion is limited, a bump is placed under the opposite hip. Both bipolar and unipolar cauteries are available.

A posteromedial incision is made midway between the posterior edge of the medial malleolus and the medial edge of the tendo Achilles. Unless there is a proximal medial Tinel sign, the incision is begun just above the tip of the malleolus (**Fig. 5**). The incision is carried distally and anteriorly to cross the midpoint of the medial "soft spot" and

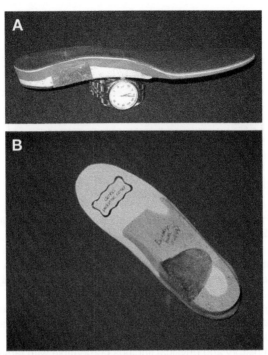

Fig. 4. Total contact insert with posteromedial nerve relief channel (dark blue) filled with viscoelastic polymer for tarsal tunnel syndromes. (*A*) Lateral view. (*B*) Plantar view. (*Courtesy of* John S. Gould, MD, Birmingham, AL.)

then continues across the sole of the foot just distal to the heel pad about three-quarters of the width of the sole.

The laciniate ligament is divided over the visible vascular structures followed by the superficial fascia of the abductor hallucis. The entire plantar fascia is released from the abductor hallucis to the abductor digiti quinti. (The total release is done as patients with partial releases or partial ruptures frequently have residual ongoing plantar fascia pain. The problem with dorsal arch and lateral border pain, which prompted

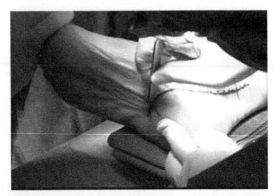

Fig. 5. Photo of the skin incision for the extensile exposure for tarsal tunnel release. (*From* Gould JS. Tarsal tunnel syndrome. Foot Ankle Clin 2011;16:275–86; with permission.)

the notion of a partial release, is managed by the postoperative protocol.) The deep surface of the abductor muscle is swept from the deep fascia and the fascia is released, working from above and then below the muscle. With the fasciae released, the abductor hallucis and flexor digitorum brevis are easily mobilized and the interval between the 2 is visualized. The lateral plantar nerve is found on the anterior end of the space surrounded by loose areolar tissue (**Fig. 6**). It is gently retracted and the superficial fascia of the quadratus plantae muscle palpated with the forceps. As the nerve turns into the foot from the ankle, there are frequently rigid tendinous bands beneath it. These and the quadratus fascia itself are released. This is the only time in the primary release that a nerve is actually manipulated. If there is a septum under the abductor that isolates the nerve, it is also divided. The abductor hallucis is left intact and the wound closed using subcutaneous sutures in the ankle portion and skin-only sutures for the plantar glabrous skin. This skin is closed with 3-0 nylon suture using locking horizontal mattress individual sutures to produce a perfectly coapted closure. The skin incision in the weight-bearing area typically becomes essentially invisible.

In a primary case, the abductor hallucis is sometimes divided with a cutting unipolar cautery. If the surgeon cannot visualize the lateral plantar nerve clearly either because the incision is not properly centered over the "soft spot" or there is a septum hiding the nerve, or there is an anomaly of the nerve anatomy, dividing the abductor makes visualization and the potential for a successful procedure much more likely. In addition, if, during the dissection under the abductor or in the abductor-flexor interval, a vascular structure is lacerated, the abductor may need to be divided to properly cauterize or "ligaclip" the vessel and obtain perfect hemostasis. Finally, if there is a need to see or release more extensively the medial plantar nerve or the first branch of the lateral plantar, dividing the abductor provides better access. The first branch is posterior to the lateral plantar and has multiple small vessels crossing the structure that need to be carefully ligated or cauterized for visualization. Only ligaclips or unipolar cautery is used for this delicate maneuver.

Postoperatively, the patient is placed in a soft dressing, allowed to move the foot and ankle within the dressing to promote gliding of the nerve, but weight bearing is delayed for 1 month. Sutures are removed at 2 weeks. At 1 month, the patient is allowed to ambulate using the custom orthotic device.

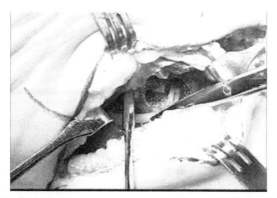

Fig. 6. Photo of the lateral plantar nerve (at the tip of the scissors) in the muscle interval between the abductor hallucis and the flexor digitorum brevis. (*From* Gould JS. Tarsal tunnel syndrome. Foot Ankle Clin 2011;16:275–86; with permission.)

REASONS FOR THE FAILED PROCEDURE
Inaccurate Diagnosis

To make this assessment, the surgeon must review the history of onset of symptoms, their presentation, and the alleged physical findings. If the history and physical findings, when collated, do not clearly indicate a tarsal tunnel diagnosis and ancillary testing was not confirmatory, the surgeon must reassess the complaint. The diagnosis may become more difficult at this point, as postsurgical issues are added to the original findings. Understanding the differential diagnosis of plantar heel pain and, in addition, the potential symptomatology resulting from a surgical misadventure, may lead to the conclusion that the current diagnosis could be a combination of both conditions.

Chhabra and colleagues[21] have pointed out the value of high-resolution magnetic resonance (MR) neurography in assessing these failed cases providing the visualization of nerve damage, neuromas, local fibrosis, and regional muscle denervation before reoperation. An MR image (MRI) also is useful to assess the status of the plantar fascia, lesions within the heel or tarsal tunnel, and the possibility of a foreign body or a stress fracture of the calcaneus. Tedder and colleagues[14] have reported a neurolemmoma within the tunnel, and Yoo and colleagues[22] a tarsal coalition as a cause of failure of tarsal tunnel release.

An Inadequate Release Due a Lack of Understanding of the Tarsal Tunnel Anatomy and Variations in the Neuroanatomy

This is a likely reason for failure and may be anticipated by observing the location and extent of the skin incision. It is helpful to determine if the current findings are primarily medial or lateral plantar, which would help direct remedial surgery. Barker and colleagues[23] have emphasized the importance of recognizing septa within the tunnel and failure to do a proper release. Sammarco and Conti[24] reported on an anomaly of the tibial nerve in which the nerve failed to divide within the tunnel and had multiple anomalous vulnerable branches. The author describes his own experience with a failed release due to a tibial nerve anomaly in a later section of this article.

A Failure to Properly Perform the Procedure

In some cases, a less-experienced surgeon may understand the basics of the procedure, but may become "lost in the anatomy." This is most likely to occur with an inaccurate skin incision: placed too posteriorly, did not bisect the "soft spot," or, distally, the incision followed the posteromedial tendons rather than the course of the nerves. The critical anatomy was simply not found.

Inadequate Hemostasis During the Release, Leading to Scarring and Subsequent Traction Neuritis

Failure to manage hemostasis may be due to a poorly functioning tourniquet or inadequate exsanguination. It is essential to have an adequate tourniquet for the size of a thigh and to drape in such a manner as to allow exsanguination all the way up to the tourniquet to prevent back bleeding early in the procedure. In a large thigh, a double tourniquet used simultaneously may be needed to have adequate width. A sterile tourniquet distal to the drape also may assist in avoiding back bleeding. Excellent visualization with good lighting, loupe magnification, and careful soft tissue handling are essential, as well as the use of proper ligation equipment and bipolar cautery.

Persistent Hypersensitivity of the Nerve

A nerve with long-standing compression or traction, as well as rough handling during surgery, may lead to long-standing hypersensitivity of the nerve. As a consequence, minimal handling of the nerves is the usual rule in a primary surgery. Further discussion on the management of this condition follows.

Damage to the Nerve and Its Branches During the Primary Release

Variations in nerve anatomy, as indicated previously, may lead to damage of branches of the nerves. Careful dissection with good visualization, as well as knowledge of the nerve anatomy, should avoid this possibility. The anticipated takeoff of the calcaneal nerve(s) and the first branch of the lateral plantar should be appreciated and care taken to avoid any damage to these structures.

Preexisting Intrinsic Damage to the Tibial Nerve and Branches

When the history and physical examination, as well as electrodiagnostic studies, indicate intrinsic damage before the primary surgery, the surgeon should be prepared to deal with these findings at the time of the procedure. This surgery will be discussed in the "Revision Surgery" section.

INDICATIONS FOR REVISION SURGERY

Some surgeons decry revision surgery,[25] essentially emphasizing prevention of such outcomes and recommend relegating the patients to pain control measures and clinics. Others,[25] including the author, in referral practices (often "of last resort") have made an effort to sort out the bad outcomes with some success in these difficult cases. As one attempts to determine the likely reason for the failed surgery, some etiologies have a good chance at remediation, such as an inaccurate diagnosis or inadequate procedure. Significant scarring around the nerve can be difficult, and nerve damage is the most problematic. When the latter conditions probably exist, every effort at conservative measures is used, including manual desensitization, mobilization, and systemic medication for chronic neuropathy.

When these efforts fail and the patient faces only pain clinic measures, such as the implantation of nerve stimulators, pain pumps, chronic pain medication regimens, psychotherapeutic efforts with relaxation, hypnosis, and the like; or quackery, the author believes that an effort to deal with the primary diagnosis, namely the peripheral nerve, is indicated.

THE BASIC SURGICAL APPROACH TO A FAILED TARSAL TUNNEL RELEASE

After the updated history of the past and current status and a physical examination looking for points of tenderness, hypersensitivity, and a Tinel sign, and an assessment of the placement of the old incision with a decision on how one might deal with it, further studies are often obtained. A detailed EMG may be done to help assess the specific nerve branch or branches involved.[19] Ultrasonography performed by an experienced neurosonographer may be helpful to study the nerve, looking for areas where the nerve is enlarged or narrowed, or has a neuroma or signal change indicating localized fibrosis in or around the nerve. This study should be done by or in the presence of the surgeon, the skin marked where lesions may exist, or the report should include measurements and reference points to help the surgeon localize the relevant findings.[26] An MRI or a neuro MR may assist this effort. The surgeon needs to be prepared to deal with potential findings, including nerve repair instruments, conduits, and wraps. In addition, and foremost, the surgeon must allot enough time for the potential findings and not be compromised by the need to do other following cases.

The surgical approach is essentially the same as for the primary procedure described earlier. Some of the original incision may be incorporated into the new one even if this means dissecting in the deep subcutaneous anterior or posterior to the skin incision. It is also essential to start proximally to the old scar to find the uninvolved nerve in normal territory. The new incision should bisect the "soft spot" if this will not compromise the intervening skin, and the distal incision should extend farther than the original to again find normal nerve. A vessel loupe is placed around the tibial nerve proximally and the lateral plantar distally. The abductor hallucis is dissected from its deep fascia and divided carefully by a unipolar cautery in cutting mode. The entire plantar fascia is divided and the flexor digitorum brevis is also often divided with cutting cautery to gain better access. (The author strongly believes that releasing the entire plantar fascia is not harmful, as indicated earlier, and eliminates the likelihood of chronic plantar fascial pain. In addition, the author believes that the complete plantar fascial release produces superior results to those done with a partial plantar fascial release.[27,28]) The deep fascia (or scar of the fascia) of the abductor and flexor brevis is divided, as well as the superficial fascia of the quadratus. Working from distal to proximal and proximal to distal, the surgeon dissects from the normal to the abnormal, approaching the area of pathology. The posterior tibial artery and plantar arteries and the main venous comitans are maintained intact, but crossing small arteries and veins are ligated with ligaclips and the smaller vessels with bipolar cautery to gain access to the tibial nerve and medial and lateral plantar. All septa are divided. If further dissection of the medial plantar nerve is indicated, its exact course is delineated and the skin marked over the course of the nerve. A curved incision is then made from the initial curvilinear one down to the course of the medial plantar through the abductor muscle. Unless there are symptoms to suggest tenosynovitis of the flexor digitorum or flexor hallucis, the main area of entrapment of the medial plantar is where it turns to run horizontally under the muscle. With this extensive exposure to the tibial nerve and its branches, all marked with vessel loops, the remaining maneuvers depend on the findings, as discussed later in this article. If an inadequate decompression was the issue and there is no nerve damage or fibrosis, this basic procedure is sufficient and closure proceeds.

ATTEMPTED RESOLUTION OF SPECIFIC SOURCES OF FAILURE WITH CITATION OF SPECIFIC CASES
Unsuspected Lesions in the Tunnel

A middle-aged physician with vague tarsal tunnel symptoms treated his symptomatology with analgesics and anti-inflammatories and inserts for 2 years and avoided primary surgical intervention after negative radiographs and an MRI. An ultrasound study demonstrated a lipoma under the tibial nerve in the proximal tunnel, which had been interpreted on the MRI as a fat collection. A proximal tunnel release with excision of the lesion provided complete relief of symptoms (**Fig. 7**).

A young woman had tarsal tunnel symptoms, with the MRI showing an accessory muscle: the flexor digitorum accessorius. The proximal release with excision of the muscle belly provided no relief. A subsequent complete release of the distal tunnel in the revision surgery provided full relief.

In another young woman, after a primary proximal release, an MRI revealed a ganglion under the abductor hallucis, presumably extending from the subtalar joint. The distal release with excision of the ganglion provided full relief.

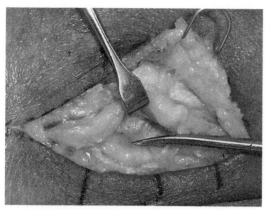

Fig. 7. Photograph of a lipoma under the tibial nerve in the tarsal tunnel. (*From* Gould JS. Tarsal tunnel syndrome. Foot Ankle Clin 2011;16:275–86; with permission.)

Scarring Around the Nerve: Generalized and Localized

This condition may be caused by any intervention that may have also not been complete, but poor hemostasis with the primary procedure may well be a factor as well as prolonged immobilization. EMG may help determine which nerve or nerves may be involved, but ultrasonography may be helpful in localizing the most problematic area of compression or traction. The author has used barrier tissues or material after neurolysis to attempt to prevent rescarring of the surrounding tissues to the nerve. Initially, autogenous greater saphenous vein was harvested and wrapped around the nerve (**Fig. 8**).[2] At this point in time, bovine collagen wraps are used for this purpose (**Fig. 9**).[2] The greater saphenous was harvested through a longitudinal medial incision, dilated, and split longitudinally. It is then wrapped barber-pole fashion loosely but securely around the nerve. The loops are connected with a few sutures and the ends are attached to the surrounding tissue as depicted in the artist drawing. The collagen wraps have the advantage of relatively unlimited supply, no morbidity of the donor site, avoiding damage to the saphenous nerve, and the potential use of a cardiac bypass graft. They are available in multiple diameters and 2.5-cm to 5.0-cm lengths. One of the available brands wraps around itself, eliminating the need for supplementary sutures. The nerve is simply laid into the wrap that coils around it. Both our studies and others[2,29] have demonstrated cleavage planes between the vein wrap and the nerves, but we also have observed that the vein does not seem to adhere to surrounding tissue as well. The outcomes with the collagen wraps are the same. The collagen wrap is eventually resorbed, but apparently remains in place long enough, 3 to 6 months, for the nerve to avoid adherence and maintain gliding.

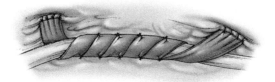

Fig. 8. Artist's rendition of vein wrapping of a nerve. (*Courtesy of* John S. Gould, MD, Birmingham, AL.)

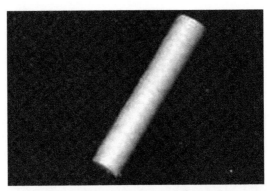

Fig. 9. A bovine collagen tube used for either a conduit or for wrapping a nerve.

An octogenarian was referred to the author with a diagnosis of persistent tarsal tunnel syndrome, and a history of multiple consultations and interventions. He presented with tarsal tunnel pain, a hypersensitive posteromedial scar, and the requirement for multiple systemic drugs, including several used for neuropathy, and narcotics. It was clear that addiction management would be required along with any potential intervention. An ultrasonic evaluation demonstrated adhesion of the tibial and both plantar nerves, but an area of proximal nerve swelling and distal narrowing with more extensive localized fibrosis was noted on the lateral plantar in the abductor-flexor interval. There were no neuromas or apparent intra-articular pathology. The extensive neurolysis was performed with collagen wrapping of the tibial and both plantar nerves. The anticipated area of severe constriction was found as expected, and an external neurolysis performed here as well. The nerve also was bathed with a long-acting local anesthetic to hopefully avoid a flare reaction. In more than a year of follow-up, the patient claims to have finally obtained relief. His drug addiction is managed by his local physician.

An early middle-aged real-estate agent presented with several failed efforts at tarsal tunnel release. She was cachectic and had not walked for more than a year and had apparently alienated most of her close acquaintances. In addition to the tarsal tunnel, she had a significant sympathetic overflow reaction that had not responded to medications and sympathetic blocks. Under spinal anesthesia, the extensile release was performed with the finding of extensive adherence of the tibial and both plantars. Collagen wrapping was performed of all 3 nerves. At 2 weeks, her sutures were removed and the wound steri-stripped. At 3 weeks, she fell with a partial wound dehiscence. The wound was reclosed but reopened a week later with the wrap visible in the wound. She was moving her foot and ankle but not weight bearing and said her pain was minimal. The wound was reopened and closed with a local rotational flap, but did not require grafting. She went on to heal her wound at this point. She began walking with her insert and complained that she now had pain. Her postoperative narcotics were resumed along with a neuropathy medication. She progressed her walking from a 3-point gait to a single crutch to no support. By 3 months, she was walking quickly without support, allegedly without medications, had resumed her work and had regained a social life.

Persistent Hypersensitivity of the Nerve

When this condition is mononeural without evidence of a more generalized sympathetic overflow reaction and manual desensitization has been unsuccessful, the author has used collagen wrapping to attempt to ameliorate this condition. Although there has been no study to confirm its efficacy, the author's impression is that this effort has frequently been successful.

Finding of Neuromas, Apparently Iatrogenic

The possibility of damage to the calcaneal nerves or the first branch of the lateral plantar is a very likely finding in this salvage surgery. Dellon has simply excised the neuromas, but the author has had more success using conduits for this problem.[2,23,30] The neuroma is excised and the nerve end drawn into the conduit (**Fig. 10**) with sutures placed between the edge of the conduit and the epineurium of the nerve; 8-0 monofilament nylon is used and 2 sutures are typically placed approximately 180° apart. The conduit should easily fit over the nerve without redundancy.

A neuroma of the calcaneal nerve was found in a young woman along with marked scarring of the tibial nerve and lateral plantar. Wrapping of the nerves was performed along with placement of a conduit on the calcaneal nerve. The conduit was laid parallel to the other nerves (**Fig. 11**).

A young woman with trauma to her heel had clinically central heel pad pain. This was not a recurrent tarsal tunnel, but the extensile approach was used to explore the nerves and a neuroma found of the first branch of the lateral plantar. The neuroma was excised with the end of the nerve placed within a conduit, which was subsequently directed into the retrocalcaneal space. Her symptoms were relieved (**Fig. 12**).

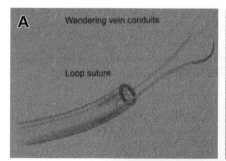
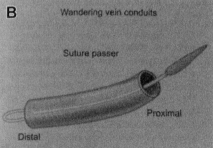
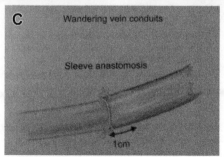

Fig. 10. Artist's rendition of the technique for using a vein or collagen conduit. (*A*) A nylon suture is placed through the end of the nerve. (*B*) A Hewson suture passer is inserted through the tube with the suture passed through the loop. (*C*) The nerve is drawn into the conduit and the edge is sewn to the epineurium with 8-0 nylon sutures placed 180° apart. The 4-0 nylon suture is withdrawn from the nerve. (*Courtesy of* John S. Gould, MD, Birmingham, AL.)

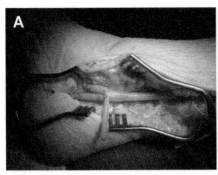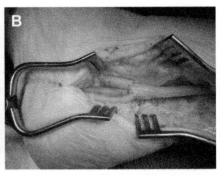

Fig. 11. The tibial and medial and lateral plantar nerves have been wrapped with bovine collagen with a collagen conduit placed over the calcaneal branch. (*A*) The calcaneal conduit projects from the other nerves at 90°. (*B*) The conduit has been laid alongside the other nerves. (*From* Gould JS. The failed tarsal tunnel release. Foot Ankle Clin 2011;16:287–93; with permission.)

Variation in Nerve Anatomy

A young woman in her 30s presented almost a year after a tarsal tunnel release. Her symptoms and findings on preliminary examination appeared to be reasonably classic for the diagnosis, and the surgery performed appeared to be done in the manner described by the author. The incision was in the proper location. The patient had no relief at any point in time from the procedure. The history, however, suggested more symptomatology in the medial plantar distribution, as well as the heel. EMG confirmed primarily medial plantar involvement. A standard MRI was not helpful and ultrasonography was not done.

The plan was to do the extensile approach and to decompress the medial plantar as well. With full exposure of the tibial nerve, there was no division of the nerve into the

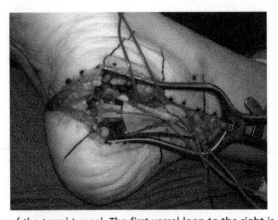

Fig. 12. Dissection of the tarsal tunnel. The first vessel loop to the right is around the tibial nerve. The next 2 are around the medial and lateral plantar nerves. The more posterior nerve is the lateral plantar and the branch seen to the right, going to the subcutaneous is the calcaneal. The more distal one is the first branch going to the abductor digiti quinti. To the far left on this nerve is a neuroma of the first branch of the lateral plantar. (*Reprinted* with permission from Orthopaedic Knowledge Online Journal. © American Academy of Orthopaedic Surgeons.)

medial and lateral plantar. The calcaneal branch and the first branch going to the central heel and abductor digiti quinti emerged from the main tibial nerve. The entrance to the medial plantar tunnel under the abductor hallucis appeared somewhat constricted as the entire tibial nerve passed through this site. Following the release, the patient had recovery from her symptoms.

Dealing with Intrinsic Damage to the Nerve

The most problematic issue to deal with in recurrent tarsal tunnel surgery is the finding of damage to the tibial nerve and its 2 main branches: the medial and lateral plantar. Scarring is usually abundant as well. If a plantar nerve has been cut and both ends are retrievable, repair is the treatment of choice. A 1-cm gap is amenable to use of a conduit. If longer, a graft will be needed. Although the sural nerve is close by, it does provide sensibility to the lateral heel and border of the foot, and with a deficit already, it is wise to leave it intact. Consequently, the contralateral sural is used.

If the distal end of a plantar nerve cannot be found, and the patient is now accustomed to the sensory deficit, the proximal neuroma is excised and the nerve placed into a conduit and led into the retrocalcaneal space. Adjacent intact nerves will decrease the sensory deficit and protective inserts and care to observe the area frequently will help the patient deal with this issue. If clawing of the toes occurs, this can be dealt with using typical foot and ankle reconstructive surgical maneuvers.

With a neuroma in continuity, particularly the tibial, following an epineurotomy, the neuroma can be excised and the fascicles involved repaired with an intercalary graft **(Fig. 13)**.

When there is severe pain and extensive scarring with multiple lesions in continuity of the nerves *and no sensibility* from these nerves on the plantar surface, as a last resort the author has excised the injured nerve and placed the proximal end into a conduit to provide pain relief only, treating the patient like a neuropathy patient who has lost plantar sensibility. The author has used extensive grafting for a median nerve with a similar problem in the wrist when sensibility was critical for function.

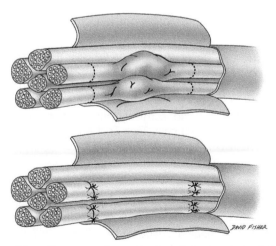

Fig. 13. Artist's rendition of neuromas in continuity within a nerve and, following the excision of the involved fascicles, the insertion of intercalary grafts. (*Reprinted* with permission from Orthopaedic Knowledge Online Journal. © American Academy of Orthopaedic Surgeons.)

When the same scenario existing in the tibial nerve in the preceding paragraph presents but *there is sensibility* in the plantar foot, the author has opted *to not excise* the nerve. Instead, the tibial nerve and branches are wrapped in an effort to decrease the hypersensitivity of the nerve and hypersensibility of the plantar foot. This has been helpful for many patients, although ongoing pain clinic care still may be needed.

THE PATIENT WITH CHRONIC PAIN

The author acknowledges that chronic pain does not dependably respond to local surgical maneuvers and that central nervous system pain responses and psychological response to pain require a multidisciplinary approach to care for these patients. At the same time, continued efforts to find solutions for the local peripheral nerve problem are warranted, as described previously, if a significant amelioration of pain can be achieved in many cases. With many comorbid factors, and poor evaluative tools, it is difficult to assess the statistical significance of many pain studies in the literature. As a consequence, the success of any methodology advocated must be viewed with reservations and the understanding that nerve pain does not reliably respond favorably on all occasions. Systemic medications dispensed and followed by specialists in this area, and nerve stimulators, have a role in the care of these patients. The peripheral nerve stimulators have been used by the author but abandoned because of problems with continued nerve-electrode contact, electrical leaks at connectors, and patient complaints of shocking when passing through metal detectors. Dorsal column simulators have a role and are placed and followed by neurosurgeons or anesthesiologists who specialize in this area.

SUMMARY

The usual reasons for a failed tarsal tunnel release given in the literature and in the author's experience have been presented. The author's extensile surgical approach to the nerves and treatment for specific findings during these procedures is discussed and illustrated.

REFERENCES

1. Davies MS, Weiss GA, Saxby TX. Plantar fasciitis: how successful is surgical intervention? Foot Ankle Int 1999;20:803–7.
2. Gould JS. The failed tarsal tunnel release. Foot Ankle Clin 2011;16(2):287–93.
3. DiGiovanni BF, Abuzzahab FS, Gould JS. Plantar fasciitis release with proximal and distal tarsal tunnel release: surgical approach to chronic disabling plantar fasciitis with associated nerve pain. Tech Foot Ankle Surg 2003;2:254–61.
4. Gould JS, DiGiovanni BF. Plantar fascia release in combination with proximal and distal tarsal tunnel release. In: Wiesel SW, editor. Operative techniques in orthopaedic surgery. Philadelphia: Wolters Kluwer/Lippincott Williams and Wilkins; 2011. p. 3911–9.
5. Gould JS. Entrapment syndromes. In: Gould JS, editor. The handbook of foot and ankle surgery: an intellectual approach to complex problems. New Delhi (India); London; Philadelphia; Panama: Jaypee Bros; 2013. p. 247–69.
6. Kopell HP, Thompson AL. Peripheral entrapment neuropathies of the lower extremity. N Engl J Med 1960;262:56–60.
7. Keck C. The tarsal tunnel syndrome. J Bone Joint Surg Am 1962;44:180–2.
8. Lam SJ. A tarsal tunnel syndrome. Lancet 1962;2:1354–5.

9. Heimkes B, Posel P, Stots S, et al. The proximal and distal tarsal tunnel syndromes: an anatomic study. Int Orthop 1987;11:193–6.
10. Williams EH, Rosson GD, Hagan RR, et al. Soleal sling syndrome (proximal tibial nerve compression): results of surgical decompression. Plast Reconstr Surg 2012;129(2):454–62.
11. Baxter DE, Thigpen CM. Heel pain: operative results. Foot Ankle 1984;5:16–25.
12. Rask MR. Medial plantar neurapraxia (jogger's foot): a report of three cases. Clin Orthop Relat Res 1978;(134):93–5.
13. Gould JS. Tarsal tunnel syndrome. Foot Ankle Clin 2011;16(2):275–86.
14. Tedder JL, Insler HP, Antoine R. Tarsal tunnel syndrome secondary to neurilemmoma. Orthop Rev 1992;21(5):613–4, 616–7.
15. Gould N, Alvarez R. Bilateral tarsal tunnel syndrome caused by varicosities. Foot Ankle 1983;3(5):290–2.
16. Lau TC, Daniels TR. Effects of tarsal tunnel release and stabilization procedures on tibial nerve tension in a surgically created pes planus foot. Foot Ankle Int 1998; 19:770–6.
17. Gould JS. Chronic plantar fasciitis. Am J Orthop 2003;32:11–3.
18. Labib SA, Gould JS, Rodriguez del Rio FA, et al. Heel pain triad; the combination of plantar fasciitis, posterior tibial tendon dysfunction, and tarsal tunnel syndrome. Foot Ankle Int 2002;23:212–20.
19. Roy PC. Electrodiagnostic evaluation of lower extremity neurogenic problems. Foot Ankle Clin 2011;16(2):225–42.
20. Gould JS, Ford D. Orthoses and insert management of common foot and ankle problems. In: Schon LC, Porter DA, editors. Baxter's the foot and ankle in sport. Chapter 27. Philadelphia: Elsevier; 2008. p. 587–93.
21. Chhabra A, Subhawong TK, Williams EH, et al. High-resolution MR neurography: evaluation before repeat tarsal tunnel surgery. Am J Roentgenol 2011;197(1): 175–83.
22. Yoo JH, Kim EH, Kim BS, et al. Tarsal coalition as a cause of failed tarsal tunnel release for tarsal tunnel syndrome. Orthopedics 2009;32(4). pii:orthosupersite.com/view.asp?rID=38347.
23. Barker AR, Rosson GD, Dellon AL. Outcome of neurolysis for failed tarsal tunnel surgery. J Reconstr Microsurg 2008;24(2):111–8.
24. Sammarco GJ, Conti SF. Anomalous tibial nerve. A case report. Clin Orthop Relat Res 1994;(305):239–41.
25. Raikin SM, Minnich JM. Failed tarsal tunnel syndrome surgery. Foot Ankle Clin 2003;8(1):159–74.
26. Lopez-Ben R. Imaging of nerve entrapment in the foot and ankle. Foot Ankle Clin 2011;16(2):213–24.
27. Watson TS, Anderson RB, Davis WH, et al. Distal tarsal tunnel release with partial plantar fasciotomy for chronic heel pain: an outcome analysis. Foot Ankle Int 2002;23(6):530–7.
28. Mook WR, Gay T, Parekh SG. Extensile decompression of the proximal and distal tarsal tunnel combined with partial plantar fascia release in the treatment of chronic plantar heel pain. Foot Ankle Spec 2013;6(1):27–35.
29. Campbell JT, Schon LC, Burkhardt LD. Histopathologic findings in autogenous saphenous vein graft wrapping for recurrent tarsal tunnel syndrome: a case report. Foot Ankle Int 1998;19(11):766–9.
30. Gould JS, Naranje SM, McGwin G Jr, et al. Use of collagen conduits in management of painful neuromas of the foot and ankle. Foot Ankle Int 2013; 34(7):932–40.

The Midfoot Is Really Deformed After Hindfoot Arthrodesis: How to Salvage?

Paul T. Fortin, MD

KEYWORDS

- Foot deformity • Equinus • Hindfoot fusion

KEY POINTS

- Recognition of common patterns of combined midfoot and hindfoot deformity helps prevent unanticipated midfoot surgery after hindfoot fusion.
- Familiarity with a variety of osteotomy techniques is necessary to treat multiplanar foot deformities.
- Equinus is probably the most common cause of midfoot deformity following hindfoot fusion.

Concomitant hindfoot and midfoot deformity is not uncommon. Hindfoot fusion is associated with prolonged recovery and significant disability. Unanticipated midfoot deformity after a debilitating recovery from hindfoot correction often leaves the patient distraught. Not uncommonly, further surgery is required to obtain a plantigrade foot. Understanding normal structural and kinematic relationships between the midfoot and hindfoot, as well as recognizing common combined patterns of midfoot and hindfoot deformity, can help minimize these unanticipated consequences of hindfoot fusion. Treatment of residual or resultant midfoot deformity requires a thorough analysis of the deformity and familiarity with a variety of operative techniques for correction.

CAUSES OF UNANTICIPATED MIDFOOT DEFORMITY

- Malpositioned hindfoot fusion
- Unrecognized equinus or muscle imbalance
- Compensatory midfoot deformity
- Unrecognized neuropathy

Disclosure: None.
Department of Orthopaedic Surgery, School of Medicine, Oakland University William Beaumont, 30575 Woodward Avenue, Royal Oak, MI 48073, USA
E-mail address: ptf@oakland-ortho.com

Recurrent or residual deformity following hindfoot fusion can be the result of soft tissue imbalance and/or bony malalignment that is either preexisting or consequent to the hindfoot procedure. One of the most common causes of midfoot deformity is a malpositioned hindfoot fusion. Often, a patient with a fixed hindfoot deformity will have a fixed compensatory midfoot deformity that, despite proper hindfoot realignment, results in an unbalanced nonplantigrade foot. Similarly, soft tissue conditions such as muscle imbalance and soft tissue contracture are common with hindfoot deformity and can become more apparent after hindfoot repositioning. Unrecognized hindfoot equinus from gastrocsoleus contracture leads to increased bending forces through the midfoot. In a cadaveric study, Thordarson and colleagues[1] showed that the triceps surae had the most significant arch-flattening effect in the sagittal plane and contributed significantly to forefoot abduction in the axial plane. Unrecognized neuropathy is another cause of unanticipated midfoot collapse after hindfoot arthrodesis.

Triple arthrodesis is one of the most commonly performed procedures for the correction of hindfoot deformity. Since Hoke[2] first described triple arthrodesis in 1921, it has been used successfully in several degenerative, traumatic, developmental, and neuromuscular conditions.[3–5] Analysis of long-term follow-up of triple arthrodesis provides some insight into subsequent midfoot problems. In a long-term review of triple arthrodesis, Angus and Cowell[6] reported a 62% incidence of residual deformity and a high incidence of midfoot degenerative change. Equinus, cavus, and supination were among the residual midfoot deformities. Rigid preoperative equinovarus deformity was associated with the poorest outcome and highest incidence of reoperation. Saltzman and colleagues[5] reported 25-year and 40-year follow-ups on subjects undergoing triple arthrodesis primarily for neuromuscular conditions. Following triple arthrodesis, 78% of subjects had residual deformity and more than half required additional surgery within 8 weeks. Tendon transfers within 8 weeks following the initial procedure were required in 40% of cases. These series underscore the inextricable interplay between the midfoot and hindfoot in complex deformity, as well as the somewhat unpredictable nature of hindfoot fusion in patients with deformity. Several investigators have pointed out that triple arthrodesis provides very limited correction of fixed forefoot deformity.[7,8]

Normally, there is kinematic coupling of hindfoot and midfoot motion that allows the foot to go from a flexible structure at heel strike to a propulsive rigid structure at toe off. This mechanism is irreversibly altered by hindfoot arthrodesis. Because of this, even subtle residual midfoot deformity following hindfoot fusion can result in significant disability from aberrant weight transfer, leading to painful overloading and gait alteration.

The Modern Triple Arthrodesis

Problems such as these have led to significant modifications of the traditional triple arthrodesis to minimize unanticipated midfoot or forefoot deformity. Several investigators have pointed out the importance of meticulous joint preparation, avoiding large bone resection, precise joint reduction instead of in situ fusion, soft tissue balancing, and correction of concomitant deformity.[3–6,9–12] Lateral column overload is a common consequence triple arthrodesis. It has been suggested that fusion of the talonavicular and subtalar joints alone, leaving the calcaneal-cuboid joint intact, may help lessen lateral column pain because of the small remaining motion in this joint.[13,14] Other procedures such as cuboid osteotomy and plantar- flexion medial column osteotomy have also been described as methods to diminish lateral overload.[15,16]

Simultaneous or staged correction of both the hindfoot and midfoot in patients with severe multiplanar deformity is more likely to result in a plantigrade foot compared with triple arthrodesis alone (**Fig. 1**). Den Hartog and Kay[11] proposed a step-wise

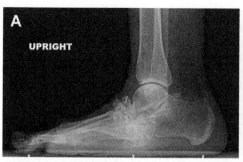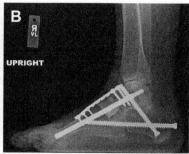

Fig. 1. (*A*) Sagittal plane collapse of the hindfoot and midfoot with significant hindfoot equinus. (*B*) Failure to address hindfoot equinus will result in ongoing stress through the midfoot.

approach working from proximal to distal using a combination of osteotomies and selective arthrodesis for correction of severe multiplanar deformity. They point out that hindfoot deformity cannot be addressed in isolation and concomitant treatment of midfoot malalignment and any soft tissue imbalance is required.

PATTERNS OF DEFORMITY AND ASSOCIATED CONDITIONS
Commonly Associated Hindfoot and Midfoot Deformities

- Hindfoot equinus: midfoot or sagittal axial plane collapse
- Valgus hindfoot: fixed midfoot or forefoot varus
- Varus hindfoot: midfoot cavus or forefoot valgus
- Valgus hindfoot: midfoot or forefoot abduction
- Varus hindfoot: midfoot or forefoot adduction
- External tibial torsion: hindfoot varus metatarsus adductus

An understanding of commonly associated hindfoot and midfoot deformities helps identify patients that will need simultaneous or staged midfoot correction and, therefore, limit unanticipated secondary surgery. Knowledge of normal radiographic parameters that delineate hindfoot–midfoot relationships can aid in identifying abnormal hindfoot–midfoot relationships. Angular measurements (lateral talometatarsal angle, calcaneal pitch angle, talonavicular, coverage angle), as well as linear measurements (hindfoot alignment, metatarsal-cuneiform height), are reliable indicators of flatfoot and cavovarus deformity but provide indirect information about relationships between hindfoot, midfoot, and forefoot. Arunakul and colleagues[17] pointed out that these single radiographic measurements are not able to quantify the additive effect of combined and compensatory deformity such as metatarsus adductus and cavovarus or planovalgus and forefoot abduction. They have proposed the "Tripod Index" that measures the relationship of the subtalar axis and foot tripod, which potentially provides a radiographic summation of hindfoot, midfoot, and forefoot deformity in multiple planes. Investigators showed excellent reliability of the index, which correlated highly with currently used radiographic parameters.[18]

Hindfoot Equinus and Midfoot Rocker-bottom

Probably one of the most commonly associated conditions is equinus and midfoot collapse. This can result in sagittal plane rocker-bottom–type deformity as well as axial plane abduction-type deformity. Equinus is often very subtle and easily unrecognized. On examination, ankle dorsiflexion can be normal but associated with significant hindfoot equinus. This is best seen on the standing lateral radiograph that shows a diminished calcaneal pitch angle and a plantar flexed talus (**Fig. 2**). Because of significant individual radiographic variation, however, these radiographic findings can be overlooked. Untreated hindfoot equinus either from insufficient reduction of the hindfoot or inadequate soft tissue release leads to ongoing bending stress through the midfoot leading to sagittal and/or axial plane collapse.

Coronal Hindfoot–Coronal Forefoot Relationships

Another common deformity association that is difficult to quantify with a radiograph is coronal plane hindfoot and forefoot–midfoot relationships. Hindfoot valgus, whether from tibial, ankle, or peritalar deformity, often results in a compensatory varus forefoot posture as the foot rotates in the coronal plane to strike the ground in plantigrade manner (**Fig. 3**). This foot posture is flexible and inconsequential once the hindfoot valgus has been corrected; however, in long-standing cases of fixed hindfoot valgus, this can result in a fixed compensatory deformity that leaves the foot in a nonplantigrade position after the hindfoot is repositioned. Not only is this difficult to assess with a radiograph, it also clinically difficult to assess flexibility and the likelihood of spontaneous correction. Therefore, in all cases of long-standing hindfoot valgus the clinician should anticipate the need for coronal plane midfoot or forefoot correction.

Similarly, patients with long-standing hindfoot varus often have compensatory forefoot or midfoot valgus or pronation that results in an unbalanced foot with excessive weight transfer through the first metatarsal head after hindfoot varus is corrected (**Fig. 4**). Cavovarus and equinovarus deformity can also be associated with excessive external tibial torsion that is believed to be caused by overpull of the posterior tibial tendon. This is more often seen in neuromuscular conditions such as Charcot-Marie-Tooth disease but it can be a developmental or idiopathic phenomenon. When present, it can result in an abducted or externally rotated foot posture once the hindfoot is corrected. Hansen[19] has suggested careful assessment of the transmalleolar axis with the patient prone and knees flexed to 90°. External tibial torsion between 10° and 15° of is considered normal in an adult.

Coronal Hindfoot–Axial Forefoot Relationships

Coronal plane deformity is also seen in combination with axial plane deformity. Hindfoot valgus or forefoot abduction and hindfoot varus or forefoot adduction are the

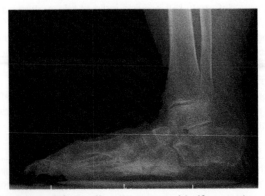

Fig. 2. When concomitant midfoot collapse is present, hindfoot equinus is not easily recognized. Standing lateral radiograph demonstrates loss of calcaneal pitch.

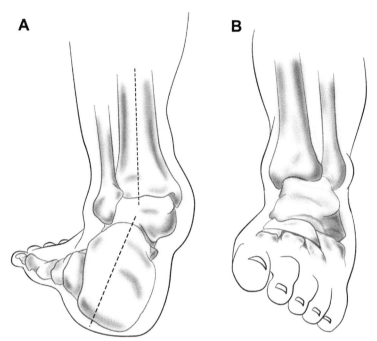

Fig. 3. (*A, B*) Hindfoot valgus is often associated with compensatory forefoot varus or supination.

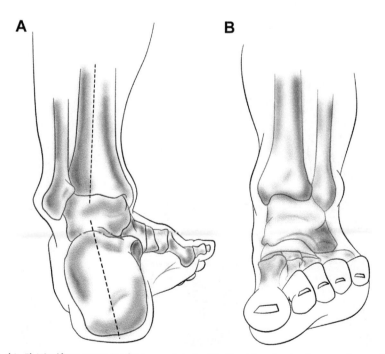

Fig. 4. (*A, B*) Hindfoot varus is often associated with fixed forefoot valgus or plantar flexion of the first metatarsal.

most commonly associated malalignment in these planes. Rarely are these combined deformities strictly biplanar and complex multiplanar deformity makes it even more difficult to predict the consequences of a particular hindfoot correction on the remainder of the foot and its overall alignment (**Fig. 5**).

EVALUATION

It is hoped that identifying patterns of associated midfoot and hindfoot deformity before any surgical endeavors will prevent unnecessary surgery. However, when faced with the need for subsequent midfoot correction, it is important to be systematic in the evaluation of these patients. Multiple clinical and radiographic factors need to be addressed to fully characterize the deformity:

- Cause of the deformity
- Fixed or flexible
- Location, magnitude, and direction of the deformity
- Bone loss
- Muscle imbalance or soft tissue contracture
- Comorbid factors (neuropathy, vasculopathy, poor skin)

Determine the cause of the midfoot deformity. Is it from a poorly positioned hindfoot fusion, a preexisting primary midfoot deformity, or degenerative collapse of the midfoot despite a well-positioned hindfoot? Is it fixed or flexible? Some flexible midfoot deformities are well managed with orthotics and shoe modification. Where is the patient's primary source of pain and what aspect of the deformity is causing the greatest disability? These are often complex deformities with numerous clinical manifestations that cannot be made normal and identifying the chief complaint is a necessity. What are the anatomic and radiographic components of the deformity? This involves a

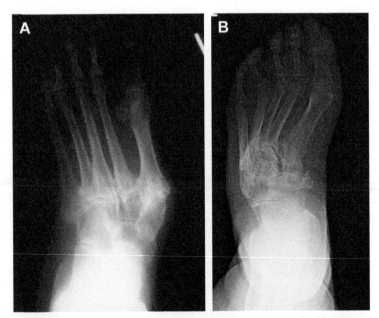

Fig. 5. (*A, B*) Axial plane malalignment with forefoot abduction and adduction can be the cause of ongoing deformity and discomfort after hindfoot fusion.

careful assessment of overall limb alignment, as well as sagittal, axial, and coronal plane alignment of the hindfoot, midfoot, and forefoot. Where is the apex of the deformity in each plane at each of these areas? Usually, midfoot collapse is associated with significant bone loss that may be underestimated on plain radiograph because midfoot bone structure is often ill-defined in the face of arthritic change and collapse (see **Fig. 1A**). Bone loss may require structural grafting or compensatory wedge resection to realign the foot. Muscle imbalance and soft tissue contracture is important to evaluate. Gastrocsoleus contracture is invariably present in conjunction with sagittal and axial plane collapse. Other muscle imbalances include peroneus brevis contracture with forefoot abduction, tibialis posterior, peroneus longus contracture or overpull with cavovarus deformity, and tibialis anterior overpull with forefoot supination. Recurrent deformity despite proper bony alignment can occur if these muscle imbalances are not recognized. Finally, comorbid variables such as neuropathy, vasculopathy, and skin status can sometimes determine if further surgery should be considered. These variables also may dictate what means of surgical intervention is most appropriate, such as conventional open fixation versus limited open or percutaneous techniques.

TREATMENT

Nonoperative treatment with appropriate shoe wear modification and orthotic management is often successful in achieving comfortable ambulation. In particular, axial plane deformity such as residual forefoot abduction or metatarsus adductus is reasonably well tolerated and a wait-and-see approach is sometimes the most appropriate. Full-length carbon or steel shanks, along with rocker-bottom shoe modification, can be helpful in alleviating midfoot bending stress. Braces such as ankle-foot orthoses can also be used in patients who are not operative candidates but can be poorly tolerated when fixed deformity is present.[20] Custom off-loading orthotics can be extremely helpful in relieving pressure points from medial or lateral column overload.

Because of the complexity of these deformities, surgical treatment requires familiarity with a variety of techniques to facilitate correction. Surgical intervention typically involves a combination of osteotomies, selective arthrodesis, and soft tissue balancing. Several osteotomy and realignment techniques have been described that can be useful depending on the individual situation (**Table 1**). The magnitude of bone loss and soft tissue tolerance for acute deformity correction often dictate which method is used. For instance, severe fixed deformity, particularly when soft tissue tolerance for acute correction is questionable, may require bone shortening or gradual distraction techniques to safely realign the foot.

Although most of these deformities are multiplanar, it is helpful to group them according to cardinal planes based on the direction of maximal deformity. The apex of each plane of deformity is determined, as well as the structures at greatest risk with correction (skin, neurovascular structures). With open realignment procedures, correction typically proceeds from proximal to distal and medial to lateral. Provisional pin fixation facilitates sequential correction and repositioning as necessary before definitive fixation. Incisions need to be carefully planned and meticulous soft tissue handling is necessary. Tracing paper cut outs preoperatively is extremely helpful to plan the osteotomies and predict the final foot position.

Axial and Coronal Plane Correction

Forefoot valgus or pronation deformities isolated to the first metatarsal can be treated with isolated dorsiflexion osteotomy of the first metatarsal. More commonly, however,

Table 1
Surgical procedures: midfoot correction after hindfoot fusion

	Indications	Advantages	Disadvantages	Risks	Reference
Joint reduction with fusion	Multiplanar deformities Preserved bone stock	Immediate correction or no shortening	Limited ability to correct severe deformities	Wound healing Inadequate correction	1
Closing midfoot wedge osteotomy	Axial sagittal plane deformity	Rapid healing Immediate correction	Foot shortening	Overcorrection or undercorrection	3
Rotational midfoot osteotomy	Coronal plane deformity	Rapid healing	Can lead to unleveling of metatarsal heads	Overcorrection or undercorrection	4
Biplanar midfoot wedge osteotomy	Rocker-bottom deformity	Limits foot shortening	Potential soft tissue compromise	Nonunion Wound healing	5
Staged distraction midfoot fusion	Severe multiplanar deformity or soft tissue compromise	Allows correction of severe deformities	Technically demanding Prolonged recovery	Infection	—
Percutaneous midfoot osteotomy (single or staged)	Severe multiplanar deformity or soft tissue compromise	Can be used in cases of compromised soft tissue	Technically demanding Prolonged recovery	Infection	6,7
Supramalleolar tibial osteotomy	Sagittal coronal plane deformity	Useful in select cases Refractory equinus	Mechanical axis deviation	Nonunion or malunion	6

the entire midfoot must be derotated. In cases of malpositioned triple arthrodesis, osteotomy through the fusion mass is required. A medial incision centered between the anterior and posterior tibial tendons and a lateral incision from the tip of the fibula in line with the fourth metatarsal allows adequate exposure. Subperiosteal dissection is carried out around the entire fusion mass, malleable retractors facilitate protection of tendinous and neurovascular structures. After osteotomy, the forefoot is rotated into the desired position and provisionally pinned to assess overall foot posture with simulated weight bearing. Axial plane alignment can then be evaluated and biplanar correction with opening or closing wedge osteotomy may be required (**Fig. 6**). The choice between opening or closing wedge osteotomy should be based on soft tissue tolerance and the amount of shortening that would result to effect the desired amount of angular correction. With nonneuropathic patients, shortening is less well tolerated and maintenance of medial column length is desirable. When the apex of the deformity is more distal in the midfoot between the navicular and metatarsal bases, correction is performed through these joints. Midfoot bone loss is common in this scenario and must be planned for. Restoration of medial column length is difficult even with structural bone grafting. Correction starts with mobilization and multiplanar reduction of each of the midfoot joints that are malaligned. Typically, this is accomplished through two or three longitudinal incisions on the dorsum of the foot. In most circumstances, the lateral-most rays reduce spontaneously once the medial three rays are repositioned. Tarsometatarsal, intertarsal, and naviculocuneiform joints should all be

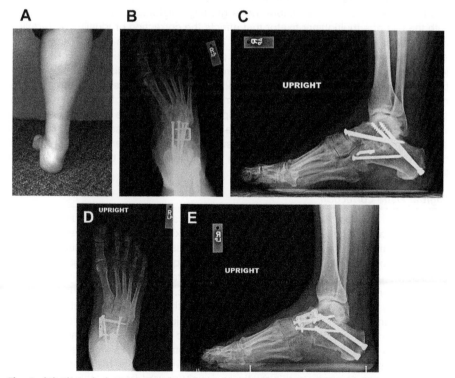

Fig. 6. (*A*) Clinical photograph of a patient 3 years after triple arthrodesis complaining of lateral forefoot pain. (*B*) Anteroposterior and (*C*) lateral radiographs of forefoot supination and hindfoot varus. (*D*) Anteroposterior and (*E*) lateral radiographs following opening wedge and rotational midfoot osteotomy and closing wedge calcaneal osteotomy.

evaluated for stability and meticulously prepared for fusion as necessary. With forefoot abduction and rocker-bottom collapse in the sagittal plane, there is usually significant dorsolateral bone loss that often requires structural grafting. Rigid fixation is then carried out with solid core screws or plating of the medial three rays. Plate and screw constructs are variable depending on the amount of bone loss, bone quality, and soft tissue conditions. Although some investigators have suggested that the lateral rays should be included in the fusion, this is rarely necessary unless there is fixed deformity of these joints such as with neuropathic rocker-bottom deformity.[21] In circumstances of painful arthritic involvement of the lateral tarsometatarsal joints, resection arthroplasty of these joints may be beneficial.

In some patients, long-standing and extensive medial column bone loss can make acute correction difficult or impossible. Gradual distraction and staged reconstruction can be used in select patients with midfoot deformities that are difficult to correct with conventional methods. A percutaneous or limited-open osteotomy is performed through the apex of the deformity.[22–24] Corticotomy, as well as percutaneous Gigli saw techniques, have been described.[23] The Gigli saw technique works well for osteotomies in the region from the transverse tarsal joints to the base of the metatarsals. Two small medial incisions and two small lateral incisions are made and a small blunt elevator is used to perform a subperiosteal dissection along the plane of the osteotomy and the Gigli saw or passing suture is then routed along the plane of the osteotomy. The osteotomy is typically made after the fixator has been placed. Advantages of this technique are that it allows multiplanar deformity correction, minimizes shortening, and obviates structural bone grafting. Historically, this has been done with the use of a multiplanar fixator that effects the correction gradually and remains in place until healing is complete. External fixation on the foot is usually poorly tolerated and the longer the fixator remains in place, the greater the chance of pin tract infection. An alternative is to use a multiplanar fixator to accomplish deformity correction until provisional healing of the regenerate bone takes place. The fixator is then removed and, if pin sites are remote from the involved area of the midfoot, joints are prepared for arthrodesis through an open incisions and the midfoot is spanned with plate or intramedullary fixation. If there is any pin site in close proximity to where an incision is planned, definitive fixation is staged, the fixator is removed until pin sites have healed (usually 7–10 days), and plate fixation follows after the soft tissue envelope is completely healed.

Sagittal Plane Correction

Equinus after hindfoot fusion is poorly tolerated. Because residual equinus after hindfoot fusion can result in compensatory sagittal and axial plane deformity, surgical procedures usually have to address the cause for equinus as well as the resultant midfoot deformity. For example, an ankle fusion placed in equinus can lead to sagittal plane breakdown of the transverse tarsal or tarsometatarsal joints resulting abduction and/or rocker-bottom deformity through these areas. Surgical treatment in this situation not only involves revision ankle arthrodesis with supramalleolar osteotomy but also treatment of the midfoot deformity. In this situation, the midfoot and hindfoot deformities are addressed individually. Reduction and provisional pin fixation of both areas allows fine-tuning of each site to facilitate obtaining a plantigrade foot before definitive fixation. Supramalleolar osteotomy is a powerful means of correcting uniplanar and biplanar deformity and is relatively straightforward from a technical point of view but there are some important nuances. Osteotomies remote from the deformity apex will result in translation through the osteotomy, which may or may not be desirable. For example, a closing wedge osteotomy for a malunited ankle arthrodesis in which the apex of the sagittal plane deformity is through the ankle joint will result in anterior translation of the foot and deviation of the sagittal plane mechanical axis. In addition, shortening that occurs with closing wedge osteotomies must be anticipated. Dome osteotomy of the distal tibia performed from lateral to medial or vice versa minimizes translation, shortening, and mechanical axis deviation.

Neuropathic patients can have severe combined deformity of the hindfoot and midfoot. Stabilization of ankle and hindfoot deformity often leaves the midfoot decompensated and the foot in a nonplantigrade alignment. Hindfoot equinus and midfoot rocker-bottom collapse can be addressed simultaneously with double level correction using gradual distraction. Percutaneous or limited open osteotomy of the calcaneus and midfoot followed by gradual restoration of calcaneal pitch and midfoot alignment can successfully restore the foot to a plantigrade position and resolve refractory plantar ulceration that is so often seen with this type of deformity (**Fig. 7**).

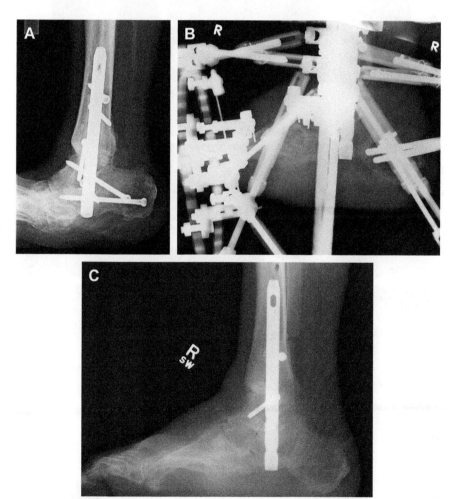

Fig. 7. (*A*) Rocker-bottom collapse of the midfoot following ankle and hindfoot fusion. (*B*) Failure to adequately address equinus leads to progressive sagittal plane midfoot breakdown. (*C*) Limited incision osteotomy through the midfoot and hindfoot with gradual correction using a spatial frame.

Open acute correction of multiplanar deformity through extensile exposure in patients with multiple operations can be risky, especially when there is more than one anatomic site that requires significant angular or rotational correction. An alternative is staged reconstruction with gradual distraction followed by definitive fixation (**Fig. 8**). This technique has the advantage of preserving bone stock and allowing

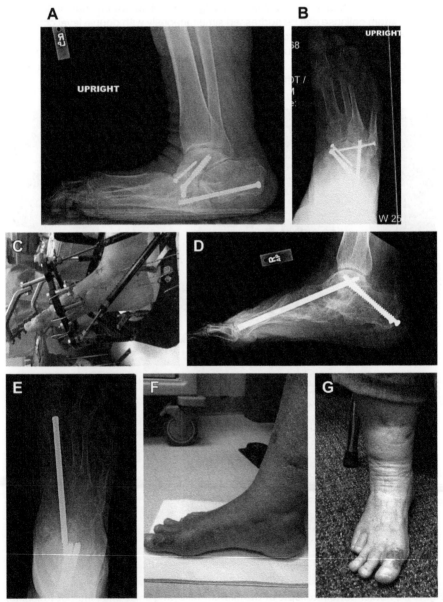

Fig. 8. (*A–G*) Multiple operated foot with multiplanar deformity after hindfoot fusion. Staged reconstruction with gradual distraction followed by definitive internal fixation through limited incision techniques.

multiplanar correction through areas of compromised skin. Disadvantages include prolonged recovery, stiffness of unfused joints, and infection.[22,25] Floerkemeier and colleagues[22] reported on a series of seven subjects with severe multiplanar equino-varus or pes cavus deformities treated with the Taylor spatial frame and gradual correction techniques. Six of seven subjects had good results with no recurrent deformity. Osteotomy of the calcaneus and/or midfoot was performed in all subjects. Complications were frequent and all of the subjects experienced at least one pin tract infection. Other complications included deep infection, wound healing issues, and neuropraxia. Although complication rates are high, gradual correction tech-niques are often the only alternative to amputation in severe fixed multiplanar deformity.

In addition to bony correction, consideration must also be given to soft tissue contracture and imbalance. If muscle balancing is not addressed, it can result in recur-rent deformity. The need for gastrocnemius or Achilles lengthening should be evalu-ated in all patients with midfoot collapse. This is sometimes difficult to accurately assess when rocker-bottom midfoot deformity exists because the midfoot deformity gives the false sense of adequate ankle dorsiflexion. In patients with cavovarus defor-mity, consideration should be given to tendon balancing with transfers such as pero-neus longus to peroneus brevis transfer. When there is unopposed plantar flexion inversion or impaired dorsiflexion strength, posterior tibial lengthening and/or medial midfoot capsular release may be necessary. Transfer of the posterior tibialis through the interosseous membrane to the dorsum of the foot may be indicated in patients with impaired ankle dorsiflexion strength. In cases of fixed forefoot abduction, lengthening or release of the peroneus brevis is sometimes necessary.

REFERENCES

1. Thordarson DB, Schmotzer H, Chon J, et al. Dynamic support of the human longitudinal arch. A biomechanical evaluation. Clin Orthop Relat Res 1995;(316): 165–72.
2. Hoke M. An operation for stabilizing paralytic feet. J Orthop Surg 1921;3: 494–505.
3. Graves SC, Mann RA, Graves KO. Triple arthrodesis in older adults. Results after long-term follow-up. J Bone Joint Surg Am 1993;75:355–62.
4. Tisdel CL, Marcus RE, Heiple KG. Triple arthrodesis for diabetic peritalar neuro-arthropathy. Foot Ankle Int 1995;16:332–8.
5. Saltzman CL, Fehrle MJ, Cooper RR, et al. Triple arthrodesis: twenty-five and forty-four-year average follow-up of the same patients. J Bone Joint Surg Am 1999;81:1391–402.
6. Angus PD, Cowell HR. Triple arthrodesis. A critical long-term review. J Bone Joint Surg Br 1986;68:260–5.
7. Barg A, Brunner S, Zwicky L, et al. Subtalar and naviculocuneiform fusion for extended breakdown of the medial arch. Foot Ankle Clin 2011;16:69–81.
8. Van Boerum DH, Sangeorzan BJ. Biomechanics and pathophysiology of flat foot. Foot Ankle Clin 2003;8:419–30.
9. Mäenpää H, Lehto MU, Belt EA. What went wrong in triple arthrodesis? An analysis of failures in 21 patients. Clin Orthop Relat Res 2001;(391):218–23.
10. Kadakia AR, Haddad SL. Hindfoot arthrodesis for the adult acquired flat foot. Foot Ankle Clin 2003;8:569–94.
11. Den Hartog BD, Kay DB. Non-neuropathic midfoot multiplanar deformity: surgical strategies for reconstruction. Foot Ankle Clin 2009;14:383–92.

12. Knupp M, Stufkens SA, Hintermann B. Triple arthrodesis. Foot Ankle Clin 2011;16: 61–7.

13. Sammarco VJ, Magur EG, Sammarco GJ, et al. Arthrodesis of the subtalar and talonavicular joints for correction of symptomatic hindfoot malalignment. Foot Ankle Int 2006;27:661–6.

14. Taylor R, Sammarco VJ. Minimizing the role of fusion in the rigid flatfoot. Foot Ankle Clin 2012;17:337–49.

15. Haddad SL. Surgical strategies: use of the cuboid osteotomy in combination with the triple arthrodesis with lateral column overload. Foot Ankle Int 2009;30:904–11.

16. Hirose CB, Johnson JE. Plantarflexion opening wedge medial cuneiform osteotomy for correction of fixed forefoot varus associated with flatfoot deformity. Foot Ankle Int 2004;25:568–74.

17. Arunakul M, Amendola A, Gao Y, et al. Tripod index: a new radiographic parameter assessing foot alignment. Foot Ankle Int 2013;34(10):1411–20.

18. Arunakul M, Amendola A, Gao Y, et al. Tripod index: diagnostic accuracy in symptomatic flatfoot and cavovarus foot: part 2. Iowa Orthop J 2013;33:47–53.

19. Hansen ST. The cavovarus/supinated foot deformity and external tibial torsion: the role of the posterior tibial tendon. Foot Ankle Clin 2008;13:325–8, viii.

20. Patel A, Rao S, Nawoczenski D, et al. Midfoot arthritis. J Am Acad Orthop Surg 2010;18:417–25.

21. Raikin SM, Schon LC. Arthrodesis of the fourth and fifth tarsometatarsal joints of the midfoot. Foot Ankle Int 2003;24:584–90.

22. Floerkemeier T, Stukenborg-Colsman C, Windhagen H, et al. Correction of severe foot deformities using the Taylor spatial frame. Foot Ankle Int 2011;32:176–82.

23. Paley D. The correction of complex foot deformities using Ilizarov's distraction osteotomies. Clin Orthop Relat Res 1993;(293):97–111.

24. Eidelman M, Keren Y, Katzman A. Correction of residual clubfoot deformities in older children using the Taylor spatial butt frame and midfoot Gigli saw osteotomy. J Pediatr Orthop 2012;32:527–33.

25. Ferreira RC, Costo MT, Frizzo GG, et al. Correction of neglected clubfoot using the Ilizarov external fixator. Foot Ankle Int 2006;27:266–73.

Triple Arthrodesis
Tips and Tricks to Navigate Trouble

Nathan J. Kiewiet, MD[a], Stephen K. Benirschke, MD[b], Michael E. Brage, MD[b,*]

KEYWORDS

- Triple arthrodesis • Talonavicular arthrodesis • Subtalar arthrodesis
- Calcaneocuboid arthrodesis

KEY POINTS

- The goal of triple arthrodesis is to restore a stable, plantigrade foot.
- Keys to success are predicated on thorough preoperative evaluation of the patient, meticulous surgical technique, and the use of adjunctive procedures to help correct other preoperative deformities to achieve one's goal.
- Salvage options may include revision triple arthrodesis or other procedures involving the midfoot to reconcile a plantigrade foot.

BACKGROUND

Triple arthrodesis was first described by Ryerson[1] in 1923, as a dual-incision approach to arthrodesis of the talonavicular (TN), subtalar (ST), and calcaneocuboid (CC) joints for correction of rigid deformity secondary to paralytic conditions. While paralytic conditions resulting in rigid hindfoot deformity have become less prevalent, triple arthrodesis has been adapted to treat hindfoot deformity related to trauma, inflammatory arthropathies, and long-standing peritalar subluxation with posterior tibial tendon dysfunction or cavovarus deformity with arthritic changes.

Triple arthrodesis can be a powerful corrector of hindfoot deformity and a reliable procedure for pain relief in patients with hindfoot arthritis; however, it is not without complications.[2,3] Postoperative complications may include malunions and nonunions (**Fig. 1**A), lateral wound breakdown, and induction of adjacent joint arthritis.[4–6] Residual deformity (see **Fig. 1**B) may also accompany even a successful triple arthrodesis if remaining deformities of the foot are not considered and addressed at the time of initial evaluation and operative intervention.

The authors have nothing to disclose regarding this publication.

[a] Drisko, Fee & Parkins Orthopaedics, PC, 19550 East 39th Street, Suite 410, Independence, MO 64057, USA; [b] Department of Orthopaedics, University of Washington, 325 9th Avenue, Box 359798, Seattle, WA 98104, USA
* Corresponding author.
E-mail address: bragem@uw.edu

Foot Ankle Clin N Am 19 (2014) 483–497
http://dx.doi.org/10.1016/j.fcl.2014.06.008
foot.theclinics.com

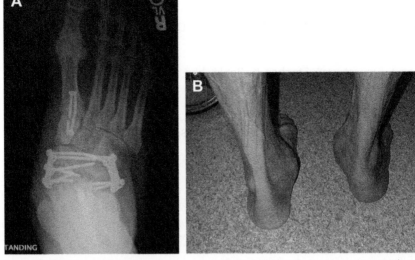

Fig. 1. (*A*) AP foot radiograph showing nonunion of talonavicular joint along with under-correction of underlying peritalar subluxation. (*B*) Clinical photo of patient with residual deformity following attempted triple arthrodesis.

The goal of providing the patient with a stable, plantigrade foot to maximize function utilizing a triple arthrodesis can be maximized through meticulous preoperative evaluation, surgical planning, and surgical technique, including joint preparation and rigid fixation. The goal of this article is to provide pathways to maximize this goal through the use of cases to illustrate tips to avoid the common complications. Cases to illustrate salvage options for residual deformity following triple arthrodesis are also discussed.

PREOPERATIVE EVALUATION AND PLANNING

As with any encounter, the initial evaluation begins with a thorough history taking and physical examination of the patient. Patient medical comorbidities, medications, or social factors that may affect bone or wound healing require special attention, such as diabetes, steroid use, or tobacco use. Medical optimization of comorbidities and tobacco cessation may help to maximize risk reduction. Examination should include a thorough assessment of the entire lower extremity. Special attention should be given to lower extremity alignment proximally to assure that correction of the hindfoot will not exacerbate proximal deformity. Hindfoot alignment must be assessed in a weight-bearing position, and the rigidity of the deformity should be evaluated. Compensatory or contributory alignment of the midfoot and forefoot must also be assessed (**Fig. 2**), along with the status of the musculotendinous units driving foot alignment. Equinus deformity and whether it is an isolated gastrocnemius contracture or tendoachilles contracture, as well as contracture of other musculotendinous units and joint capsules, must be assessed.

Radiological examination begins with weight-bearing views of the foot and ankle in the anteroposterior, lateral, and oblique planes to assess deformity and plan for surgical correction. Weight-bearing radiographs allow for more accurate assessment of deformity, alignment, and loss of joint space (**Fig. 3**).[7] A simulated weight-bearing computed tomography (CT) protocol has been designed and implemented at the

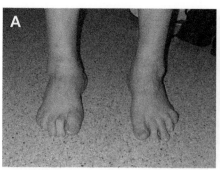
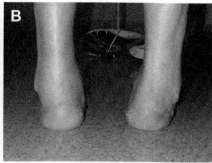

Fig. 2. (*A*) Anterior and (*B*) posterior clinical photos assessing alignment of a cavovarus deformity. Note the varus position of the hindfoot and weight bearing on the lateral border of the foot.

senior author's institution and is an invaluable adjunct to assess hindfoot arthritis and deformity. CT allows for assessment of further structural deformity that may prevent appropriate reduction, particularly of the subtalar joint prior to arthrodesis (**Fig. 4**). Attention should be centered on reliably identifying the apex of deformity and whether any other adjunctive procedures are required to fully correct the deformity or to prevent residual deformity after triple arthrodesis. These residual deformities and adjunctive procedures will be discussed later in this article.

If concern arises for deformity of the proximal lower extremity, full-length limb alignment radiographs may be warranted. Correction of proximal deformity may be warranted at the time of or prior to the triple arthrodesis; however, this subject is beyond the scope of the current article.

CLASSIC TRIPLE AND BONE GRAFT

The traditional approach for a triple arthrodesis involves a combined medial and lateral approach.[8] The CC and ST joints are approached through the lateral incision. The TN joint is approached through both the medial and lateral approaches to allow for adequate debridement of cartilage. Bono and Jacobs[9] showed in a cadaver model that only 38% of cartilage could be removed from the TN joint through an isolated lateral incision. Joint preparation is performed by removing all cartilage with a combination of osteotomes and curettes. The subchondral bone is then perforated with a 2 mm drill.

Reduction begins with either the ST or TN joint; however, adjunctive procedures, which will be illustrated in more detail later in this article, may be required to allow for reduction. The ST joint is placed in approximately 5° of valgus, and fixation is achieved with a varying number of partially threaded cancellous screws that are at least 5.5 mm in diameter. The senior author prefers 2 or 3 partially threaded screws. Reduction of the TN joint is performed by varying amounts of inversion or eversion and plantarflexion or dorsiflexion depending on the deformity that exists. For lateral peritalar subluxation, a combination of inversion and plantarflexion is required to correct the underlying deformity, while the opposite may be true for cavovarus deformity. Fixation of the TN joint is achieved either through 2 or 3 partially threaded screws for compression or with a compression-type plate construct.[10–12] Following fixation of the ST and TN joints, little reduction should be needed at the CC joint. Depending on the preoperative deformity, hindfoot correction may leave the lateral column fairly intact or with gapping. If no more than a minimal gap exists, the CC joint can be fused

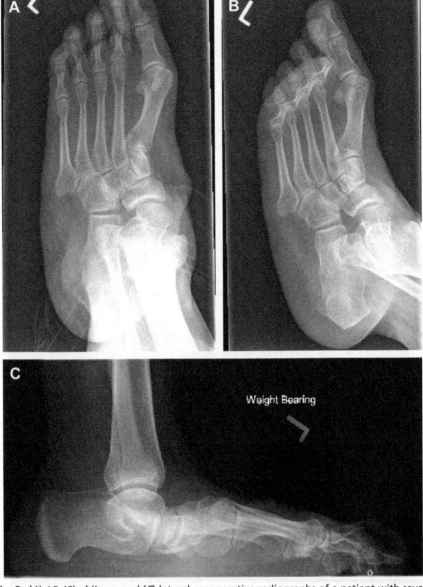

Fig. 3. (*A*) AP, (*B*) oblique, and (*C*) lateral preoperative radiographs of a patient with severe lateral peritalar subluxation. Note the near dislocation of the subtalar joint and extreme pes planus deformity through the midfoot. Correction of the hindfoot only would leave residual deformity through the midfoot and forefoot.

in situ; however, if gapping exists, bone graft may be required to provide apposition.[13] CC joint fixation may consist of screws or plate constructs (**Fig. 5**).[14] Following correction, the remainder of the foot must be assessed for residual deformity and the need for adjunctive procedures, which will be discussed in further detail later in this article.

Although bone graft may be necessary to fill gaps in at least 1 of the 3 joints, the routine use of bone graft does not appear to be warranted when adequate compression can be

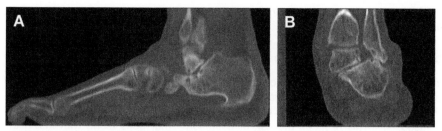

Fig. 4. (*A*) Sagittal and (*B*) coronal CTs scan showing bottoming out of the sinus tarsi, subtalar joint incongruity, and arthritis.

achieved after meticulous joint preparation. Rosenfeld and colleagues,[15] reported a nonunion rate as low as 4% in 100 triple arthrodesis cases performed with graft from resected subchondral bone alone. If minimal deformity exists, joint preparation and compression may achieve adequate bony apposition. However, if bony resection is required to correct the underlying deformity, particularly in the ST joint, or if gapping

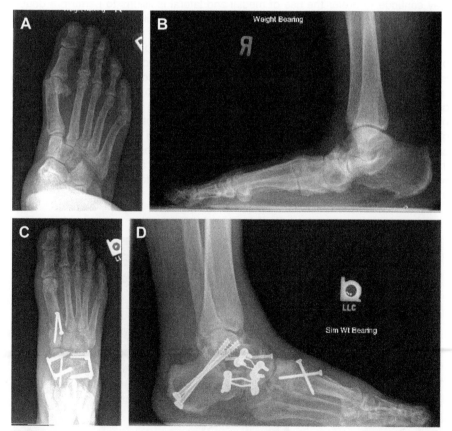

Fig. 5. (*A*) Preoperative AP and (*B*) preoperative lateral foot radiographs showing severe lateral peritalar subluxation. (*C*) Postoperative AP and (*D*) postoperative lateral foot radiographs showing standard construct triple arthrodesis with good correction of underlying lateral peritalar subluxation deformity. First tarsometatarsal (TMT) fusion was added to help correct residual deformity after correction of the hindfoot.

exists following correction, the senior author routinely uses local autograft to fill any gaps that remain.

DOUBLE ARTHRODESIS (TN AND ST)

In an effort to reduce the risk of complications such as nonunions, lateral wound breakdown, and induction of adjacent joint arthritis, several authors have recommended performing an arthrodesis of the TN and ST joints and leaving the CC joint unfused.[16–18] This reduces the risk of nonunion[18] that goes along with fusing the CC joint and also retains some movement through the CC joint,[19] which may diminish the loading of adjacent joints. Others have also recommended performing this double arthrodesis through an isolated medial incision to avoid lateral wound breakdown.[20,21]

Although arthrodesis of the TN and ST joints alone can correct most hindfoot deformities, caution must be exercised. A formal triple arthrodesis may be more beneficial when there is underlying CC joint arthritis or if shortening the lateral column will help with deformity correction. The authors do agree that sparing the CC joint may allow for retention of some movement and reduce the risk of adjacent joint arthritis, but they continue to prefer the use of medial and lateral incisions to perform a double arthrodesis. The use of a smaller lateral incision may be utilized, which may decrease the risk of associated breakdown.

Depending on the hindfoot deformity, it may be difficult to fully visualize the joints for preparation, and it can be even more difficult to obtain adequate reduction through an isolated medial incision. **Figs. 6** and **7** illustrate a reduction maneuver utilizing a laminar spreader in the sinus tarsi to restore the relationship of the talus and calcaneus during correction of lateral peritalar subluxation. One arm of the laminar spreader is placed on the anterior process of the calcaneus and the other on the lateral process of the talus, which provides a rotational reduction of the underlying deformity and correction of the normal relationship. Once the relationship has been corrected through use of the laminar spreader, it can be held with an axially directed wire. It would be difficult to obtain adequate reduction of this deformity through an isolated medial incision.

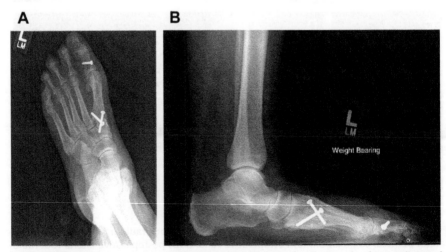

Fig. 6. (*A*) Preoperative AP foot radiograph and (*B*) lateral preoperative foot radiograph showing lateral peritalar subluxation. Note the change in the normal relationship of the talus and calcaneus.

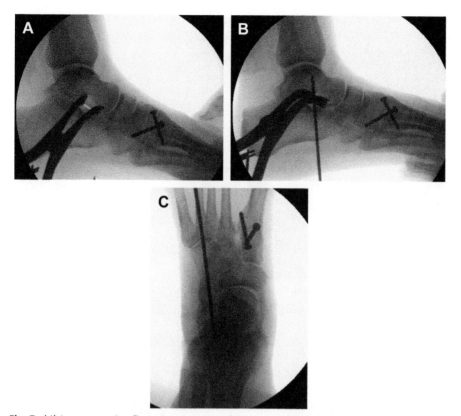

Fig. 7. (A) Intraoperative fluoroscopic image showing placement of the laminar spreader in the sinus tarsi. (B) Intraoperative fluoroscopic image showing reduction and placement of an axially directed wire to hold the reduction. (C) Intraoperative fluoroscopic AP image showing reduction of the relationship of the talus to the calcaneus and navicular.

ADJUNCTIVE PROCEDURES

Triple arthrodesis is a powerful corrector of hindfoot deformity. To achieve full correction of deformity, adjunctive procedures such as soft tissue releases and tendon lengthening may be required.[22] Procedures such as midfoot fusions or metatarsal osteotomies may also be required to correct residual deformity that exists after correction of the hindfoot.[23,24]

The first case illustrates the need for both soft tissue and bony corrections in conjunction with triple arthrodesis in a patient with a seizure disorder and left-sided hemiparesis secondary to a right frontotemporal craniotomy. She had a severe equinocavovarus foot deformity that the family noted was progressing over the past several years. She had limited ambulatory capacity and was having increasing difficulty with brace wear. Her examination showed a rigid equinocavovarus deformity with severe gastroc-soleus and posterior tibialis contractures and minimal peroneal functioning. Preoperative radiographs showed a severe equinocavovarus deformity (**Fig. 8**). She elected for operative intervention and underwent a corrective triple arthrodesis with several adjunctive procedures to help correct her rigid deformity. Multiple soft tissue procedures were performed to allow for adequate correction of the deformity prior to triple arthrodesis, including an Achilles lengthening, posterior ankle

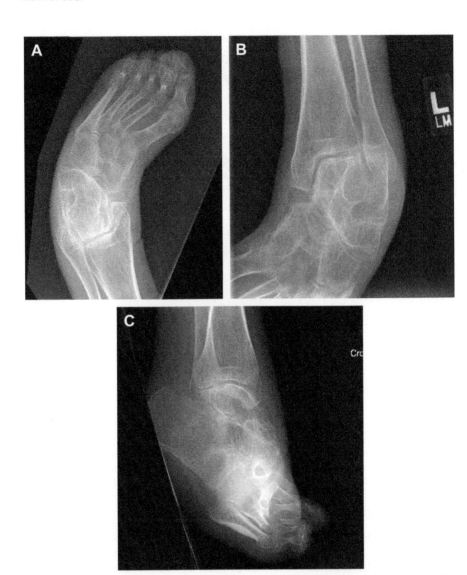

Fig. 8. (*A*) AP foot, (*B*) AP ankle, and (*C*) lateral radiographs of severe equinocavovarus foot deformity. Note the significant varus deformity through the talonavicular joint and amount of equinus.

capsular release, posterior tibialis tendon lengthening, and midfoot capsular release. Midfoot arthrodesis was performed following triple arthrodesis to correct her residual forefoot pronation after correction of her hindfoot. Adequate correction to position the foot in a near-plantigrade position and allow for easier brace wear was obtained (**Fig. 9**).

SALVAGE

Even after successful healing of a triple arthrodesis, deformity may persist, secondary to malunion or residual uncorrected deformity of the midfoot. Recurrent deformity may

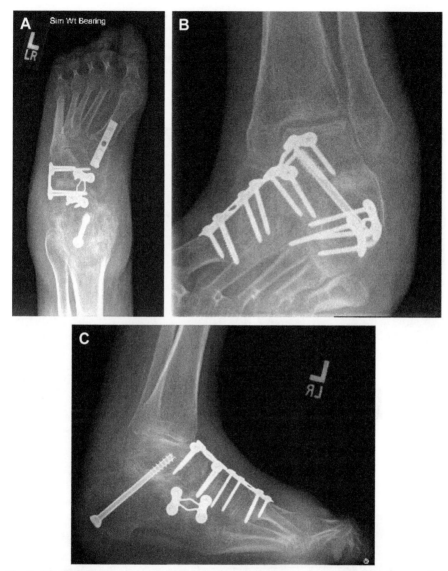

Fig. 9. (*A*) AP foot, (*B*) AP ankle, and (*C*) lateral radiographs of same patient after surgical correction. Note the near plantigrade position. Midfoot fusion was also performed at the time of surgery to help correct residual pronation deformity by dorsiflexing the first ray.

also occur through the midfoot after successful triple arthrodesis. Salvage options depend on the deformity. For malunions, one may consider a revision of the triple arthrodesis; however, for residual deformity of the midfoot, midfoot fusion or osteotomy would be more beneficial.

The next case illustrates correction of a triple arthrodesis malunion in a patient born with clubfoot deformity, initially treated with casting. He continued to have some residual or recurrent deformity, and a triple arthrodesis was performed approximately 7 years prior to presentation to the authors' clinic. He continued to have difficulty with deformity and pain after his triple arthrodesis. **Fig. 10** shows his initial radiographs on presentation to the author's clinic. He has a well healed fusion but continues to have significant deformity secondary to undercorrection during his initial operation. He continued to have significant pain along the lateral border of his foot secondary to overload with weight bearing and elected for operative intervention. He underwent a revision triple arthrodesis for correction of his residual clubfoot deformity.

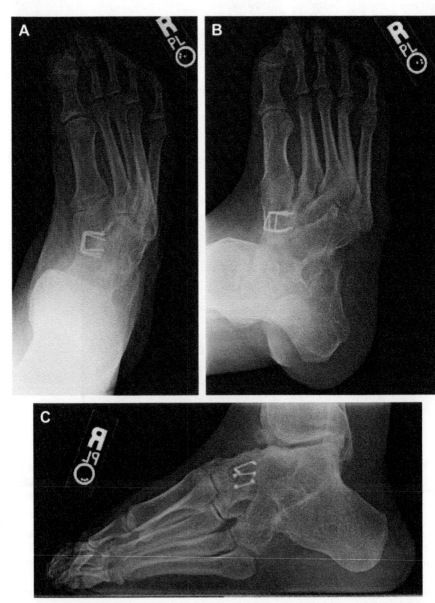

Fig. 10. (*A*) AP, (*B*) oblique, and (*C*) lateral preoperative radiographs of triple arthrodesis malunion. Note the significant cavus, varus, and supination deformities that remain between the hindfoot and midfoot.

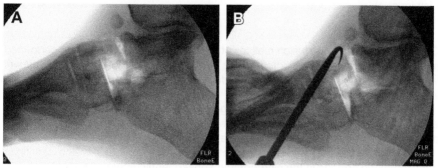

Fig. 11. (*A*) Intraoperative fluoroscopic picture showing osteotomies through TN, CC, and ST joints. (*B*) Intraoperative fluoroscopic picture showing reduction maneuver with a bone hook to pronate the midfoot on the hindfoot.

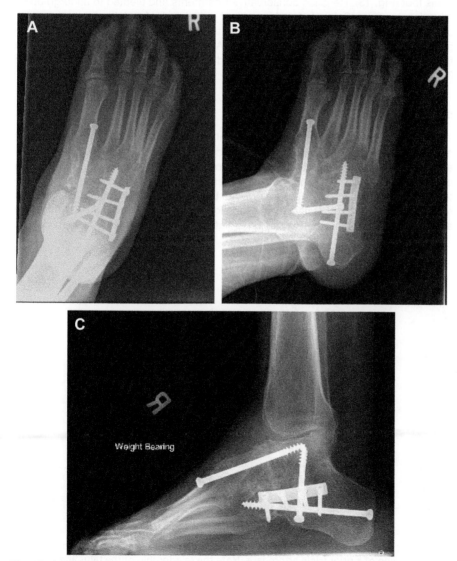

Fig. 12. (*A*) AP, (*B*) oblique, and (*C*) lateral radiographs at nearly 12 weeks postoperatively showing well healed revision fusion and plantigrade position.

Osteotomies through the fusion masses of the TN, CC, and ST joints were performed, and the relationship of the hindfoot to the midfoot was corrected and stabilized with internal fixation (**Fig. 11**). A plantigrade foot was restored, and the patient healed without difficulty (**Fig. 12**).

The last case illustrates another salvage option for correction of a triple arthrodesis malunion in a patient who underwent a triple arthrodesis for post-traumatic arthritis. The patient initially sustained a misdiagnosed calcaneus fracture in the remote past and was treated nonoperatively. He went on to develop significant post-traumatic arthritis in the hindfoot and subsequently underwent a triple arthrodesis, which healed uneventfully. However, he had continued pain secondary to varus malunion of his triple arthrodesis and weight bearing on the lateral border of his foot (**Fig. 13**). He failed conservative treatments and elected to undergo operative intervention. Salvage for this patient consisted of a lateralizing calcaneal osteotomy to correct his hindfoot varus and a midfoot closing and rotational osteotomy to correct his midfoot varus (**Fig. 14**). Adequate correction was obtained with the calcaneal and midfoot osteotomies, and a near plantigrade foot was obtained (**Fig. 15**).

DISCUSSION

Triple arthrodesis continues to be a powerful procedure to address severe hindfoot malalignment or arthritis due to several underlying pathologies. The goal of triple arthrodesis is to provide pain relief while providing a stable, plantigrade foot to optimize function for the patient. Several methods can be utilized to help maximize this goal. Limiting the arthrodesis to the talonavicular and subtalar joints may reduce the risk of nonunion and the development of adjacent joint arthritis. The authors caution against the use of an isolated medial incision to perform double

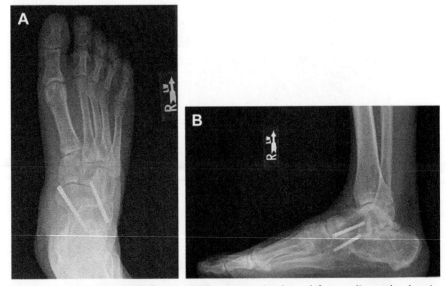

Fig. 13. (*A*) Preoperative AP foot and (*B*) preoperative lateral foot radiographs showing varus malunion of a prior triple arthrodesis. Note the relationship of the talus and navicular and the stacked lateral metatarsals.

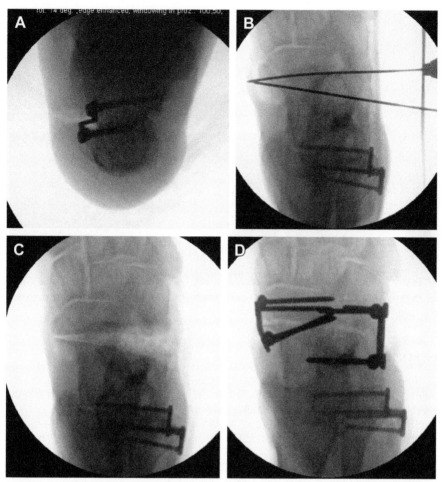

Fig. 14. (*A*) Intraoperative fluoroscopic image showing lateralizing calcaneal osteotomy. (*B*) Intraoperative fluoroscopic image showing wires outlining the proposed lateral closing wedge midfoot osteotomy. (*C*) Intraoperative fluoroscopic image showing midfoot osteotomy. (*D*) Intraoperative fluoroscopic image showing reduction after closing the midfoot osteotomy.

arthrodesis, as the visualization of the joints and reduction of the deformity can be compromised.

Adjunctive procedures may also be an integral part of providing a stable, plantigrade foot. Soft tissue releases and tendon lengthening prior to triple arthrodesis may aid in reduction of the deformity. Subsequent procedures of the midfoot, such as fusion or osteotomy, may be required after reduction of the hindfoot to prevent residual deformity. Careful preoperative assessment and planning will allow the surgeon to assure that all adjunctive procedures are being performed.

Underlying meticulous surgical technique, including joint preparation and the use of rigid internal fixation, along with appropriate reduction of deformity, will help prevent malunion and the need for salvage operations. If salvage is needed, the surgeon must again assess the deformity and perform the appropriate correction.

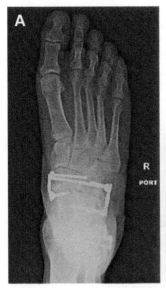
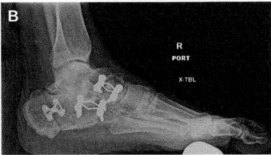

Fig. 15. (*A*) AP foot and (*B*) lateral foot radiographs showing correction of previous varus malunion to a near plantigrade foot position.

REFERENCES

1. Ryerson E. Arthrodesing operations of the feet. J Bone Joint Surg Am 1923;5:453–71.
2. Pell RF 4th, Myerson MS, Schon LC. Clinical outcome after primary triple arthrodesis. J Bone Joint Surg Am 2000;82(1):47–57.
3. Smith RW, Shen W, Dewitt S, et al. Triple arthrodesis in adults with non-paralytic disease. A minimum ten-year follow-up study. J Bone Joint Surg Am 2004; 86A(12):2707–13.
4. Figgie MP, O'Malley MJ, Ranawat C, et al. Triple arthrodesis in rheumatoid arthritis. Clin Orthop Relat Res 1993;(292):250–4.
5. Knupp M, Skoog A, Tornkvist H, et al. Triple arthrodesis in rheumatoid arthritis. Foot Ankle Int 2008;29(3):293–7.
6. Maenpaa H, Lehto MU, Belt EA. What went wrong in triple arthrodesis? An analysis of failures in 21 patients. Clin Orthop Relat Res 2001;(391):218–23.
7. Wapner KL. Triple arthrodesis in adults. J Am Acad Orthop Surg 1998;6(3):188–96.
8. Johnson JE, Yu JR. Arthrodesis techniques in the management of stage II and III acquired adult flatfoot deformity. Instr Course Lect 2006;55:531–42.
9. Bono JV, Jacobs RL. Triple arthrodesis through a single lateral approach: a cadaveric experiment. Foot Ankle 1992;13(7):408–12.
10. Chen CH, Huang PJ, Chen TB, et al. Isolated talonavicular arthrodesis for talonavicular arthritis. Foot Ankle Int 2001;22(8):633–6.
11. Harper MC. Talonavicular arthrodesis for the acquired flatfoot in the adult. Clin Orthop Relat Res 1999;(365):65–8.
12. Weinraub GM, Heilala MA. Isolated talonavicular arthrodesis for adult onset flatfoot deformity/posterior tibial tendon dysfunction. Clin Podiatr Med Surg 2007; 24(4):745–52, ix.
13. Horton GA, Olney BW. Triple arthrodesis with lateral column lengthening for treatment of severe planovalgus deformity. Foot Ankle Int 1995;16(7):395–400.

14. Kann JN, Parks BG, Schon LC. Biomechanical evaluation of two different screw positions for fusion of the calcaneocuboid joint. Foot Ankle Int 1999;20(1):33–6.

15. Rosenfeld PF, Budgen SA, Saxby TS. Triple arthrodesis: is bone grafting necessary? The results in 100 consecutive cases. J Bone Joint Surg Br 2005;87(2): 175–8.

16. Graves SC, Mann RA, Graves KO. Triple arthrodesis in older adults. Results after long-term follow-up. J Bone Joint Surg Am 1993;75(3):355–62.

17. Knupp M, Schuh R, Stufkens SA, et al. Subtalar and talonavicular arthrodesis through a single medial approach for the correction of severe planovalgus deformity. J Bone Joint Surg Br 2009;91(5):612–5.

18. Sammarco VJ, Magur EG, Sammarco GJ, et al. Arthrodesis of the subtalar and talonavicular joints for correction of symptomatic hindfoot malalignment. Foot Ankle Int 2006;27(9):661–6.

19. Astion DJ, Deland JT, Otis JC, et al. Motion of the hindfoot after simulated arthrodesis. J Bone Joint Surg Am 1997;79(2):241–6.

20. Jackson WF, Tryfonidis M, Cooke PH, et al. Arthrodesis of the hindfoot for valgus deformity. An entirely medial approach. J Bone Joint Surg Br 2007;89(7):925–7.

21. Jeng CL, Vora AM, Myerson MS. The medial approach to triple arthrodesis. Indications and technique for management of rigid valgus deformities in high-risk patients. Foot Ankle Clin 2005;10(3):515–21, vi–vii.

22. DiGiovanni CW, Langer P. The role of isolated gastrocnemius and combined Achilles contractures in the flatfoot. Foot Ankle Clin 2007;12(2):363–79, viii.

23. Hirose CB, Johnson JE. Plantarflexion opening wedge medial cuneiform osteotomy for correction of fixed forefoot varus associated with flatfoot deformity. Foot Ankle Int 2004;25(8):568–74.

24. Thompson IM, Bohay DR, Anderson JG. Fusion rate of first tarsometatarsal arthrodesis in the modified Lapidus procedure and flatfoot reconstruction. Foot Ankle Int 2005;26(9):698–703.

Nonunion of Fifth Metatarsal Fractures

Matthew Solan, FRCS Tr&Orth[a,b,*], Mark Davies, FRCS Tr&Orth[c]

KEYWORDS

- Metatarsal • Fracture • Nonunion • Internal fixation

KEY POINTS

- Fractures of the 5th metatarsal require careful evaluation and classification to ensure selection of the optimum treatment plan. Distal fractures rarely require fixation, even when displacement is wide.
- Type 1 fractures are best managed functionally, without cast immobilization and heal reliably.
- Type 2 fractures have a high union rate when managed nonoperatively but a period of cast immobilization is advised and both clinical and radiological follow-up is required.
- Type 3 fractures should be considered for operative fixation, particularly if there is any cavus posture of the foot, neuropathy, or if the patient is a competitive sportsperson; this is because of the risk of delayed or nonunion.
- Cases of established nonunion or refracture require fixation. The authors do not routinely use bone graft. The screw head should be countersunk (and washers avoided) because of the risk of symptomatic metalwork.
- A cannulated 4.5-mm screw is the authors' implant of choice unless the patient is very large. In such cases a 6.5-mm screw is preferred.

INCIDENCE

These injuries are common.[1] Metatarsal fractures are those most frequently encountered in the foot.[2] More than half of these are of the 5th metatarsal.[3] The incidence is increasing, along with the activity levels of the general population. In a large study of fractures in older female subjects, Hasselman and colleagues[3] found that of all foot fractures those of the 5th metatarsal are the most common, accounting for nearly 60% of injuries. Reduced bone mineral density was associated with these fractures, whereas ankle fractures were more likely in overweight subjects of normal bone density.

[a] Surrey Foot and Ankle Clinic, Mount Alvernia Hospital, Harvey Road, Guildford, Surrey GU1 3LX, UK; [b] Royal Surrey County Hospital, Egerton Road, Guildford, Surrey GU2 5XX, UK; [c] London Foot and Ankle Centre, Hospital of St John and St Elizabeth, 80 Grove End Road, London NW8 9NH, UK
* Corresponding author. London Foot and Ankle Centre, Hospital of St John and St Elizabeth, 80 Grove End Road, London NW8 9NH, UK.
E-mail address: Matthewsolan1@aol.com

Foot Ankle Clin N Am 19 (2014) 499–519
http://dx.doi.org/10.1016/j.fcl.2014.06.009
foot.theclinics.com

Injuries in athletes may cause prolonged periods away from sport, and fractures distal to the 5th metatarsal diaphyseal-metaphyseal junction excite particular debate[4–6] due to the high risk of delayed union, nonunion, and refracture.[7] In a large study of National Football League players, Low and colleagues[8] noted an incidence (over a 14 year period) of 1.8%. There are reports that the type of stud or cleat used by soccer players is partly responsible for the increasing number of affected professional sportspersons.[9] Playing surface has also been implicated and with more use of all-weather surfaces some investigators believe that the incidence of fracture will increase further.[10]

Nonathletes suffer prolonged symptoms as well, and this can still lead to significant periods of time lost from work.[11]

By way of contrast, distal 5th metatarsal fractures in active individuals heal reliably and usually without sequelae.[12] The authors of this study report results in 35 professional dancers. Four were treated operatively. However, the results of nonoperative management for even widely displaced fractures were so good that they recommend nonoperative treatments. Pain-free walking was possible at 6 weeks and dance training resumed after 11 weeks. There were no long-term problems and only one delayed union. Surgical treatment of these injuries may occasionally be required (**Fig. 1**) but offers no advance over nonoperative treatment, even for active patients.

AMALGAMATING EVIDENCE FOR TREATMENT OF FRACTURES OF THE 5TH METATARSAL BASE

The available evidence on the best way to manage fractures of the 5th metatarsal base is limited and consists mostly of case series and retrospective reviews. Recent attempts to draw useful conclusions through systematic reviews and meta-analyses are potentially confusing.[13,14] In spite of the increasing number of such orthopedic papers, the authors struggle to really understand how lumping together a heterogeneous series of poor-quality papers can lead to "scientifically proved" conclusions!!

CLASSIFICATION OF BASE FRACTURES

The 5th metatarsal, in its more proximal part, is commonly classified into 3 zones.[15] The Lawrence and Botte classification was largely based on the observation that more distal fractures, beyond the tuberosity, are prone to delayed union or nonunion. Some investigators offer dogmatic recommendations regarding the role of operative treatment.[16] There are, nevertheless, several areas of controversy.

Robert Jones's name has been associated with the 5th metatarsal fracture because he reported his own injury as part of a small case series.[17] Stewart called injuries distal to the 4th-5th junction "Jones fractures"[18] but Dameron used the same eponym for tuberosity fractures that extend into the 4th-5th junction.[19,20] The rationale for these classifications was to try and recognize those injuries that present the greatest risk of delayed or nonunion; this has long been recognized as a clinical problem.[21]

A recent paper by Polzer and colleagues[22] argues that only 2 zones need to be considered because they believe that the prognosis of fractures in the 2 more proximal zones is identical. Styloid process fractures (Zone 1) and those involving the joint between the bases of the 4th and 5th metatarsal bases (Zone 2)—the so-called Jones fracture—can thus be managed functionally. Only the fractures more distal still (in Lawrence and Botte's Zone 3) need to be managed differently. Assuming that a classification system is of use to surgeon or patient if it informs the decision regarding treatment, this new and more straightforward 2-part classification would appear to be helpful.

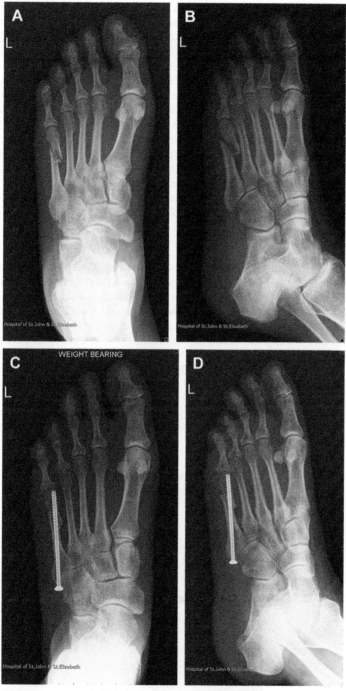

Fig. 1. (*A–D*) Fifth metatarsal shaft facture treated operatively.

However, Chuckpaiwong and colleagues[23] made a similar case for simplification of the classification from 3 to 2 zones, but chose to lump Jones fractures with diaphyseal fractures (ie, Zones 2 and 3 together). The argument was based on their findings that both of these more distal fracture types have a higher rate of complications when compared with styloid fractures.

These 2 papers present conflicting advice about how Zone 2 injuries should be reclassified and treated. Polzer and colleagues have based their argument on a critical appraisal of all the available literature (Level II evidence), whereas Chuckpaiwong and colleagues' work is based on a retrospective case series (Level IV evidence).

Based on our experience (Level V evidence) we prefer that Zone 2 injuries, which are not as benign as styloid process fractures, are treated with functional treatment after a period of immobilization. Although styloid fractures do not require routine follow-up, treatment of Zone 2 fractures should be supplemented with formal clinical and radiographic follow-up. Thus we recommend that the Zone 3 classification still be considered the best for guiding treatment (**Figs. 2–4**).

ZONE 1 FRACTURES

Zone 1 (styloid process) fractures are treated functionally. The only real debate in the literature is in relation to how much splintage is required and for how long it should be retained. Zenios and colleagues[24] published a randomized study of 50 patients and concluded that an elastic bandage is preferable to cast immobilization. Weiner had previously demonstrated that cast immobilization is associated with slower recovery.[25] Vorlat and colleagues[26] used regression analysis in a group of 38 patients to show that prolonged periods of non–weight bearing are associated with poor outcome. The mean period of non–weight bearing in that study was 17 days and of casting was 38 days.

Children's fractures are often managed rather differently to similar injuries in adults. The largest series on the subject of pediatric 5th metatarsal fractures reviewed 103 cases and concluded that they should be managed just like their adult counterparts.[27]

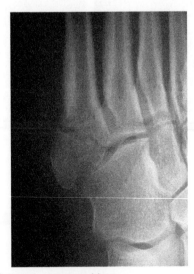

Fig. 2. Type 1 fracture of the 5th metatarsal base.

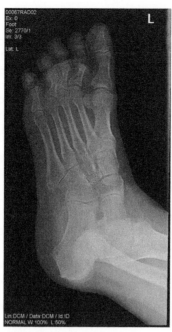

Fig. 3. Type 2 fracture of the 5th metatarsal base.

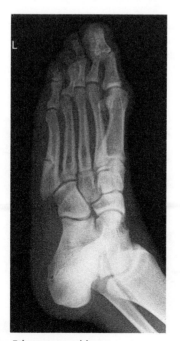

Fig. 4. Type 3 fracture of the 5th metatarsal base.

It is extremely rare for fractures of the styloid process of the base of the 5th metatarsal to remain painful because of fracture nonunion. It is more common to encounter patients, often skeletally immature, who have been given poor and conflicting advice about their injury. The normal radiographic appearances of the apophysis at the base of the 5th metatarsal are not well understood in Emergency Departments. Many youngsters with no fracture are immobilized in a cast, told to use crutches, and bear no weight. A proportion of these patients then develop disuse problems including chronic regional pain syndrome. Check radiographs still show the "fracture" and so anxiety is redoubled and rehabilitation is further delayed (**Fig. 5**).

The epiphysis at the base of the 5th metatarsal begins to ossify at the age of 9 to 11 years in girls and 11 to 14 years in boys. The physis closes 2 to 3 years later.[15]

In the skeletally mature patient, a similar unfortunate chain of events can occur when an accessory bone is misrepresented as a fracture (**Fig. 6**).[28,29]

Accessory bones at the 5th metatarsal base include the os vesalianum. An os peroneum is present in all patients but often cartilaginous rather than bony. One study found the incidence of ossification to be 4.7%.[30] Given the relative proximity to the metatarsal base this is a further cause of diagnostic error.[30–32]

STYLOID FRACTURE FIBROUS UNION

Radiographic appearances can be misleading in this situation, and it is advisable to avoid routine re-X-ray of these injuries in the absence of any specific bony tenderness. There is a significant rate of painless fibrous union, which requires no treatment (**Fig. 7**). Patients cannot easily comprehend that painless fibrous union is a satisfactory outcome. When confronted with a radiograph where the fracture line remains visible, some lose confidence and this perpetuates symptoms that would otherwise have resolved as normal function and activities resumed. The authors do not routinely re-X-ray these injuries.

Consensus on the precise definition of delayed union remains elusive. In the authors' view, intrusive symptoms beyond 3 months require investigation but, in the absence of major displacement of the proximal fragment, continued symptomatic management is preferred. Although nonoperative treatment modalities such as

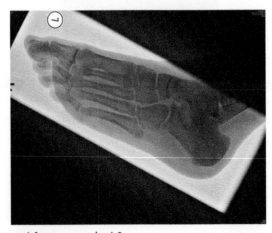

Fig. 5. Fifth metatarsal fracture or physis?

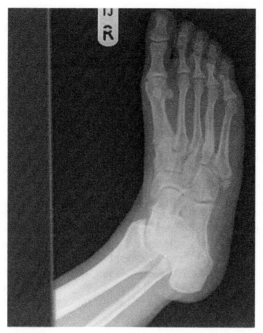

Fig. 6. Os vesalianum.

Exogen or extracorporeal shockwave therapy (ESWT) are useful but where there remains a large fracture gap, their efficacy is not well documented.

Surgery for styloid process fracture nonunion is very rarely required. Even large fragments, where the fracture line extends into the articulation with the cuboid, heal well. There is therefore very little written regarding treatment of this particular eventuality.

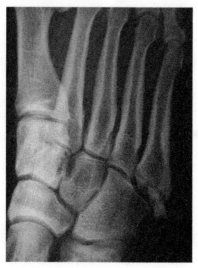

Fig. 7. Displaced fracture not requiring surgery.

Should nonunion occur then the authors recommend internal fixation after reduction of the fracture. Debridement of the fibrous tissue is performed and bone graft may be required (**Fig. 8**).

ZONE 2 (OF 3) FRACTURES

Lawrence and Botte Zone 2 injuries heal just as reliably as styloid fractures and so the case for classifying the 2 types together[22] is a strong one. The potential for degenerative joint disease developing between the 4th and 5th metatarsal bases because of malunion is a potential concern. Any practicing foot and ankle surgeon will, however, have to think extremely hard to recall such a problem presenting clinically, except after major trauma or a crush injury (**Fig. 9**). Cases like these are managed in the same way as other patients with tarsometatarsal joint arthritis. Fusion of the (4th and) 5th tarsometatarsal joint is avoided where possible. Nevertheless, just as for other joints that are painful enough to require surgery, fusion provides excellent pain relief. Fixation is more difficult than for tarsometatarsal 1 to 3 but the outcomes after excision or interposition arthroplasty are, in the authors' experience, generally disappointing.

The argument for managing Zone 2 (Jones) fractures nonoperatively should not be extended too far. Unlike Zone 1 injuries, an elastic support is not sufficient. Symptomatic management, including use of a stiff shoe, is preferred for Zone 1 injuries. But for Zone 2 the authors prefer formal support in a protective short Aircast boot or similar. Zone 1 injuries usually require no formal clinical and radiological follow-up, not least because the sight of an asymptomatic fibrous union can cause concern to the patient. Nonunion after Zone 2 injury is extremely rare, but repeat radiographs and clinical examination is advisable at 8 weeks. Physiotherapy is helpful for both fracture types but deferred until after the 8-week review in Zone 2 injuries.

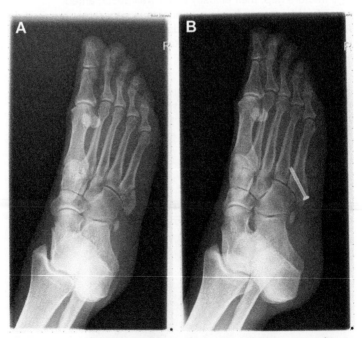

Fig. 8. (*A, B*) Nonunion of type 1 fracture treated with debridement, grafting, and screw fixation.

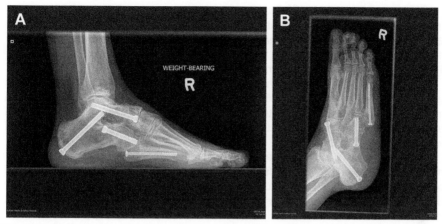

Fig. 9. Stress fracture in 5th MT after triple arthrodesis with mild residual cavus posture.

ZONE 3 FRACTURES

Fractures confined to the region of the proximal 5th metatarsal that are distal to the 4–5 articulation are those that cause patients and their orthopedic surgeons the most difficulty. The goals of treatment are to achieve fracture healing and return to normal function as safely and rapidly as possible. Secondary prevention of refracture through identification of any predisposing factors is also desirable. Cast treatment and non-weight bearing will allow many fractures to unite, but successful treatment of cases where there is delayed or nonunion has lowered the threshold for primary fixation. However, the amount of good evidence in the literature is disappointing.

A recent analysis of the published literature by Roche and Calder[14] included 26 previous papers of which only one was a randomized controlled trial. The overall union rate for delayed unions managed nonoperatively was 44%, whereas cases treated with screw fixation healed in 97% of cases. Although careful to acknowledge that the evidence base is mainly Level IV studies and that complications of surgery must be considered, the investigators concluded that screw fixation is superior to nonoperative management.

Reviewing some of the case series and biomechanical studies regarding screw fixation of Zone 3 injuries is worthwhile.

Outcome scores for metatarsal fractures are generally good. Cakir and colleagues[2] studied 322 nonoperatively managed patients. Half had 5th metatarsal fractures. All united. High body mass index, diabetes, female gender, and wider fracture displacement were discriminators for a less good outcome.

A prospectively studied cohort of 100 patients with 5th metatarsal fractures was followed-up by Clapper and colleagues.[33] They found that nonoperative treatment of Zone 3 fractures was successful in 72% of cases. Those subsequently managed operatively all united rapidly and reported higher satisfaction with the rapid rehabilitation after surgery when compared with the prolonged period of protected weight-bearing during nonoperative treatment.

Zogby and Baker[5] achieved excellent results in 9 active patients treated in cast and then with a period of activity modification. Some patients took more than 22 weeks to unite, but previous levels of athletic activity were resumed at an average of 12 weeks.

Josefsson and colleagues[34] published the long-term results of nonoperative treatment of a series of 40 cases treated nonoperatively. At an average of 17 years (11–26 years) after *"transversal or short oblique fractures of the proximal shaft of the fifth metatarsal bone (Jones fracture)"*, there was only one patient with residual symptoms. The investigators did, however, find 7 cases of delayed union.

The same investigators published another series where a proportion of patients were treated operatively.[35] After 5 years of follow-up there were no nonunions. The investigators emphasized that late surgery was required in 12% of acute fractures and in 50% of those chronic fractures where sclerosis narrowing the medullary canal was evident.

These older case series therefore suggest that nonoperative management is, mostly, reliable. Recovery periods are, however, slow. The particular requirements of professional athletes (early return to competitive sport) are the rationale for early operative stabilization. Some investigators, such as Portland,[36] even advocate fixation of all Zone 3 fractures in both athletic and nonathletic patients.

There is only one prospective randomized controlled study of operative versus nonoperative treatment of acute fractures in Zone 3. Mologne and colleagues[37] studied, at an average of 25-month follow-up, 37 athletic patients of whom 19 were randomized to screw fixation. In this group there was one failure, whereas in the 18 patients randomized to cast immobilization there were 2 refractures, 1 delayed union, and 5 symptomatic nonunions; this made a total of 44% significant problems in the cast group.

Primary fixation should therefore be considered for fractures in Zone 3 (and maybe 2), particularly where biomechanics and/or activity levels demand. Fixation for these higher-risk patients is not a new concept.[38]

Basketball players are a particularly high-risk group for ankle and 5th metatarsal injuries. Fernandez and colleagues[39] studied 17 cases and concluded that operative treatment was more reliable than nonoperative management, with faster return to sport (within 12 weeks).

Other investigators have studied American Football players and reached a consensus that it is best to fix these fractures in athletes.[8,40] Porter and colleagues reported excellent results in 23 successive athletic patients treated with cannulated screw fixation. There were no refractures. Clinical union was 100%. Return to sport was at a mean of 7.5 weeks (10 days–12 weeks).

The abnormal loading of the lateral column of the foot seen in patients with a cavus posture means that this foot shape is prone to stress fracture and subsequent refracture. There is a strong case for early surgery in this group (see **Fig. 9**; **Fig. 10**).

Raikin and colleagues[41] reported a case series of 20 patients (21 fractures) with a cavus foot posture who were managed by early surgical fixation. Union was achieved in 100% and the surgical treatment supplemented by use of a corrective foot orthotic.

Weinfeld and colleagues[42] also emphasize that a cavus deformity, or functional supination of the foot due to for example hallux rigidus, should be identified and treated at the same time as screw fixation for 5th metatarsal stress fracture.

MANAGEMENT OF DELAYED OR NONUNION

Glasgow and colleagues[43] undertook an analysis of failure in a series of patients who had been managed surgically with either screw fixation or in-lay bone grafting for Jones fractures. The 11 cases (1 nonunion, 7 refracture, and 3 delayed union) were all considered to have been treated with undersized bone graft, insufficient reaming of the medullary cavity, too small a screw, or too rapid a return to sport.

Nonoperative management of cases of nonunion has a high failure rate.

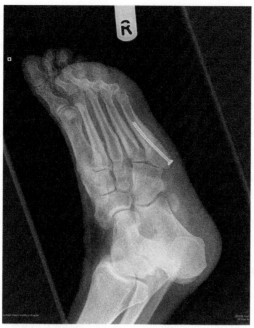

Fig. 10. Fixation of delayed union in cavus foot.

Reports in the literature pertaining to the alternative treatments of 5th metatarsal fracture nonunions are few and far between. They also tend to be at the lower end of the Levels of Evidence spectrum.

Griffin and colleagues[44] recently reviewed the evidence for ultrasound and ESWT in fracture nonunion and concluded that the existing evidence is insufficient to recommend routine use of these modalities.

Exogen: The authors have been able to find no literature pertaining specifically to the use of this modality to help with the management of 5th metatarsal fractures.

Pulsed electromagnetic field: Holmes studied 9 cases of delayed union and reported that all fractures united, at a mean of 4 months. They recommend this as a useful alternative to prolonged cast immobilization or inlay bone grafting.[45]

ESWT: Furia[46] is credited with providing good evidence that ESWT is beneficial in the treatment of nonunion of 5th metatarsal fractures. His randomized controlled trial showed fewer side effects and equal efficacy when ESWT was compared with screw fixation. Union rates were determined at 3 months.

The author's own experience with these modalities is extremely limited. The nonoperative healing adjuncts all have a low-risk profile, but are of uncertain efficacy. Furthermore, any improvement will be measured over months. Surgery is, in most cases, rewarded by rapid symptom resolution. As long as attention is paid to technical detail, the risks of surgical complication are very low. On the basis of the highly scientific "what would I want if this was my foot" test, the authors recommend surgery when functional treatment is insufficient.

SURGICAL TREATMENT

Surgery produces good results, but there remains debate about surgical technique, the need for bone graft (or other adjuncts to fixation), and the problems associated with surgical hardware.

Some of the early reports of operative intervention used bone grafting alone[47] or in combination with intramedullary curettage.[48] When fixation was deemed necessary, crossed wire fixation,[49] tension band wiring,[50] modified tension band wiring,[51] external fixation,[52] and bicortical screw fixation[53] have all been advocated. The advantages of intramedullary screw fixation have been appreciated for many years now.[38,54]

Habbu and colleagues[55] followed 14 patients for 2 years after screw fixation for nonunion. The mean time between injury and surgery was 28 weeks. Mean time to union was 13 (8–20) weeks. All patients were able to fully weight bear without pain at mean 10.2 weeks. They concluded that closed intramedullary screw fixation is an excellent treatment.

Many other investigators have reported good outcomes,[8,22,36,37,40,41,52,56–71] and recent refinements in technique focus on the type and size of screw that is required, whether hardware should be removed, and whether supplementary grafting is required.

Reports of screw breakage prompted investigation into the size and type of screw required.[59,64,65,68,72–74]

SCREW SIZE AND MATERIAL

Reese and colleagues[72] studied the fatigue strength of different screws and found that solid stainless steel screws were resistant to failure when compared with cannulated screws, which were in turn stronger than titanium screws. In the clinical part of their study, however, all fractures united irrespective of the type of screw used. They nevertheless concluded that the largest practical screw should be chosen. In a retrospective study of 53 patients, DeVries and colleagues[63] found no differences in union rates or complications when either titanium or stainless steel screws were used.

Porter and colleagues[74] compared 2 cohorts of patients. One was treated with 4.5-mm screw fixation. In the second group a 5.5-mm screw was used. There were excellent union rates in both groups, and although 3 bent screws were observed in the radiographs of patients fixed with the smaller screws, the conclusion of this study was that size does not matter. This conclusion reaffirmed the same investigators' earlier report of excellent outcomes with a 4.5-mm screw.[75]

Kelly and colleagues[65] further investigated different screw sizes in a cadaveric model. The 5th metatarsal was found to accommodate a 6.5-mm screw. Resistance to bending did not differ but the pullout strength was higher in the group fixed with the larger diameter screw. The clinical relevance of this is unclear.

Sides and colleagues[64] drew the same conclusions when experimentally comparing 6.5-mm screws with variable pitch headless compression screws.

Nunley and Glisson[60] compared a variety of screws in a biomechanical study, including their own design of solid screw with a low-profile head, which is available in a variety of sizes. The smallest screw from this Charlotte set had a bending strength exceeding that of all of the alternatives that were tested. The investigators concluded that there are advantages to the use of a purpose-designed implant that is available in a range of sizes.

Wright and colleagues[76] critically reviewed 6 instances of refracture after screw fixation. They recommend large screws for heavy sportsmen, bracing, or orthotic use on return to sport and consideration of computed tomography (CT) scanning rather than plain radiographs to determine whether the bone is united.

The authors' preference is to use a 4.5-mm cannulated screw (**Fig. 11**). They have not seen implant failure with this choice of hardware, but they do not often deal with extremely large athletes. Where there are concerns, a 6.5-mm cannulated

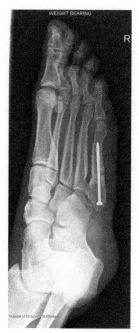

Fig. 11. Cannulated 4.5-mm screw fixation of recurrent stress fracture.

screw is the chosen implant (**Fig. 12**). Individuals with extremely high body mass and high functional demands are probably best managed with the biggest screw that will fit.

BONE GRAFT

The literature provides wide views on whether supplementary bone grafting is required. Thomas[66] found that all fractures in a small case series healed without grafting. Weinfeld and colleagues[42] advocated drilling of the fracture site at the time of intramedullary screw fixation. Tsukada and colleagues recommends grafting in all cases.[58]

The type of bone graft was investigated in a clinical study[57] comparing autogenous bone graft with demineralized bone matrix plus bone marrow aspirate. The study of 21 athletes was not sufficiently large to detect any differences between groups.

Murawski and Kennedy[77] prefer bone marrow aspirate, and when used in combination with the stainless steel solid Charlotte screw felt able to report healing at a mean of 5 weeks (no CT scan confirmation) with only one subsequent refracture in their group of 26 athletic patients.

If bone graft is preferred then it can be harvested locally and conveniently.[78] Enthusiastic arthroscopists will be interested in the paper by Lui, who describes a technique[79] that allows grafting with minimal periosteal dissection using endoscopy. Although this may be a useful method in selected cases, it seems something of a triumph for technology over reason and seems unlikely to become standard practice.

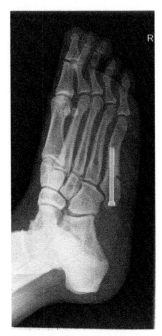

Fig. 12. Fixation for the larger patient (6.5-mm screw).

REMOVAL OF METAL

When screw insertion has been through the styloid tip, there is a significant incidence of discomfort from the hardware necessitating subsequent reoperation for screw removal. Use of a washer makes this even more likely (**Fig. 13**). The technique described by the developers of the Charlotte screw system advocates a "high and inside" entry point on the dorsomedial aspect of the base of the metatarsal.[57,60] Inspection of a dry-bone specimen reveals that this entry point permits the straight, solid screw a direct line into the medullary cavity. When cannulated screws are passed via the styloid process, there is either bending of the screw (see **Fig. 13**) or passage through the far cortex and consequent stress-riser (**Fig. 14**). Removal of metal is less frequent when the "high and inside" entry-point is used for screw fixation.

Screw head prominence may necessitate hardware removal, with further time away from sport and concern about the risk of refracture. If a screw is prominent then footwear modification may suffice,[43,54,62,76] and if surgery is required then consideration could be given to exchange for a better countersunk (or headless) screw (see **Fig. 13**).

Nagao and colleagues[80] looked at the clinical results after a headless screw was used to treat 60 athletic patients. One patient required reoperation with grafting, but the results were otherwise excellent with no hardware prominence. The authors currently have no experience using headless screws, but a reduction in the necessity for hardware removal makes this an interesting development of the technique.

SUMMARY

Fractures of the 5th metatarsal require careful evaluation and classification to ensure selection of the optimum treatment plan. Distal fractures rarely require fixation, even when displacement is wide. Fractures of the base are classified into the 3 types

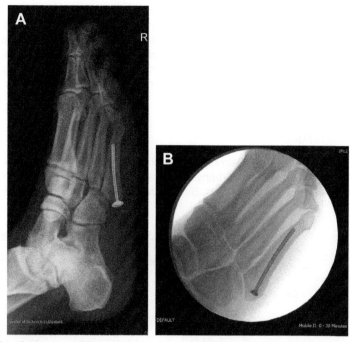

Fig. 13. (*A, B*) Fixation with screw and washer that was symptomatic. Revised rather than removed.

described by Lawrence and Botte. Type 1 fractures are best managed functionally, without cast immobilization and heal reliably. Type 2 fractures have a high union rate when managed nonoperatively but a period of cast immobilization is advised and both clinical and radiological follow-up is required. Type 3 fractures should be

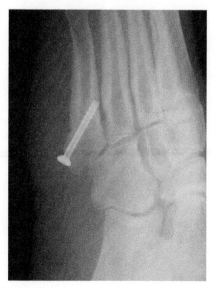

Fig. 14. Bicortical fixation.

considered for operative fixation, particularly if there is any cavus posture of the foot, neuropathy, or if the patient is a competitive sportsperson; this is because of the risk of delayed or nonunion. Cases of established nonunion or refracture require fixation. The authors do not routinely use bone graft. The screw head should be countersunk (and washers avoided) because of the risk of symptomatic metalwork. A cannulated 4.5-mm screw is our implant of choice unless the patient is very large. In such cases a 6.5-mm screw is preferred.

SURGICAL TECHNIQUE

Fig. 15 highlights the surgical technique. General or regional anesthesia is used. No tourniquet is needed. Antibiotic prophylaxis. Image intensifier control. Mark the entry point, proximal to the styloid process. Small skin incision then blunt dissection. Pass

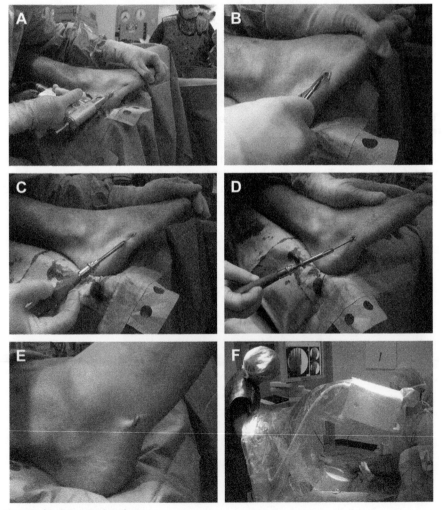

Fig. 15. (*A–I*) Surgical technique.

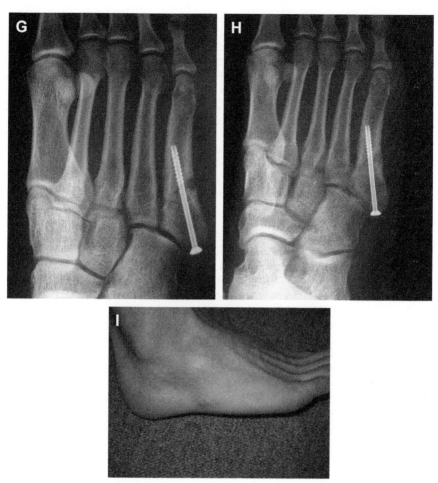

Fig. 15. (*continued*)

wire under fluoroscopic control, with images in 2 planes. Measure, drill, and counter-sink. Insert screw and confirm placement with fluoroscopy. Post-operative rehabilitation will depend on whether this is a fresh fracture, nonunion, or refracture. For the former immediate weight-bearing in a boot is allowed.

REFERENCES

1. Petrisor BA, Ekrol I, Court-Brown C. The epidemiology of metatarsal fractures. Foot Ankle Int 2006;27(3):172–4.
2. Cakir H, Van Vliet-Koppert ST, Van Lieshout EM, et al. Demographics and outcome of metatarsal fractures. Arch Orthop Trauma Surg 2011;131(2):241–5.
3. Hasselman CT, Vogt MT, Stone KL, et al. Foot and ankle fractures in elderly white women. Incidence and risk factors. J Bone Joint Surg Am 2003;85-A(5):820–4.
4. Quill GE Jr. Fractures of the proximal fifth metatarsal. Orthop Clin North Am 1995;26(2):353–61.

5. Zogby RG, Baker BE. A review of nonoperative treatment of Jones' fracture. Am J Sports Med 1987;15(4):304–7.

6. Nunley JA. Fractures of the base of the fifth metatarsal: the Jones fracture. Orthop Clin North Am 2001;32(1):171–80.

7. Lehman RC, Torg JS, Pavlov H, et al. Fractures of the base of the fifth metatarsal distal to the tuberosity: a review. Foot Ankle 1987;7(4):245–52.

8. Low K, Noblin JD, Browne JE, et al. Jones fractures in the elite football player. J Surg Orthop Adv 2004;13(3):156–60.

9. Smeets K, Jacobs P, Hertogs R, et al. Torsional injuries of the lower limb: an analysis of the frictional torque between different types of football turf and the shoe outsole. Br J Sports Med 2012;46(15):1078–83.

10. Williams S, Hume PA, Kara S. A review of football injuries on third and fourth generation artificial turfs compared with natural turf. Sports Med 2011;41(11): 903–23.

11. Egol K, Walsh M, Rosenblatt K, et al. Avulsion fractures of the fifth metatarsal base: a prospective outcome study. Foot Ankle Int 2007;28(5):581–3.

12. O'Malley MJ, Hamilton WG, Munyak J. Fractures of the distal shaft of the fifth metatarsal. "Dancer's fracture". Am J Sports Med 1996;24(2):240–3.

13. Smith TO, Clark A, Hing CB. Interventions for treating proximal fifth metatarsal fractures in adults: a meta-analysis of the current evidence-base. Foot Ankle Surg 2011;17(4):300–7.

14. Roche AJ, Calder JD. Treatment and return to sport following a Jones fracture of the fifth metatarsal: a systematic review. Knee Surg Sports Traumatol Arthrosc 2013;21(6):1307–15.

15. Lawrence SJ, Botte MJ. Jones' fractures and related fractures of the proximal fifth metatarsal. Foot Ankle 1993;14(6):358–65.

16. Zwitser EW, Breederveld RS. Fractures of the fifth metatarsal; diagnosis and treatment. Injury 2010;41(6):555–62.

17. Jones RI. Fracture of the base of the fifth metatarsal bone by indirect violence. Ann Surg 1902;35(6):697–700.2.

18. Stewart IM. Jones's fracture: fracture of base of fifth metatarsal. Clin Orthop 1960;16:190–8.

19. Dameron TB Jr. Fractures and anatomical variations of the proximal portion of the fifth metatarsal. J Bone Joint Surg Am 1975;57(6):788–92.

20. Dameron TB Jr. Fractures of the Proximal Fifth Metatarsal: Selecting the Best Treatment Option. J Am Acad Orthop Surg 1995;3(2):110–4.

21. Carp L. Fracture of the fifth metatarsal bone: with special reference to delayed union. Ann Surg 1927;86(2):308–20.

22. Polzer H, Polzer S, Mutschler W, et al. Acute fractures to the proximal fifth metatarsal bone: development of classification and treatment recommendations based on the current evidence. Injury 2012;43(10):1626–32.

23. Chuckpaiwong B, Queen RM, Easley ME, et al. Distinguishing Jones and proximal diaphyseal fractures of the fifth metatarsal. Clin Orthop Relat Res 2008; 466(8):1966–70.

24. Zenios M, Kim WY, Sampath J, et al. Functional treatment of acute metatarsal fractures: a prospective randomised comparison of management in a cast versus elasticated support bandage. Injury 2005;36(7):832–5.

25. Wiener BD, Linder JF, Giattini JF. Treatment of fractures of the fifth metatarsal: a prospective study. Foot Ankle Int 1997;18(5):267–9.

26. Vorlat P, Achtergael W, Haentjens P. Predictors of outcome of non-displaced fractures of the base of the fifth metatarsal. Int Orthop 2007;31(1):5–10.

27. Herrera-Soto JA, Scherb M, Duffy MF, et al. Fractures of the fifth metatarsal in children and adolescents. J Pediatr Orthop 2007;27(4):427–31.
28. Riccardi G, Riccardi D, Marcarelli M, et al. Extremely proximal fractures of the fifth metatarsal in the developmental age. Foot Ankle Int 2011;32(5):S526–32.
29. Kose O. Os vesalianum pedis misdiagnosed as fifth metatarsal avulsion fracture. Emerg Med Australas 2009;21(5):426.
30. Coskun N, Yuksel M, Cevener M, et al. Incidence of accessory ossicles and sesamoid bones in the feet: a radiographic study of the Turkish subjects. Surg Radiol Anat 2009;31(1):19–24.
31. Shortt CP. Magnetic resonance imaging of the midfoot and forefoot: normal variants and pitfalls. Magn Reson Imaging Clin N Am 2010;18(4):707–15.
32. Cheung J, Au-Yong I. Anatomy of the bones of the foot. BMJ 2011;343:d7830.
33. Clapper MF, O'Brien TJ, Lyons PM. Fractures of the fifth metatarsal. Analysis of a fracture registry. Clin Orthop Relat Res 1995;(315):238–41.
34. Josefsson PO, Karlsson M, Redlund-Johnell I, et al. Closed treatment of Jones fracture. Good results in 40 cases after 11-26 years. Acta Orthop Scand 1994; 65(5):545–7.
35. Josefsson PO, Karlsson M, Redlund-Johnell I, et al. Jones fracture. Surgical versus nonsurgical treatment. Clin Orthop Relat Res 1994;(299):252–5.
36. Portland G, Kelikian A, Kodros S. Acute surgical management of Jones' fractures. Foot Ankle Int 2003;24(11):829–33.
37. Mologne TS, Lundeen JM, Clapper MF, et al. Early screw fixation versus casting in the treatment of acute Jones fractures. Am J Sports Med 2005;33(7):970–5.
38. Kavanaugh JH, Brower TD, Mann RV. The Jones fracture revisited. J Bone Joint Surg Am 1978;60(6):776–82.
39. Fernandez Fairen M, Guillen J, Busto JM, et al. Fractures of the fifth metatarsal in basketball players. Knee Surg Sports Traumatol Arthrosc 1999;7(6):373–7.
40. Leumann A, Pagenstert G, Fuhr P, et al. Intramedullary screw fixation in proximal fifth-metatarsal fractures in sports: clinical and biomechanical analysis. Arch Orthop Trauma Surg 2008;128(12):1425–30.
41. Raikin SM, Slenker N, Ratigan B. The association of a varus hindfoot and fracture of the fifth metatarsal metaphyseal-diaphyseal junction: the Jones fracture. Am J Sports Med 2008;36(7):1367–72.
42. Weinfeld SB, Haddad SL, Myerson MS. Metatarsal stress fractures. Clin Sports Med 1997;16(2):319–38.
43. Glasgow MT, Naranja RJ Jr, Glasgow SG, et al. Analysis of failed surgical management of fractures of the base of the fifth metatarsal distal to the tuberosity: the Jones fracture. Foot Ankle Int 1996;17(8):449–57.
44. Griffin XL, Smith N, Parsons N, et al. Ultrasound and shockwave therapy for acute fractures in adults. Cochrane Database Syst Rev 2012;(2):CD008579.
45. Holmes GB Jr. Treatment of delayed unions and nonunions of the proximal fifth metatarsal with pulsed electromagnetic fields. Foot Ankle Int 1994;15(10): 552–6.
46. Furia JP, Juliano PJ, Wade AM, et al. Shock wave therapy compared with intramedullary screw fixation for nonunion of proximal fifth metatarsal metaphyseal-diaphyseal fractures. J Bone Joint Surg Am 2010;92(4):846–54.
47. Hens J, Martens M. Surgical treatment of Jones fractures. Arch Orthop Trauma Surg 1990;109(5):277–9.
48. Torg JS, Balduini FC, Zelko RR, et al. Fractures of the base of the fifth metatarsal distal to the tuberosity. Classification and guidelines for non-surgical and surgical management. J Bone Joint Surg Am 1984;66(2):209–14.

49. Arangio G. Transverse proximal diaphysial fracture of the fifth metatarsal: a review of 12 cases. Foot Ankle 1992;13(9):547–9.

50. Sarimo J, Rantanen J, Orava S, et al. Tension-band wiring for fractures of the fifth metatarsal located in the junction of the proximal metaphysis and diaphysis. Am J Sports Med 2006;34(3):476–80.

51. Lee KT, Park YU, Young KW, et al. Surgical results of 5th metatarsal stress fracture using modified tension band wiring. Knee Surg Sports Traumatol Arthrosc 2011;19(5):853–7.

52. Lombardi CM, Connolly FG, Silhanek AD. The use of external fixation for treatment of the acute Jones fracture: a retrospective review of 10 cases. J Foot Ankle Surg 2004;43(3):173–8.

53. Mahajan V, Chung HW, Suh JS. Fractures of the proximal fifth metatarsal: percutaneous bicortical fixation. Clin Orthop Surg 2011;3(2):140–6.

54. DeLee JC, Evans JP, Julian J. Stress fracture of the fifth metatarsal. Am J Sports Med 1983;11(5):349–53.

55. Habbu RA, Marsh RS, Anderson JG, et al. Closed intramedullary screw fixation for nonunion of fifth metatarsal Jones fracture. Foot Ankle Int 2011;32(6):603–8.

56. Rosenberg GA, Sferra JJ. Treatment strategies for acute fractures and nonunions of the proximal fifth metatarsal. J Am Acad Orthop Surg 2000;8(5):332–8.

57. Hunt KJ, Anderson RB. Treatment of Jones fracture nonunions and refractures in the elite athlete: outcomes of intramedullary screw fixation with bone grafting. Am J Sports Med 2011;39(9):1948–54.

58. Tsukada S, Ikeda H, Seki Y, et al. Intramedullary screw fixation with bone autografting to treat proximal fifth metatarsal metaphyseal-diaphyseal fracture in athletes: a case series. Sports Med Arthrosc Rehabil Ther Technol 2012;4(1):25.

59. Orr JD, Glisson RR, Nunley JA. Jones fracture fixation: a biomechanical comparison of partially threaded screws versus tapered variable pitch screws. Am J Sports Med 2012;40(3):691–8.

60. Nunley JA, Glisson RR. A new option for intramedullary fixation of Jones fractures: the Charlotte Carolina Jones Fracture System. Foot Ankle Int 2008; 29(12):1216–21.

61. Mindrebo N, Shelbourne KD, Van Meter CD, et al. Outpatient percutaneous screw fixation of the acute Jones fracture. Am J Sports Med 1993;21(5):720–3.

62. Larson CM, Almekinders LC, Taft TN, et al. Intramedullary screw fixation of Jones fractures. Analysis of failure. Am J Sports Med 2002;30(1):55–60.

63. DeVries JG, Cuttica DJ, Hyer CF. Cannulated screw fixation of Jones fifth metatarsal fractures: a comparison of titanium and stainless steel screw fixation. J Foot Ankle Surg 2011;50(2):207–12.

64. Sides SD, Fetter NL, Glisson R, et al. Bending stiffness and pull-out strength of tapered, variable pitch screws, and 6.5-mm cancellous screws in acute Jones fractures. Foot Ankle Int 2006;27(10):821–5.

65. Kelly IP, Glisson RR, Fink C, et al. Intramedullary screw fixation of Jones fractures. Foot Ankle Int 2001;22(7):585–9.

66. Thomas JL, Davis BC. Treatment of Jones fracture nonunion with isolated intramedullary screw fixation. J Foot Ankle Surg 2011;50(5):566–8.

67. Smith JW, Arnoczky SP, Hersh A. The intraosseous blood supply of the fifth metatarsal: implications for proximal fracture healing. Foot Ankle 1992;13(3): 143–52.

68. Shah SN, Knoblich GO, Lindsey DP, et al. Intramedullary screw fixation of proximal fifth metatarsal fractures: a biomechanical study. Foot Ankle Int 2001;22(7): 581–4.

69. Sammarco GJ. The Jones fracture. Instr Course Lect 1993;42:201–5.
70. McBryde AM Jr. The complicated Jones fracture, including revision and malalignment. Foot Ankle Clin 2009;14(2):151–68.
71. Fetzer GB, Wright RW. Metatarsal shaft fractures and fractures of the proximal fifth metatarsal. Clin Sports Med 2006;25(1):139–50, x.
72. Reese K, Litsky A, Kaeding C, et al. Cannulated screw fixation of Jones fractures: a clinical and biomechanical study. Am J Sports Med 2004;32(7): 1736–42.
73. Pietropaoli MP, Wnorowski DC, Werner FW, et al. Intramedullary screw fixation of Jones fractures: a biomechanical study. Foot Ankle Int 1999;20(9):560–3.
74. Porter DA, Rund AM, Dobslaw R, et al. Comparison of 4.5- and 5.5-mm cannulated stainless steel screws for fifth metatarsal Jones fracture fixation. Foot Ankle Int 2009;30(1):27–33.
75. Porter DA, Duncan M, Meyer SJ. Fifth metatarsal Jones fracture fixation with a 4.5-mm cannulated stainless steel screw in the competitive and recreational athlete: a clinical and radiographic evaluation. Am J Sports Med 2005;33(5): 726–33.
76. Wright RW, Fischer DA, Shively RA, et al. Refracture of proximal fifth metatarsal (Jones) fracture after intramedullary screw fixation in athletes. Am J Sports Med 2000;28(5):732–6.
77. Murawski CD, Kennedy JG. Percutaneous internal fixation of proximal fifth metatarsal jones fractures (Zones II and III) with Charlotte Carolina screw and bone marrow aspirate concentrate: an outcome study in athletes. Am J Sports Med 2011;39(6):1295–301.
78. Lawrence SJ. Technique tip: local bone grafting technique for Jones fracture management with intramedullary screw fixation. Foot Ankle Int 2004;25(12): 920–1.
79. Lui TH. Endoscopic bone grafting for management of nonunion of the tuberosity avulsion fracture of the fifth metatarsal. Arch Orthop Trauma Surg 2008;128(11): 1305–7.
80. Nagao M, Saita Y, Kameda S, et al. Headless compression screw fixation of jones fractures: an outcomes study in Japanese athletes. Am J Sports Med 2012;40(11):2578–82.

The Treatment of Calcaneal Malunion

Prof. Roger M. Atkins, MA (Oxon), MB BS (London), DM (Oxon), FRCS (England)

KEYWORDS

- Calcaneal malunion • Bone block distraction arthrodesis • Subtalar fusion
- Chevron osteotomy • Foot biomechanics

KEY POINTS

- Do not undertake an isolated subtalar fusion in the presence of abnormal foot anatomy and biomechanics.
- Do not simply excise the lateral impinging bone in the presence of dynamic lateral impingement. In addition, correct the abnormal anatomy by a calcaneal osteotomy.
- Warn the patient of the risk of amputation.
- The extended lateral approach is a dissection of the posterior peroneal angiosome; it is a very radical exposure.
- It is better to have an incomplete correction than to close the incision under tension.
- The bone-block distraction arthrodesis only corrects talar rotation; it does not require a bone distractor.

INTRODUCTION

Calcaneal fractures continue to present a therapeutic challenge and, although operative fixation has become standardized and has its champions,[1–5] many thoughtful surgeons are unconvinced of its efficacy,[6,7] and some injuries are considered to be so severe as to defy primary surgical treatment. Therefore a significant number of calcaneal fractures will continue to be treated conservatively for the foreseeable future, and the surgical treatment of calcaneal malunion will continue to be necessary.

It is important to realize that the surgery of calcaneal malunion is very difficult and should not be performed by the occasional surgeon. The price of error is usually amputation.

A key issue in determining whether a reconstruction should be undertaken is whether an associated alteration of hindfoot biomechanics is compromising the Chopart joint and the ankle joint (**Fig. 1**). If this is the case, over time these joints will fail and the outcome of reconstruction will become progressively worse.

Disclosures: None.
Department of Orthopaedic Surgery, Bristol Royal Infirmary, Marlborough Street, Bristol BS2 8HW, England
E-mail address: roger.atkins@sneydwood.co.uk

Foot Ankle Clin N Am 19 (2014) 521–540
http://dx.doi.org/10.1016/j.fcl.2014.06.016
1083-7515/14/$ – see front matter © 2014 Elsevier Inc. All rights reserved.

foot.theclinics.com

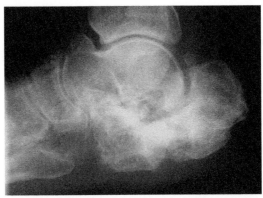

Fig. 1. Altered hindfoot biomechanics resulting from a calcaneal malunion. The ankle and talonavicular joints are compromised owing to dorsal rotation of the talus, and secondary changes are occurring.

PATIENT ASSESSMENT

The assessment and treatment of disability is made difficult by the many sources of symptoms, which cause overlapping syndromes. Patients will complain of pain, limitation of walking ability, and derangement of their lifestyle. A careful, detailed clinical assessment backed by extensive radiologic investigation will usually reveal one or more of the following problems.

Subtalar Joint Derangement

Subtalar joint derangement can be either angular (**Fig. 2**) or, less commonly, the result of subtalar joint depression (**Fig. 3**).[8] Angular malalignment causes pain on walking, particularly on uneven ground, with late rest pain.

Subtalar joint depression causes a sense of insecurity on taking a step, followed by a feeling that the foot has given way and severe pain. There is usually lateral impingement with a late valgus hindfoot.

It is important not to undertake an isolated subtalar fusion in patients who have a calcaneal malunion and associated abnormal hindfoot biomechanics, as this may worsen their condition by destroying one of their compensatory mechanisms.

Heel Boss

Heel boss is usually the late result of a conservatively treated tuberosity fracture (**Fig. 4**).[9] The patient has difficulty in shoe wear and a weak calf, but the biomechanics of the foot are unaltered and the condition does not deteriorate.

Lateral Impingement

Lateral impingement can be either static, owing to laterally displaced bone fragments (see **Fig. 12**) or dynamic, resulting from lateral displacement of the body of the calcaneus (see **Fig. 13**). Most cases of dynamic lateral impingement also have static impingement caused by lateral shards of bone, and it is important not to simply resect the lateral impinging bone in these cases because this will simply make the problem worse as the laterally disposed calcaneus sinks into the space left by the resected bone.

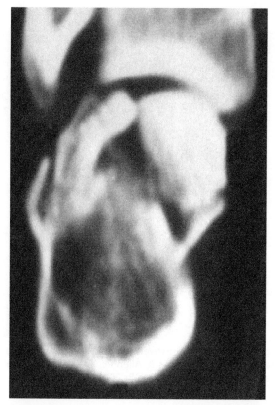

Fig. 2. Semi-coronal computed tomography (CT) scan showing angular displacement of the subtalar joint.

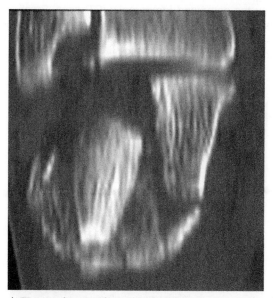

Fig. 3. Semi-coronal CT scan showing lateral joint fragment depression in a severely displaced calcaneal fracture. This condition causes more symptoms than simple angular displacement, even when it is severe as in **Fig. 2**.

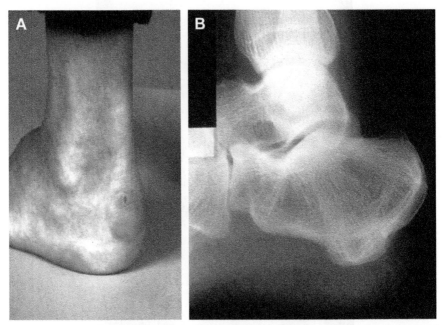

Fig. 4. (A) A heel boss caused by conservatively treated tuberosity fracture. (B) Radiographic appearance of a heel boss. (*From* Squires B, Allen PE, Livingstone J, et al. Fractures of the tuberosity of the calcaneus. J Bone Joint Surg Br 2001;83-B:55–61.)

Plain radiographs are very poor indicators of the severity of lateral impingement. The patient shown in **Fig. 12** was barely able to walk. The full extent of the lateral impingement is revealed by the computed tomography (CT) scan. Small amounts of lateral impinging bone can cause severe disability if they compromise the peroneal tendons.

The surgery for lateral impingement is straightforward, but it is important not to delay it because this can lead to subtalar and ankle joint arthritis with peroneal tendon dislocation.

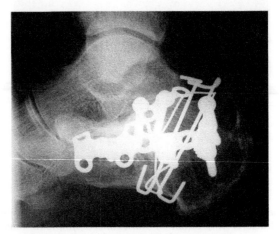

Fig. 5. Prominent metal work should be removed if symptomatic.

Peroneal Tendon Dislocation

Peroneal tendon dislocation is the late result of severe lateral impingement (see **Figs. 15** and **16**), and may occur de novo after reconstruction.

Bone in the Sole of the Foot

This condition is excruciatingly painful, and the pain usually worsens inexorably with time (see **Fig. 18**). There is little point in simply resecting the protuberant bone; a full reconstruction is needed.

In severe cases all of the aforementioned problems occur together, which produces an ascending ladder of surgery for a "standard" calcaneal malunion.

CONSERVATIVE TREATMENT OF CALCANEAL MALUNION

Provided the biomechanics of the foot are not severely deranged, a trial of conservative treatment with wide-fitting shoes, stout soles, and orthotics may minimize symptoms. However, when there is severe derangement of the foot, problems progress and secondary changes occur in other joints and the soft tissues. In these cases, there is rarely any point in temporizing.

SURGICAL TREATMENT
Patient Assessment

This treatment involves major surgery. The patient must understand that if the wound breaks down, the salvage will probably require a free flap, and there is a real risk of amputation, usually for reasons of deep infection. The bone-graft donor site may cause morbidity, and the patient will be non–weight bearing and in plaster for some time.

The results of reconstruction are reasonable but by no means perfect.[10]

The vascular status of the foot must be excellent, and the patient should stop smoking.

Careful clinical examination includes testing for dynamic lateral impingement.

Radiographic assessment includes plain radiographs and CT scanning in sagittal, axial, and semi-coronal planes. Many surgeons find 3-dimensional (3D) reconstructions helpful.

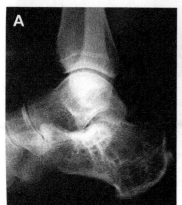 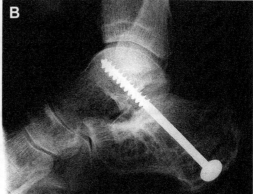

Fig. 6. (*A*) This patient continued to have pain after removal of metalwork. There is sclerosis of the calcaneus below the subtalar joint and marginal loss of calcaneal height, which compromises the talonavicular joint. (*B*) After fusion using a bone block to restore calcaneal height and bypass the sclerotic bone in the calcaneus. In today's practice, no washer would have been used.

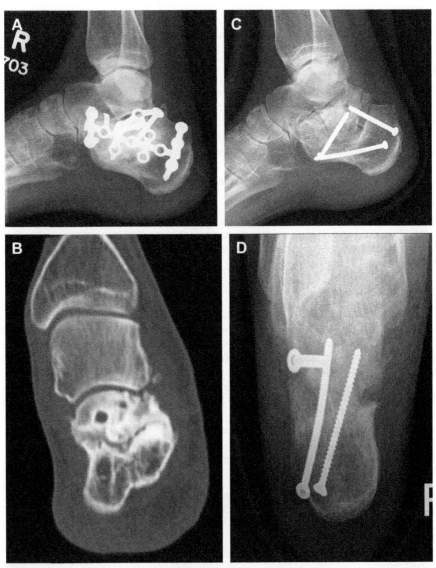

Fig. 7. (*A*) A severe calcaneal fracture in which healing has been accompanied by loss of height and subluxation of the talonavicular joint. (*B*) Semi-coronal CT scan after metalwork removal showing the well-preserved subtalar joint, which had been confirmed at the time of metalwork removal. (*C*) Lateral radiograph showing the central elevation osteotomy. At 6 weeks after surgery, the anterior osteotomy is almost united and the inferior bone block is incorporating well. Calcaneal height has been restored. The lower screw is prophylactic to prevent fracture of the inferior part of the calcaneus during the surgery. (*D*) Axial radiograph showing screw position and incorporation of the posterior bone block.

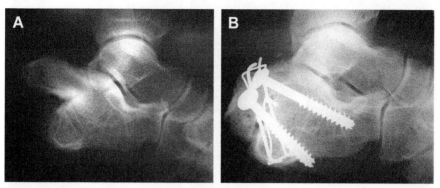

Fig. 8. (*A*) A severe heel boss in a conservatively treated tuberosity fracture. (*B*) The case shown in Fig. 8A after a triangular excision osteotomy and reconstruction.

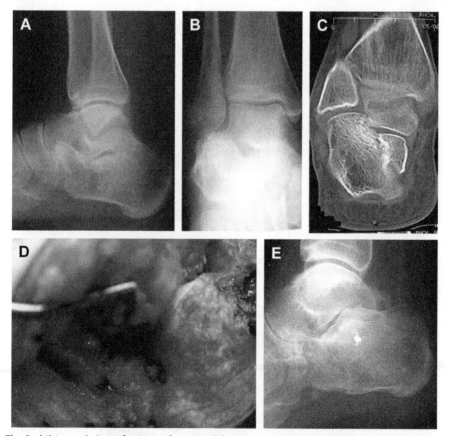

Fig. 9. (*A*) Lateral view of a 2-part fracture dislocation showing the characteristic lateral part of the calcaneus abutted against the fibula, 6 months after injury. (*B*) The abnormal position of the calcaneal body is confirmed on the lateral view. (*C*) A CT scan confirms the derangement. (*D*) At surgery, normal cartilage is confirmed on the lateral facet. This appearance indicates that a reconstruction of the subtalar joint rather than a fusion may be undertaken. (*E*) Two-year follow-up. The subtalar joint is narrowed but functional.

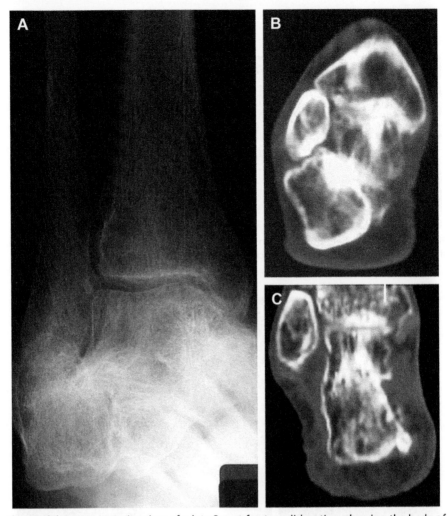

Fig. 10. (*A*) Anteroposterior view of a late 2-part fracture dislocation, showing the body of the calcaneus below the fibula. The body of the calcaneus is fused to the lateral part of the talus. Note the subluxation of the ankle joint. (*B*) Semi-coronal CT scan showing the body of the calcaneus eroding the fibula. (*C*) After reconstructive fusion. Normal hindfoot anatomy has been restored.

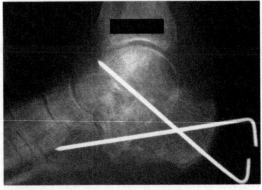

Fig. 11. Two-part fracture dislocation reconstructed with a subtalar fusion in a 77-year-old woman. Note the deliberate sacrifice of calcaneal length.

Bone Graft

A mainstay of calcaneal malunion reconstruction is the insertion of tricortical ileac crest bone blocks into the hindfoot to replace lost bone. The ileac crest defect is covered with a third tubular plate, usually fixed with a single small fragment cancellous screw at each end, and the muscles reconstructed over it.

Surgical Positioning

The patient is invariably placed in the lateral position, and a tourniquet is deployed.

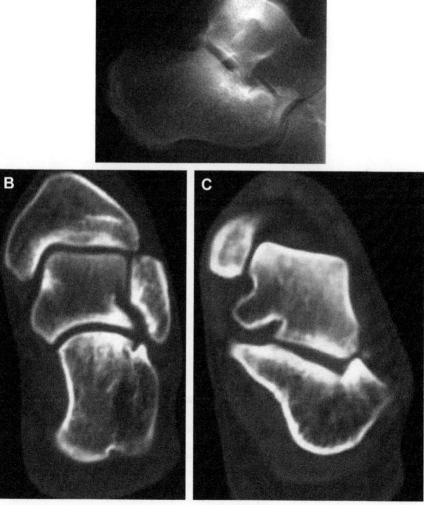

Fig. 12. (*A*) Lateral radiograph of a patient with severe lateral impingement pain. (*B*) Semi-coronal CT scan showing the lateral bone impinging on the fibula. (*C*) Semi-coronal CT scan showing the lateral bone impinging on and subluxing the subtalar joint.

Incision

The extended lateral approach[11] is used, which is a dissection of the cutaneous angiosome of the posterior peroneal nerve. A simple vertical incision does not allow sufficient exposure to access the entire surgical region. Closure is in 3 layers, the deepest layer being the periosteum, which is carefully dissected during the approach and is sutured to the fascia over abductor digiti minimi. This action keeps tension away from the skin closure and minimizes wound problems.

It is uncommon to be unable to close the wound if surgery is directed at restoring hindfoot anatomy and biomechanics, but occasionally this does occur. Under these circumstances it is important not to put tension on the wound. The reconstruction has to be taken down and a more modest correction obtained. Patients are warned preoperatively of the possibility that the reconstruction may be staged.

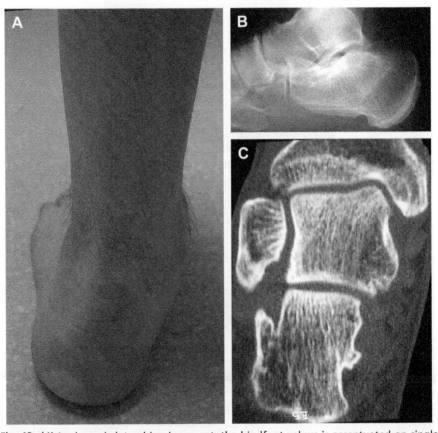

Fig. 13. (A) In dynamic lateral impingement, the hindfoot valgus is accentuated on single stance. (B) Lateral radiograph shows filling in of the crucial angle of Gissane by impinging bone. (C) Semi-coronal CT scan shows the lateral impinging piece of bone. (D) Axial CT scan shows lateral displacement of the body fragment. (E) Detail of surgery. Medial displacement chevron osteotomy has been undertaken, revealing the amount of lateral bone to be removed. (F) The chevron osteotomy is fixed with a single screw. The subtalar joint has "opened up" because the impinging bone has been removed. Note that nowadays a 6.5-mm noncannulated screw without a washer is used.

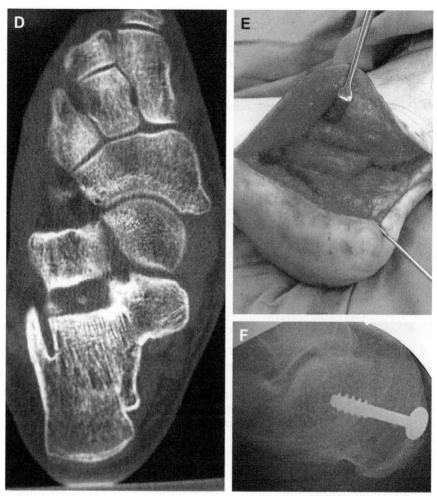

Fig. 13. (*continued*)

Suction drainage is usually used, as surgical hematoma is a severe complication. Occasionally excessive drainage requires it to be clamped for a period following surgery.

Postoperative Management

Wound healing is paramount. Elevation for 24 hours is usual, followed by application of a below-knee cast. The patient mobilizes non–weight bearing until the wound is healed and until bone healing is sufficiently advanced to allow load bearing. The plaster is maintained until bone healing is secure.

SPECIFIC SURGERIES FOLLOWING INTERNAL FIXATION
Removal of Metalwork

The metalwork is often prominent (**Fig. 5**), and removal often minimizes symptoms so that formal reconstruction is not necessary. This procedure is significantly less intrusive for the patient than a reconstruction.

Subtalar Fusion

Arthritis of the subtalar joint is often associated with some loss of calcaneal height, which compromises Chopart joint function because of talar rotation. Simple excisional subtalar joint fusion worsens this problem. In addition, there is often severe sclerosis of the calcaneus beneath the subtalar joint so that nonunion may be a problem (see **Fig. 7**). Under these circumstances, a bone-block subtalar fusion should be used to restore calcaneal height and bypass the sclerotic bone (**Fig. 6**).

Central Elevation Calcaneal Osteotomy

In patients with severe calcaneal fractures, there is often some loss of calcaneal height after internal fixation (**Fig. 7**). If the subtalar joint is in good condition, it can be preserved by elevation of the central part of the calcaneus, which is achieved by making 3 osteotomies around the subtalar joint. Anteriorly the osteotomy passes into the sinus tarsi and exits anterior to the sustentaculum. Centrally the osteotomy is horizontal beneath the sustentaculum, and posteriorly it is vertical behind the subtalar joint. These osteotomies are joined, and the central part of the calcaneus including the subtalar joint is elevated. Care must be taken not to fracture the inferior part of the calcaneus. Prophylactic screws may be used to help prevent this. Two bone blocks are placed, one inferiorly and one posteriorly.

SPECIFIC SURGERIES FOR CONSERVATIVELY TREATED FRACTURES
Heel Bossing Following a Tuberosity Fracture

At a preliminary surgery, a gastrocnemius and soleal fascial release is undertaken because the heel cord will be tight; this is followed by vigorous physiotherapy to restore full dorsiflexion.

The definitive surgery is a triangular excision osteotomy (**Fig. 8**). Key steps are the use of pelvic reduction forceps to reduce the fragments after the wedge of bone has been excised, and ensuring that the skin of the heel does not become caught up in the osteotomy closure.

Fixation of the reduced tuberosity fragment is difficult. **Fig. 8**B shows a combination of a lateral tension band and cannulated screws.

Two-Part Fracture Dislocation

If treated conservatively, these rare fractures fare very poorly.[12] Reconstruction within a year may permit retention of the subtalar joint (**Fig. 9**). Surgical dissection

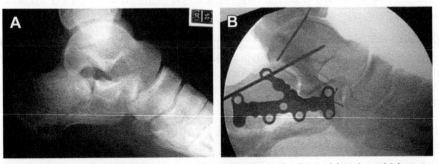

Fig. 14. (A) A calcaneal fracture is accompanied by loss of calcaneal height, which causes dorsal rotation of the talus and subluxation of the talonavicular joint. (B) Fracture reduction normalizes talar rotation and releases the Chopart joint.

is carried over the superior border of the calcaneus behind the ankle joint, and the primary fracture line is recreated using an osteotome.[13] This surgery is difficult, and great care is needed to avoid damage to medial structures. The lateral dislocated subtalar joint is then slowly eased back into place and stabilized, usually with screws placed transversely from the lateral side into the medial fragment and sustentaculum.

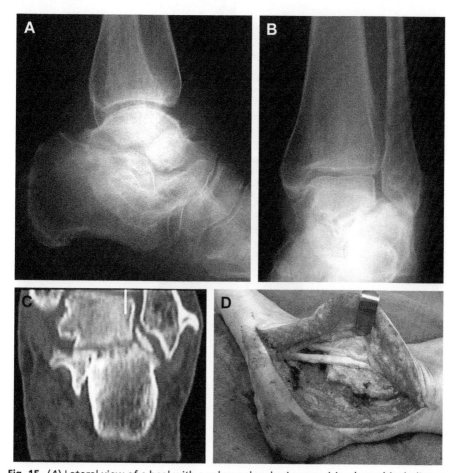

Fig. 15. (*A*) Lateral view of a heel with a calcaneal malunion requiring bone-block distraction arthrodesis. Note the dorsal rotation of the talus with secondary changes in the talonavicular joint. (*B*) Anteroposterior radiograph shows severe lateral impingement. (*C*) Semi-coronal CT scan showing severe lateral impingement, subtalar arthritis, and the peroneal tendons dislocated laterally. (*D*) Surgical detail. The extended lateral approach has been used to explore the peroneal tendons. (*E*) Bone-block distraction arthrodesis. A laminar spreader is placed between the calcaneus and talus, and opened until the required calcaneal height is restored and talar rotation is correct. (*F*) Postoperative radiograph. Note restoration of talar rotation and Chopart joint anatomy. Fixation in this case was with a single Kirschner wire. The suture anchor is part of the peroneal tendon reconstruction. (*G*) Anteroposterior view postoperatively shows the removal of lateral impingement.

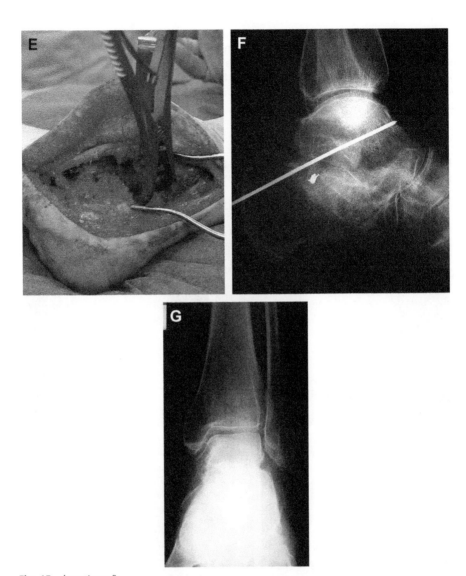

Fig. 15. (*continued*)

At a later time, the subtalar joint ceases to be salvageable and a reconstructive fusion is necessary. Surgery proceeds as for the reconstruction, but the reduced subtalar joint is fused (**Fig. 10**).

Many of these patients are elderly, but fit patients in their 70s benefit from reconstruction. In these patients calcaneal length is sacrificed to minimize the surgical insult (**Fig. 11**).

THE LADDER OF RECONSTRUCTIVE SURGERY FOR A "STANDARD" CALCANEAL MALUNION
Static Lateral Impingement

Simple resection of the protuberant bone is usually curative (**Fig. 12**). The inferior peroneal process is often osteotomized, and may require reconstruction with a suture anchor.

Dynamic Lateral Impingement

Resection of the protruding bone is accompanied by a medial displacement osteotomy to restore the hindfoot alignment (**Fig. 13**). The importance of not using simple resection of lateral protruding bone in these cases is detailed in the foregoing explanation.

Subtalar Fusion with Intra-Articular Bone-Block Placement

The bone-block distraction arthrodesis was first described by the Seattle group.[14] Although this fusion is a cornerstone of calcaneal malunion reconstruction, the name is misleading.

A calcaneal fracture is associated with loss of calcaneal height, which causes dorsal rotation of the talus and subluxation of the talonavicular joint, leading to loss of Chopart joint movement (**Fig. 14**A).

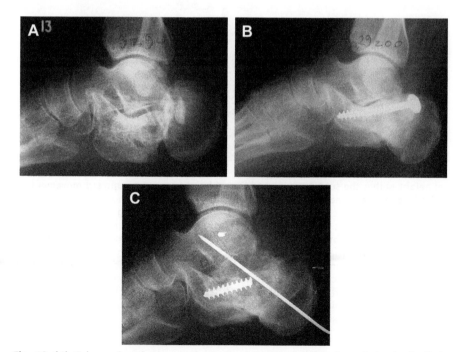

Fig. 16. (A) Calcaneal malunion with obviously upward migration of the body if the calcaneus. (B) The position after reversing the upward migration. Talar rotation has not been corrected. (C) A bone-block distraction arthrodesis then corrects talar rotation.

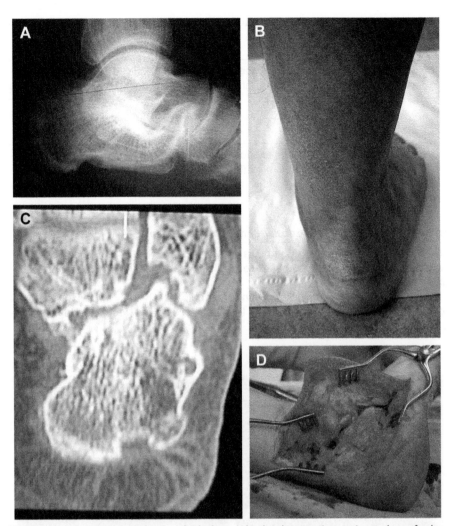

Fig. 17. (*A*) Calcaneal malunion in which there is both talar rotation owing to loss of calcaneal height within the subtalar joint and loss of height caused by upward movement of the body of the calcaneus behind the talus. (*B*) Single stance shows dynamic lateral impingement. (*C*) Semi-coronal CT scan shows severe lateral impinging bone with dislocated peroneal tendons. (*D*) Operative detail showing severe abutment of the lateral calcaneus against the fibula and dislocated peroneal tendons. (*E*) Finding and distracting the subtalar joint after lateral wall resection. (*F*) Dissection of the peroneal tendons. (*G*) Placing an intra-articular bone block (bone-block distraction arthrodesis). (*H*) Placing an extra-articular bone block into the chevron osteotomy that has been displaced medially to treat the dynamic lateral impingement. (*I*) The peroneal tendons are reconstructed into a groove fashioned in the posterior aspect of the fibula. (*J*) Postoperative radiograph showing restoration of anatomy.

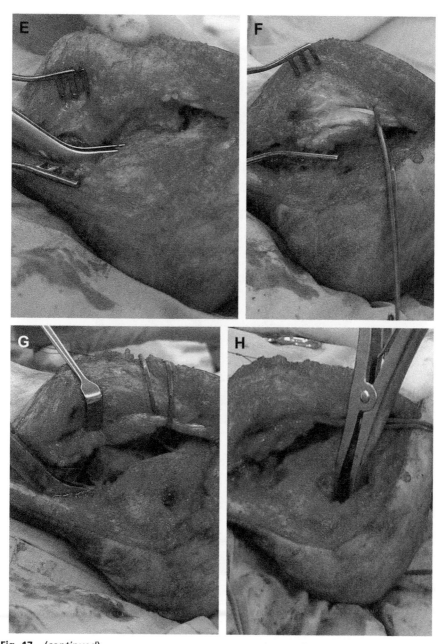

Fig. 17. (*continued*)

Reduction and fixation of the fracture corrects the abnormal talar rotation and releases the Chopart joint (see **Fig. 14**B).

The aim of a bone-block distraction arthrodesis (**Fig. 15**) is to correct the abnormal rotation of the talus and to fuse the subtalar joint. The surgery must be

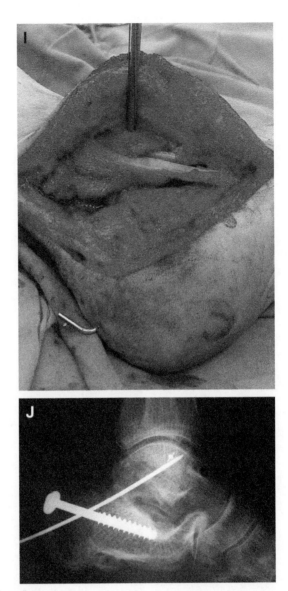

Fig. 17. (*continued*)

performed by placing a laminar spreader between the calcaneus and talus (see **Fig. 15**D), and an external distractor must not be used because it will prevent wound closure.

Surgery is undertaken using the standard extended lateral approach, and the entire lateral wall of the calcaneus is exposed to remove lateral impinging bone (see **Fig. 15**C).

Exposure of the subtalar joint in calcaneal malunion is very difficult. It should be found posteriorly, and it is all too easy to enter the ankle joint. It is helpful to remember that the subtalar joint passes inferiorly when entered posteriorly, and the ankle joint passes superiorly. If in doubt, use an image intensifier. Once entered, the subtalar joint is gradually released until a laminar spreader can be introduced, and the gentle process of derotating the talus begins.

The joint is then debrided, and on the calcaneal side this may be radical so as to expose bleeding bone of good quality. The joint is overdistracted with the laminar spreader, and an appropriately sized tricortical bone block introduced. It is stabilized with either stout Kirschner wires or screws.

Extra-Articular Bone-Block Placement

Calcaneal height may be lost outside the subtalar joint (**Fig. 16**), and this must be corrected by extra-articular bone-block placement. If the extra-articular height loss is corrected by intra-articular bone-block placement by overcorrecting talar rotation, movement of the Chopart joint is blocked.

Fig. 16 shows a case whereby initially it was not appreciated that there was loss of calcaneal height at the subtalar joint, and an attempt was made to restore hindfoot anatomy using only an extra-articular reconstruction.

The amount of calcaneal height to be restored is judged by reference to the opposite side using lateral radiographs.

The sequence of events is as described heretofore, but after the subtalar joint has been entered, debrided, and distracted, an extra-articular calcaneal chevron osteotomy is made and displaced to deal with any misalignment in the sagittal plane (**Fig. 17**). The inferior limb of the osteotomy is then distracted and the measured bone block placed. This technique can also be used to lengthen the calcaneus if indicated.

Bone in the Sole of the Foot

This condition is treated by a full reconstruction of the anatomy of the hindfoot as indicated (**Fig. 18**). At the end of the surgery, the inferior border of the calcaneus is explored through the lower part of the extended lateral approach and the displaced bone removed. It is better to avoid an incision on the sole of the foot because this causes considerable morbidity, and excising the bone through this approach is tedious.

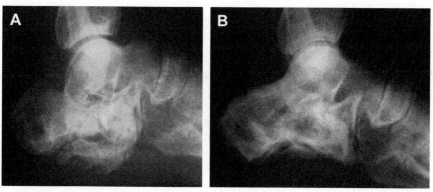

Fig. 18. (*A*) Calcaneal malunion with bone in the sole of the foot. (*B*) After reconstruction and removal of the bone.

SUMMARY

The surgical treatment of calcaneal malunion is technically very demanding and requires a careful assessment of the exact cause of the problem. The results are reasonable, and justify surgery in an otherwise disabled group of patients.[15,16]

REFERENCES

1. Eastwood DM, Langkamer VG, Atkins RM. Calcaneal fractures: an approach for open reduction and internal fixation. J Bone Joint Surg Br 1993;75:189–96.
2. Sanders R, Fortin P, Dipasquale T, et al. Operative treatment in 120 displaced intra-articular fractures of the calcaneus. Results using a prognostic computed tomography classification. Clin Orthop Relat Res 1993;(290):87–95.
3. Sanders R. Current concepts review: displaced intra-articular fractures of the calcaneus. J Bone Joint Surg Am 2000;82:225–50.
4. Zeman P, Zeman J, Matejka J, et al. Long-term results of calcaneal fracture treatment by open reduction and internal fixation using a calcaneal locking compression plate from an extended lateral approach. Acta Chir Orthop Traumatol Cech 2008;75(6):457–64.
5. Zwipp H, Tscherne H, Thermann H, et al. Osteosynthesis of displaced intraarticular fractures of the calcaneus results in 123 cases. Clin Orthop Relat Res 1993;(290):76–86.
6. Buckley R, Tough S, McCormack R, et al. Operative compared with nonoperative treatment of displaced intra-articular calcaneal fractures. J Bone Joint Surg Am 2002;84(10):1733–44.
7. Ibrahim T, Rowsell M, Rennie W, et al. Displaced intra-articular calcaneal fractures: 15-year follow-up of a randomised controlled trial of conservative versus operative treatment. Injury 2007;38(7):848–55.
8. Eastwood DM, Gregg P, Atkins RM. Calcaneal fractures: pathological anatomy and classification. J Bone Joint Surg Br 1993;75:183–9.
9. Squires B, Allen PE, Livingstone J, et al. Fractures of the tuberosity of the calcaneus. J Bone Joint Surg Br 2001;83:55–61.
10. Radnay CS, Clare MP, Sanders RW. Subtalar fusion after displaced intra-articular calcaneal fractures: does initial operative treatment matter? J Bone Joint Surg Am 2009;91(3):541–6.
11. Freeman BJ, Duff S, Allen PE, et al. The extended lateral approach to the hindfoot. The anatomical basis and surgical implications. J Bone Joint Surg Br 1998;80:139–42.
12. Eastwood DM, Maxwell-Armstrong CA, Atkins RM. Fracture of the lateral malleolus with talar tilt. Primarily a calcaneal fracture not an ankle injury. Injury 1993;24:109–12.
13. Romash MM. Reconstructive osteotomy of the calcaneus with subtalar arthrodesis for malunited calcaneal fractures. Clin Orthop Relat Res 1993;(290):157–67.
14. Carr JB, Hansen ST, Benirschke SK. Subtalar distraction bone block fusion for late complications of os calcis fractures. Foot Ankle 1988;9:81–6.
15. Banerjee R, Saltzman C, Anderson RB, et al. Management of calcaneal malunion. J Am Acad Orthop Surg 2011;19(1):27–36.
16. Clare MP, Lee WE, Sanders RJ. Intermediate to long-term results of a treatment protocol for calcaneal fracture malunions. J Bone Joint Surg Am 2005;87(5):963–73.

Ongoing Pain and Deformity After an Excision of the Accessory Navicular

Philip Vaughan, MBBS, FRCS (Tr & Orth), Dishan Singh, MBChB, FRCS (Orth)*

KEYWORDS

- Accessory navicula • Pes planus • Kidner procedure • Ongoing pain • Deformity

KEY POINTS

- Although a painful accessory navicula and a pes planus often coexist, they are not necessarily causally related, and each condition should be assessed and treated individually.
- A child or adolescent will notice the rubbing of an accessory navicula against footwear as the foot and boney swelling grows.
- Two-thirds will not have a flat foot and a simple excision of the accessory navicula will suffice if conservative measures fail. One-third will also have a flat foot; the popular Kidner procedure does not reconstitute the medial longitudinal arch but gives equally good results as a simple excision for local pain relief.
- If the patient has a concurrent or persistent flat foot, the flat foot deformity should be addressed on its own merit by means of stretching of the gastrocnemius/soleus tightness and appropriate flat foot corrective surgery. The cause of persistent local pain such as inadequate bony resection, scar pain, irritation of the tibialis posterior tendon, and so forth should be sought and addressed; management will depend on the specific presentation and previous procedure performed.
- An adult presenting with a painful accessory navicula will have had a boney prominence since adolescence; management should focus on the reason as to why the pain has developed.
- Generalized or localized hypermobility may cause flattening of the medial longitudinal arch and increased boney prominence.
- A history of trauma suggests a separation of the synchondrosis. Increasing tightness of the gastrocnemius/Achilles may make overpronation worse. The pain may not be due to the bone but due to an insertional tibialis posterior tendinopathy.
- The cause of the ongoing pain should be investigated, and the features of the adult flat foot may also need treatment.

Foot and Ankle Department, Royal National Orthopaedic Hospital, Brockley Hill, Stanmore, Middlesex, UK
* Corresponding author.
E-mail address: dishansingh@aol.com

Foot Ankle Clin N Am 19 (2014) 541–553
http://dx.doi.org/10.1016/j.fcl.2014.06.010
foot.theclinics.com

INTRODUCTION

In the management of a symptomatic accessory navicula, it is important to appreciate the individual subtypes of this developmental anomaly and, once conservative methods are rendered refractory, the surgeon can guide his/her intervention based on the pathomechanics of the medial foot pain. Although a painful accessory navicula and a flattened medial longitudinal arch often coexist, they are not necessarily causally related, and each pathologic condition should be assessed and treated individually on its own merit. When complications arise, the pathomechanics should be re-evaluated and addressed accordingly.

ANATOMY AND DEVELOPMENT OF THE FOOT AND ITS MEDIAL ARCH

In the 5th and 6th gestational weeks, the bones of the foot start their development with mesenchymal differentiation into cartilage. By the 7th week this proximal to distal sequence produces an arrangement akin to that of the adult foot. Subsequent ossification into bone is mostly completed before birth—with the navicula being the last bone to ossify, often as late as the age of 5 years. Maturation and development of the shape and architecture of the foot starts within this fetal period continuing through early childhood into adolescence, the final shape and function being influenced by both intrinsic and extrinsic factors.

The foot grows faster than the rest of the body, achieving three-quarters of its mature length by the time the child is 7 years old. A toddler's foot does not have any evidence of a medial arch but the growing foot develops a medial longitudinal arch as it matures: by 6 or 7 years old, most children have also developed their adult medial arch, whereas some take until age 10 or 11 years to complete development.[1]

The medial longitudinal arch of the foot comprises of the calcaneus, talus, navicula, the 3 cuneiforms, and the medial 3 metatarsals. The apex or keystone of this arch is the talar head that is supported by the inferior calcaneonavicular or "spring" ligament and the tendons of tibialis posterior and flexor hallucis longus. The integrity of the arch depends on these boney, ligamentous, and muscular structures alongside an intact sustentaculum tali, deltoid ligament, and a noncontracted Achilles tendon.[2]

The navicular bone (os naviculare pedis or tarsal scaphoid bone) is interposed in the medial arch between the head of the talus and the 3 cuneiforms. The anterior surface is convex and is divided, by 2 ridges, into 3 facets for the cuneiform bones. The posterior surface is concave and articulates with the rounded head of the talus forming the medial aspect of the midtarsal or Chopart joint.

The function of the tibialis posterior tendon is influenced by its tendonous insertions on the plantar medial aspect of the foot, allowing it to control the degree of pronation and act as the principal inverter of the foot. Proximal to the navicula tuberosity, the tendon usually divides into superficial and deep components. The more superficial component is the longer and is attached medially to the navicula with some fibers to the inferior surface of the medial cuneiform.[3] The deeper component passes more laterally to insert on the intermediate cuneiform and the bases of the second, third, and fourth metatarsals,[3] although insertions into the cuboid and lateral cuneiform bones, have also been described.[4]

The tibialis posterior tendon is active in the third rocker stage of gait to invert the hindfoot and convert the foot into a rigid lever on which the Achilles tendon can plantarflex the ankle. This activity is demonstrated in the supple flat foot associated with a symptomatic accessory navicula. In the second rocker, the tibialis posterior tendon acts in a closed chain kinetics to control overpronation, at a time when the ligamentous restraints are also active.

The navicular bone is a common location for an accessory bone, usually referred to as the accessory navicula but also known as the os naviculare, os tibiale externum, naviculare secundarium, bifurcated hallux, or pre-hallux. This developmental anomaly is found in approximately 1 in 8 (10%–21%) normal feet[3,5] and is bilateral[6] in most cases (50%–89%). It is inherited in an autosomal dominant trait with incomplete penetrance and through this Mendelian inheritance pattern is thought to have a single responsible gene defect.[7] However, the presence of a different subtype on either foot in a patient with bilateral accessory navicula has been reported,[8] highlighting the phenotype of this anomaly.

CLASSIFICATION AND MECHANICS OF THE ACCESSORY NAVICULA

There are 2 broad types of accessory naviculae, depending on the relationship between the primary and secondary ossification centers of the navicula.[5,8,9] The secondary ossification center can form an ossicle (accessory navicula) that is either separated (type 1, 30% of cases) or attached (type 2 and 3, 70% of cases) to the primary ossification center (body/tuberosity) of the navicula. When the navicula and accessory navicula are attached directly to each other, the connection can either be cartilaginous (type 2, 50% of cases) or bony (type 3, 20% of cases).

A Type 1 accessory navicula is usually defined as a sesamoid bone of the tibialis posterior tendon. It is a small (2–3 mm), well-defined, round- or oval-shaped ossicle[9] embedded within the substance of the tendon, located on the plantar aspect of the tendon at the level of the inferior border of the calcaeonavicular joint and is completely separated[10] by greater than 3 mm from the navicula tuberosity.

The Type 2 accessory navicula is much larger (8–10 mm) and is more triangular in shape.[9] It is a definite part of the body of the navicula but it is separated from the tuberosity by a synchondrosis. This synchondrosis is a fibrous or fibrocartilaginous joint, usually consisting of hyaline cartilage, which is irregular in outline and less than 2 mm deep.[5]

Further subclassification into Type 2A and Type 2B is described[11] according to the radiographic angle of the synchondrosis with a line drawn between the inferior border of the navicula and the talar process. A Type 2A has a more obtuse angle placing it under tension, whereas a Type 2B has a more acute angle and thus is more likely to be placed under shear.

The Type 3 accessory navicula (**Fig. 1**) is united by a bony bridge to the navicula tuberosity, which makes the shape of the navicula appear more hornlike giving rise to the name cornuate navicula or navicula beak.

The location of the accessory navicula explains its pathologic potential with both its subcutaneous (occasionally painful) prominence above the medial arch and its potential to alter the insertion and possibly function of the tibialis posterior tendon.[12] In the presence of an accessory navicula, variation in the anatomy of the insertion of the tibialis posterior tendon has been recorded.[13] The tendon may insert directly onto the accessory navicula without any apparent functional continuity to its usual plantar insertions[3] or it may be displaced inward and upward to insert onto the navicula with continuity to the medial cuneiform.[14,15] When the tendon inserts directly onto the navicula, a fibrocartilage mass can be found proximal to the insertion, which could represent attrition between a rerouted tendon and the body of the navicula.[3]

RELATIONSHIP BETWEEN THE ACCESSORY NAVICULA AND PES PLANUS

The highest incidence of accessory navicula (19%) is seen in people with flat feet.[16] Its presence is usually noted on the anteroposterior foot radiograph and, in more than

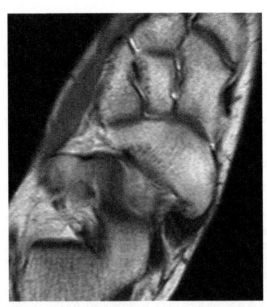

Fig. 1. A Type 3 accessory navicula causing a cornuate navicula; this only very rarely causes symptoms.

90% of cases, is asymptomatic; in the 10% minority, symptoms may relate to either localized pain over the medial navicula or clinical pes planus.[17]

Approximately 35% of patients with an accessory navicula also have a pes planus.[18] When compared with normal individuals, patients with a symptomatic accessory navicula have been shown to have a significantly lower calcaneal pitch if there is clinical evidence of flexible pes planus[19] but an equivalent calcaneometatarsal angle when there are localized symptoms only.[20]

In 1929, Kidner advocated medial advancement of the tibialis posterior tendon insertion after excision of the accessory navicula.[14] He popularized the notion that an accessory navicula displaced the insertion medially, weakening it and leading to the development of a flat foot.[15]

However, although there is evidence to support the role of an abnormal insertion of tibialis posterior tendon in some foot pathology, the literature remains inconclusive regarding a causal relationship between the accessory navicula, the altered insertion of the tibialis posterior tendon, and the cause of flexible pes planus. There is no clear evidence that the abnormal insertion of tibialis posterior tendon in patients with an accessory navicula affects the normal suspensory function of medial arch,[17] particularly in the loaded foot at rest when it is the passive structures (bony arch and ligaments) that offer primary support.[21] Indeed it has been shown[22] that a transfer of the tibialis posterior tendon for foot drop does not lead to a flattened longitudinal arch, again suggesting that Kidner's hypothesis is incorrect.

For practical purposes, it is preferable to consider the painful accessory navicula and the flattening of the medial longitudinal arch to be associated but not directly causally linked. Thus, the presence of overpronation during the second rocker may be caused by a decrease of ligamentous restraints and will predispose to both a supple flat foot and a painful accessory navicula due to rubbing of the bony prominence in the shoes. A patient with a painful accessory navicula should be assessed for the degree of flattening of the medial longitudinal arch and each condition, when coexistent, should be addressed on its own merit. The patient should be counseled appropriately.

THE SYMPTOMATIC ACCESSORY NAVICULA
Presentation

Although many patients with an accessory navicula are asymptomatic and the finding is merely incidental, a symptomatic patient will usually complain of midfoot pain and localized swelling over the medial border of the foot exacerbated by physical activity or nonaccommodative footwear. Those patients with symptoms usually have a Type 2 accessory navicula, whereas Type 3 can also be responsible for a bony prominence.[9]

Most patients, more than 80%, are female[23] usually in adolescence.[20,24] When compared with male, symptoms in adolescent female usually occur 2 years earlier, corresponding to the earlier age of ossification[23] although patients can present as late at their 6th decade.[24]

The accessory navicula most commonly becomes symptomatic in childhood or early adulthood. A child or adolescent will notice the rubbing of an accessory navicula against footwear as the foot and bony swelling grows. An adult presenting with a painful accessory navicula will have had a bony prominence because adolescence and management should focus on the reason as to why pain has developed.

Patients may present with coexistent pes planus although no definite association between an accessory navicula and the cause of the flattened arch has been identified.[9] In adults, the flattened arch is more likely to be due to posterior tibialis tendon (PTT) dysfunction, insertional PTT tendonopathy, or a separation of the synchondrosis of a Type 2 accessory navicula with a history of trauma. Conversely, PTT pathology is uncommon in young patients, and they are more likely to present due a symptomatic accessory navicula alone.[25]

Both groups may be affected by generalized or localized hypermobility or by gastrocsoleus tightness. Hypermobility may cause flattening of the medial longitudinal arch and increased bony prominence, whereas increased tightness of the gastrocsoleus may overload the forefoot or make overpronation worse.

Investigation

Once there is a clinical suspicion of an accessory navicula, its presence can be confirmed on a standard series of weight bearing plain radiographs (**Fig. 2**A) but an additional 45° external oblique (see **Fig. 2**B) delineates the accessory navicula and synchondrosis without any overlapping bones. These initial radiographs will also allow the radiographic identification of any other bony pathology including the presence and magnitude of a coexistent pes planus. Further imaging such as computed tomography or ultrasonography is advocated only when the clinical presentation remains inconclusive.[9]

Plain radiographs, however, do not confirm the role of the accessory bone in the cause of the current clinical symptoms; if the causal relationships between an accessory navicula and medial foot symptoms are unclear, a ^{99m}TcMDP bone scan[8,23] or magnetic resonance imaging (MRI) scan[26] may show evidence of a hot spot or edema in the area (**Fig. 3**).

Mechanism of Pain

Type 1 accessory naviculae are usually asymptomatic. The pain with a Type 3 accessory navicula may occasionally arise from attrition between the enlarged prominence of the navicular tuberosity/accessory navicula and footwear of inadequate width.

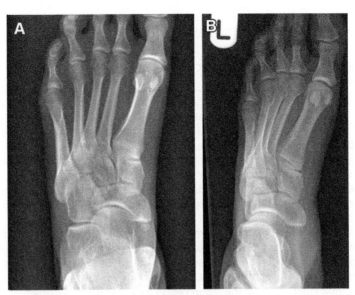

Fig. 2. Inadequate excision of a boney prominence. (*A*) The patient presented with a painful prominence due to a Type 2 accessory navicula and a boney prominence of the true navicula. (*B*) The accessory navicula was excised but the navicula was not trimmed flush with the medial cuneiform. The patient was unhappy with the persistent painful boney prominence.

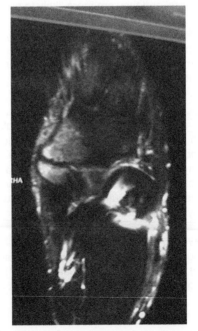

Fig. 3. A twisting injury had initially been diagnosed as a foot sprain. Persistent pain localized to the accessory navicula was investigated by an MRI scan that showed edema across the synchondrosis, indicating a traumatic separation of the bony fragments. Symptoms settled after 6 weeks of protected weight bearing.

Type 2 accessory naviculae are most likely to be symptomatic and require treatment. This synchondrosis can be exposed to compression forces in a pes planus but is usually under either tensile or shear load, from the pull of tibialis posterior in Type 2A and 2B subtypes, respectively. The chronic repetitive injury occurs at the mechanical weak spot of the synchondrosis, between the calcified and uncalcified layers and can undergo histologic changes similar to those noted in physeal injuries in children.[8,23] This initiates a normal repair and remodeling sequence that can be seen on the histologic examination of retrieved Type 2 specimens.[8,23]

As discussed earlier, an adult with an accessory navicula will have had a boney swelling since adolescence and other reasons for the new or ongoing pain should be sought.

Treatment

All treatment modalities are aimed at the relief of pain and the return to normal function and, for many patients who are in adolescence this includes a return to sports. Only once the true cause of their symptoms has been determined and conservative methods such as activity modification, footwear alteration with an orthosis, and anti-inflammatories have been deemed refractory should further intervention be considered.

Unfortunately, conservative treatments are often not effective[27] and most patients, particularly those with a Type 2 accessory navicula, progress onto surgical intervention. Surgical intervention ranges from a simple excision, Kidner procedure to arthrodesis of the ossicle to the navicula.

SURGICAL OPTIONS FOR SYMPTOMATIC ACCESSORY NAVICULA
Excision +/− Repair

The principle of simple excision is to excise the bony prominence without transfer, either whole or in part, of the tibialis posterior tendon. The tendon can either be elevated off the accessory navicula at its superior border leaving a flap of periosteum to reattach it to the navicula[28] or can be split longitudinally[29]; this then allows the ossicle to be shelled out and removed ensuring the remaining surface is flush with the medial cuneiform. Then the tendonous defect is repaired and the patient immobilized. Methods of immobilization vary with this procedure from equinovarus for 2 weeks to a neutral plantigrade cast for 6 weeks with the first 3 non–weight bearing.

Overall, removing the bony prominence leaving the tibialis tendon intact yields good or excellent results in more than 90% of patients[29] and a significant improvement in American Orthopedic Foot and Ankle Society (AOFAS) scores from 48.2 (20–75, mean 38.8) to 94.5 (83–100, mean 94.3), even in the presence of coexisting flat feet. Veitch[30] found no photographic or radiological improvement of the medial longitudinal arch in any of the 21 patients who had undergone a Kidner procedure and concluded that the success of the Kidner procedure is due to removal of the mechanical irritation caused by the bony prominence and not from a reconstruction of the medial longitudinal arch.

Kidner Procedure

The Kidner procedure[14,15] involves detaching the insertion of the tibialis posterior tendon with a thin wafer of bone, excision of the ossicle, and relocation of the tendon to the undersurface of the navicula. Its basis, as discussed earlier, is that the abnormal insertion of tibialis posterior onto the accessory navicula is associated with insufficiency of the tendon that leads to diminished dynamic stability of the foot and a progressive pes planus. Despite this concept and the success of the operation in reducing localized symptoms,[24,30] its ability to restore the medial arch of the foot either clinically or radiographically is debated.[19,28,30]

Since the original description, various modifications of the Kidner procedure have been suggested including passing the detached tendon through a drill hole,[31] suture anchors[32] or tenodesis screws to attach the tendon to the navicula,[33] or mobilization of the middle third of the tibialis posterior tendon to support the plantar aspect of the navicula.[33] However, the modifications have not been shown to provide better results than the original procedure or simple excision.

Arthrodesis of Accessory Navicula to Body of Navicula

A symptomatic synchondrosis is thought to originate as a result of a chronic repetitive injury in the form of shear or tensile forces from the tibialis posterior tendon. In such patients, arthrodesis of the synchondrosis has been proposed rather than excision of the accessory navicula.[34]

To ensure a solid arthrodesis between the ossicle and the navicula, the synchondrosis can be fused through percutaneous drilling in a process similar to that used for epiphyseodesis. When performed percutaneously, the drilling is thought to preserve the insertion of the tendon and permit earlier rehabilitation.[27] Following preparation of the synchondrosis, the ossicle is fused to the navicula in compression with lag screw fixation. However, percutaneous drilling does not address the bony prominence that is often the source of localized symptoms due to rubbing in shoes. Reducing the prominence and fusing the synchondrosis require a closing wedge excision of the synchondrosis and part of the navicula, ensuring that the bony fragment to which the tendon inserts is flush with the medial cuneiform but not advanced too far because this could potentially overtighten the tibialis posterior tendon.[34,35]

When the accessory navicula is large, excision of the accessory navicula may leave a large defect in the tibialis posterior tendon. It may be preferable in this situation to fuse the accessory navicula. However, nonunion rates of up to 20% have been reported,[34,36] which when symptomatic may require a reoperation to excise the accessory bone.[36]

Comparison of Surgical Procedures

Simple excision has been compared to the Kidner procedure in the surgical management of children or adolescents with flat feet and a symptomatic Type 2 accessory navicula.[31] In this study, immediate differences in methodology between the groups can be noted, with the simple excision group having supinating insoles only for 2 weeks post-operatively and the Kidner procedure group being immobilized in a cast for 7 weeks with the first 3 weeks non–weight bearing. Despite this there was no statistical difference in clinical or radiological outcome between the 2 groups of patients. The AOFAS midfoot scale and Visual Analog Scale scores did improve by 3 years post-operatively and both groups also experienced an improvement in their calcaneal pitch angle from 15.7 +/− 4.1 to 19.4 +/− 4.1 in the excision group and 14.6 +/− 5.1 to 19.6 +/− 4.6 in the Kidner group, but not in the talo-first metatarsal angle or the talocalcaneal angle.

This lack of benefit of the rerouting of the tibialis posterior tendon has also been reported in a study that compared arthrodesis to the modified Kidner procedure.[34] In this study, the surgeon decided intraoperatively whether to excise the ossicle or fuse it based on its size and ability to withstand instrumentation with a small fragment screw. If the fragment was excised, a modified Kidner technique was used. Their groups included adults and those who required concurrent flat foot correction but again both procedures demonstrated a significant improvement in AOFAS midfoot scores, with no difference between groups. The arthrodesis group saw AOFAS scores improve from mean 50 (range, 18–67) preoperatively to 93 (range, 81–100) post-operatively, whereas the Kidner procedure group improved from a mean AOFAS score of 52 (range, 41–67) points preoperatively to 80 (range, 52–100) post-operatively.

The results of both these comparative studies largely support other evidence[37] suggesting that rerouting the tibialis posterior tendon, as performed as part of the Kidner procedure, has no beneficial effect on either function, medial foot pain, or the medial longitudinal arch; benefits can be demonstrated with simple excision of the ossicle alone.

COMPLICATIONS OF SURGERY

The combined results from these studies[18,28–30,34,38] include 273 feet from children, adolescents, and adults with a symptomatic accessory navicula and include those with clinical pes planus. Patients underwent one of the procedures previously described, with more than 95% of patients having surgery for a Type 2 accessory navicula or synchondrosis. Every surgical procedure carries the possibility of complications that need to be fully discussed with the patient before surgical intervention. The overall rate of surgical complication was 1 in 5 patients (18%), with half of these cases being due to superficial wound infection, scar tenderness, sensitivity, or irritation.

A list of the surgical complications observed in 6 of the studies[18,28–30,34,38] highlighting the outcome of surgical treatment of accessory navicula is listed below.

- Wound/scar pain
- Persistent pain: localized
  - Residual lump (see **Fig. 2B**)
  - Neuroma
  - Osseous spur
  - Prominent metalwork
  - Nonunion/loose metalwork
  - Pain at insertion of tibialis posterior tendon (**Fig. 4A, B**)
- Persistent pain: generalized foot/lower leg
- Fatigue of muscles
- Presence or persistence of a flat foot

Approximately 45% (124/273) of these patients, operated on for their accessory navicula, also had a pes planus. Post-operatively, the pes planus was noted to clinically persist or worsen in 80 out of the 124, that is, 65%, possibly contributing to the cause of ongoing pain and/or deformity[34]; this emphasizes the need to properly identify and address the concomitant pes planus in the surgical management of the accessory navicula.

Persistent medial pain is frequently seen in patients who have undergone an arthrodesis of the synchondrosis. The nonunion rate in arthrodesis patients is reported as high as 20%, which when symptomatic leads normally to reoperation and excision. Other patients have developed pain due to screw loosening or prominence, requiring removal of the screw. This level of additional risk is unnecessary because arthrodesis offers no benefit in clinical outcome, when compared with excision alone.[34]

Another cause of medial pain is compromise (see **Fig. 4A, B**) of the distal tibialis posterior tendon attachment during simple excision or a Kidner procedure. Shelling the ossicle out for a Type 1 accessory navicula could weaken the tendon and leave a

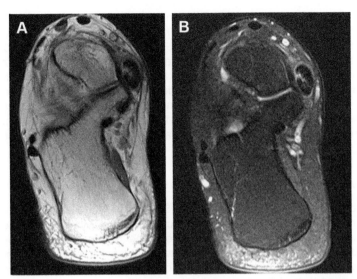

Fig. 4. Damage to the tibialis posterior tendon at surgery. (*A*) (T1 weighted) and (*B*) (T2 weighted) show a split tear in the medial aspect of an enlarged tibialis posterior tendon, which extends to an area of central, ill-defined hyperintensity within the tendon distal to the tip of the medial malleollus. The tendon becomes very poorly defined and obscured by prominent metallic artifact adjacent to the tuberosity of the navicula where a metallic anchor had been used during a Kidner-type procedure. The patient was treated by a calcaneal osteotomy and transfer of flexor digitorum longus tendon to the navicula with excision of the diseased segment of tibialis posterior tendon.

painful scarring; it is not recommended because Type 1 accessory naviculae are rarely the cause of the medial pain. The insertional tendon damage during excision of a Type 2 or Type 3 accessory navicula should be avoided by careful dissection of the tendon and repair of any defect caused intraoperatively. Detaching the insertion and transfer of the whole tendon into the body of the navicula can treat failure of conservative treatment with rest followed by supportive insoles. In adults with severe tibialis posterior insertional tendonopathy navicula (see **Fig. 4**), a transfer of the flexor digitorum longus after resection of the diseased segment of the tibialis posterior tendon can be performed.

Lateral pain after excision of an accessory navicula is usually due to subfibular impingement due to a severe persisting flat foot and is discussed later.

CONCOMITANT CORRECTION OF THE PES PLANUS

Approximately 1 in 3 adolescent patients with a symptomatic accessory navicula will have a coexistent pes planus deformity that will be persistent or worse postoperatively if not specifically addressed. Although Kidner had suggested that the accessory navicula caused a medial displacement and weakening of the tibialis posterior tendon, it is generally now agreed that the accessory navicula is not in itself an inciting cause for a flat foot deformity.

Patients who have a symptomatic accessory navicula and a symptomatic flat foot benefit from simultaneous correction of the flat foot and excision of the ossicle.[27] A thorough assessment of the patient's expectation and clinical findings as outlined in **Box 1** should be performed. The patient's expectations before and after surgery

Box 1
Assessment of a patient with an accessory navicula and co-existing or persistent flat foot

1. Patient expectation: is/was the patient expecting pain relief or reconstruction of the medial arch?
2. Generalized ligamentous laxity
3. Shortening of the gastrocnemius/soleus complex
4. Valgus hindfoot +/− subfibular impingement pain
5. Is the foot supple?
6. Hypermobile first ray
7. Overpronation
8. Tibialis posterior insufficiency (single heel raise)

should be clarified; the fact that an accessory navicula is not the cause of the flat foot should be explained.

Patients with hypermobility of the first ray may require a modified Lapidus procedure. Such hypermobility[39] may be localized or may represent generalized benign ligamentous laxity that has now been reclassified as Ehlers-Danlos syndrome Type 3. These patients do not only have multiple joint laxity and pain but also suffer from systemic symptoms of fatigue, postural hypotension, irritable bowel, and so forth, which are often missed by their treating doctors and will have a significant impact on their presentation and management.

A Silfverskiold procedure[40] will identify Achilles or isolated gastrocnemius tightness that will need to be addressed by a percutaneous Hoke or Strayer procedure if physiotherapy fails to enable the hind foot to be adequately corrected. Patients with severe hindfoot valgus and/or subfibular impingement require a calcaneal osteotomy or arthroereisis screw, whereas those with forefoot adduction may benefit from a lateral column lengthening. A medial shift calcaneal osteotomy tensions the plantar fascia while placing the heel back under the axis of the leg and reduces subfibular impingement. Middle-aged patients who have evidence of a tibialis posterior insufficiency will require a repair of the spring ligament and a flexor digitorum longus transfer in addition to a calcaneal osteotomy.

SUMMARY

The success of the surgical management of the adolescent accessory navicula and avoidance of complications appears dependant on the following factors:

- Meticulous soft tissue handling and intraoperative antibiotics to minimize the risk of post-operative wound complications.
- Adequate excision of the ossicle flush with the medial cuneiform without rerouting the tibialis posterior tendon.
- Correct identification and treatment of a coexistent and symptomatic pes planus deformity, whether or not the surgeon believes that this is due to the presence of the accessory navicula or not.

The adult/middle-aged patient presenting with a painful accessory navicula will have had a boney swelling for many years and attention should focus on the reason for the recent pain or ongoing pain after simple resection. The usually present adult flat foot deformity should also be addressed.

REFERENCES

1. Staheli LT, Chew DE, Corbett M. The longitudinal arch. A survey of eight hundred and eighty-two feet in normal children and adults. J Bone Joint Surg Am 1987;69: 426–8.
2. Gould N, Moreland M, Alvarez R, et al. Development of the child's arch. Foot Ankle 1989;9:241–5.
3. Kiter E, Günal I, Karatosun V, et al. The relationship between the tibialis posterior tendon and the accessory navicular. Ann Anat 2000;182:65–8.
4. Lewis OJ. The tibialis posterior tendon in the primate foot. J Anat 1964;98:209–18.
5. Grogan DP, Gasser SI, Ogden JA. The painful accessory navicular: a clinical and histopathological study. Foot Ankle 1989;10:164–9.
6. Mygind HB. The accessory tarsal scaphoid; clinical features and treatment. Acta Orthop Scand 1953;23:142–51.
7. Dobbs MB, Walton T. Autosomal dominant transmission of accessory navicular. I Iowa Orthop J 2004;24:84–5.
8. Sella EJ, Lawson JP, Ogden JA. The accessory navicular synchondrosis. Clin Orthop Relat Res 1986;209:280–5.
9. Leonard ZC, Fortin PT. Adolescent accessory navicular. Foot Ankle Clin 2010;15: 337–47.
10. Bareither DJ, Muehleman CM, Feldman NJ. Os tibiale externum or sesamoid in the tendon of tibialis posterior. J Foot Ankle Surg 1995;34:429–34.
11. Sella EJ, Lawson JP. Biomechanics of the accessory navicular synchondrosis. Foot Ankle 1987;8:156–63.
12. Golano P, Fariñas O, Sáenz I. The anatomy of the navicular and periarticular structures. Foot Ankle Clin 2004;9:1–23.
13. Kiter E, Erdag N, Karatosun V, et al. Tibialis posterior tendon abnormalities in feet with accessory navicular bone and flatfoot. Acta Orthop Scand 1999;70: 618–21.
14. Kidner FC. The prehallux (accessory scaphoid) in its relation to flat-foot. J Bone Joint Surg Am 1929;11:831–7.
15. Kidner FC. The prehallux in relation to flat-foot. J Am Med Assoc 1933;101: 1539–42.
16. Wood WA, Spencer AM. Incidence of os tibiale externum in clinical pes planus. J Am Podiatry Assoc 1970;60:276–9.
17. Kanatli U, Yetkin H, Yalcin N. The relationship between accessory navicular and medial longitudinal arch: evaluation with a plantar pressure distribution measurement system. Foot Ankle Int 2003;24:486–9.
18. Garras DN, Hansen PL, Miller AG, et al. Outcome of modified Kidner procedure with subtalar arthroereisis for painful accessory navicular associated with planovalgus deformity. Foot Ankle Int 2012;33:934–9.
19. Prichasuk S, Sinphurmsukskul O. Kidner procedure for symptomatic accessory navicular and its relation to pes planus. Foot Ankle Int 1995;16:500–3.
20. Sullivan JA, Miller WA. The relationship of the accessory navicular to the development of the flat foot. Clin Orthop Relat Res 1979;144:233–7.
21. Basmajian JV, Stecko G. The role of muscles in arch support of the foot. J Bone Joint Surg Am 1963;45:1184–90.
22. Yeap JS, Birch R, Singh D. Long-term results of tibialis posterior tendon transfer for drop-foot. Int Orthop 2001;25:114–8.
23. Lawson JP, Ogden JA, Sella E, et al. The painful accessory navicular. Skeletal Radiol 1984;12:250–62.

24. Ray S, Goldberg VM. Surgical treatment of the accessory navicular. Clin Orthop Relat Res 1983;177:61–6.
25. Chen YJ, Hsu RW, Liang SC. Degeneration of the accessory navicular synchondrosis presenting as rupture of the posterior tibial tendon. J Bone Joint Surg Am 1997;79:1791–8.
26. Miller TT, Staron RB, Feldman F, et al. The symptomatic accessory tarsal navicular bone: assessment with MR imaging. Radiology 1995;195:849–53.
27. Ugolini PA, Raikin SM. The accessory navicular. Foot Ankle Clin 2004;9:165–80.
28. Kopp FJ, Marcus RE. Clinical outcome of surgical treatment of the symptomatic accessory navicular. Foot Ankle Int 2004;25:27–30.
29. Bennett GL, Weiner DS, Leighley B. Surgical treatment of symptomatic accessory tarsal navicular. J Pediatr Orthop 1990;10:445–9.
30. Veitch JM. Evaluation of the Kidner procedure in treatment of symptomatic accessory tarsal scaphoid. Clin Orthop Relat Res 1978;131:210–3.
31. Cha SM, Shin HD, Kim KC, et al. Simple excision vs the Kidner procedure for type 2 accessory navicular associated with flatfoot in pediatric population. Foot Ankle Int 2013;34:167–72.
32. Dawson DM, Julsrud ME, Erdmann BB, et al. Modified Kidner procedure utilizing a Mitek bone anchor. J Foot Ankle Surg 1998;37:115–21.
33. Zinsmeister B, Edelman R. A new technique for tenodesis of the tibialis posterior in the Kidner procedure. J Foot Surg 1985;24:442–4.
34. Scott AT, Sabesan VJ, Saluta JR, et al. Fusion versus excision of the symptomatic Type II accessory navicular: a prospective study. Foot Ankle Int 2009;30:10–5.
35. Malicky ES, Levine DS, Sangeorzan BJ. Modification of the Kidner procedure with fusion of the primary and accessory navicular bones. Foot Ankle Int 1999;20: 53–4.
36. Chung JW, Chu IT. Outcome of fusion of a painful accessory navicular to the primary navicular. Foot Ankle Int 2009;30:106–9.
37. Macnicol MF, Voutsinas S. Surgical treatment of the symptomatic accessory navicular. J Bone Joint Surg Br 1984;66:218–26.
38. Micheli LJ, Nielson JH, Ascani C, et al. Treatment of painful accessory navicular: a modification to simple excision. Foot Ankle Spec 2008;1:214–7.
39. Castori M, Celletti C, Camerota F. Ehlers–Danlos syndrome hypermobility type: a possible unifying concept for various functional somatic syndromes. Rheumatol Int 2013;33:819–21.
40. Singh D. Nils Silfverskiöld (1888-1957) and gastrocnemius contracture. Foot Ankle Surg 2013;19:135–8.

Taking Out the Tarsal Coalition Was Easy

But Now the Foot Is Even Flatter. What Now?

Nikolaos Gougoulias, MD, PhD, CCT (Orth)[a],
Maurice O'Flaherty, MB BCh, BaO, MSc Sports Med, FRCSEd (Tr & Orth)[b],
Anthony Sakellariou, MBBS, BSc, FRCS (Orth)[a],*

KEYWORDS

• Tarsal coalition • Planovalgus • Calcaneal osteotomy • Arthrodesis

KEY POINTS

- After resection of a tarsal coalition, patients may present with progression of the planovalgus appearance of the foot.
- Excision of the coalition may potentially destabilize the hindfoot, by allowing any preexisting lateral ligament and peroneal tendon shortening, in combination with gastrocnemius +/− soleus tightness, to increase any valgus or equinus deformity, especially after talocalcaneal coalition bar resections.
- Joint preserving surgery (corrective calcaneal osteotomy) should be reserved for young and adolescent patients with flexible deformities.
- Fusion procedures are indicated for stiff feet, yielding predictable results.
- Gastrocnemius/gastrocsoleus/peroneal tendon releases may accompany any bony procedures.

BACKGROUND

Tarsal coalition, described for the first time in 1829 by Curveilhier,[1] presents with symptoms (hindfoot stiffness and pain) in approximately 1% of the population.[2–4] Occasionally, it is part of a more complex syndrome affecting other bones or other organs but usually it appears as an isolated condition. The 2 most common types (calcaneonavicular and talocalcaneal) account for 90% of all isolated tarsal coalitions and their

Finding Sources: None.
Conflict of Interest: None.
[a] Department of Trauma & Orthopaedics, Frimley Park Hospital NHS Foundation Trust, Portsmouth Road, Camberley, Surrey GU16 7UJ, UK; [b] Department of Trauma & Orthopaedics, Royal Surrey County Hospital and Frimley Park Hospital, Egerton Road, Guildford, Surrey GU2 7XX, UK
* Corresponding author.
E-mail address: anthony.sakellariou@fph-tr.nhs.uk

relative incidence is almost equal. Less frequently occurring coalitions are the talona-vicular, naviculocuneiform or, calcaneocuboid ones.[1] Although the cause is not fully understood, it seems to represent a failure of differentiation and segmentation of the primary mesenchyme that normally occurs in the 9th to 10th week of pregnancy.[5]

A failure to form a normal joint manifests later in life as an osseous (synostosis), cartilaginous (synchondrosis), or fibrous (syndesmosis) connection between the bones of the foot.[3] The condition causes restriction or elimination of hindfoot and, occasionally, midfoot movement (affecting hindfoot eversion/inversion and also, potentially, foot supination/pronation). The foot has a planovalgus appearance but often remains pain-free. Pain is usually the result of a "sprain" or other minor injury to the foot and may appear at the age of 8 to 12 years in children with calcaneonavicular coalitions, whereas talocalcaneal coalitions tend to become symptomatic in adolescents.[6] Nonoperative management options include physiotherapy, braces, casting, insoles and steroid injections.[7,8] Resection of the coalition with or without interposition of fat or other soft tissues, to prevent reossification, is a surgical option recommended by many investigators.[1,9–12] In recent years, technical advances have allowed these procedures to be performed endoscopically.[13,14] However, further deterioration of foot flattening and recurrence of pain and joint degeneration can complicate surgery, and some surgeons advocate the need of simultaneous hindfoot reconstruction and realignment, together with coalition excision. In this article the authors discuss salvage solutions.[15] They also refer to the pathomechanics, which leads to primary valgus alignment of the foot and the potential implications for primary surgical management to prevent this problem.

PATHOMECHANICS

Normal subtalar joint mechanics during gait involve rotation and gliding. The axis of motion of the subtalar joint is defined as a line deviated 42° from the horizontal surface and 16° internally rotated from a line extending from the center of the calcaneus, to a point between the first and second metatarsals. During the stance phase of gait, the subtalar joint rotates from 4° valgus to 6° of hindfoot varus.[16,17] When internal rotation is restricted by the coalition, the tarsal joints compensate, flattening the foot and dropping the medial arch, giving the foot its planovalgus appearance in the sagittal plane. Adaptive shortening of the peroneal tendons and reactive peroneal spasm follow,[18] which is described by some investigators as the "peroneal spastic flatfoot."[19] Prolonged restriction of motion may eventually lead to abnormal (eccentric) loading of the subtalar joint and, subsequently, to degenerative changes.

The normal gliding motion of the subtalar joint during dorsiflexion is also lost in feet with a tarsal coalition. Studies have demonstrated a "hinge joint" instead. The midfoot joints widen plantarly and become tight dorsally. Thus, the navicula "overrides" the talar head at maximum dorsiflexion, and[20] this generates a traction effect on the ligaments and capsule of the talonavicular joint and is thought to produce the "talar beaking" seen in many radiographs of feet with tarsal coalition.[4]

The pain may therefore be attributed to ligament sprain, peroneal muscle spasm, sinus tarsi, and subtalar joint posterior facet irritation and arthritic changes. The variability of the symptoms in different patients may be due to the variability of subtalar joint motion restriction. Middle facet talocalcaneal coalitions, for example, are associated with greater restriction of subtalar motion and are the most likely to generate valgus.

But why does the foot get even flatter after resection of the coalition? Should this procedure not restore normal hindfoot mechanics?

The answer may lie with the fact that we are dealing with a chronic condition and that soft tissues have "memory". The abnormal hindfoot mechanics described earlier may cause permanent shrinkage of joint capsules, ligaments, and secondary shortening of the peroneal tendons and gastrocsoleus complex. Thus, even after resection of a coalition, hindfoot stiffness remains in the same way that an arthritic ankle remains stiff even after excision of osteophytes. Furthermore, the action of the spastic, short, and less elastic peroneal tendons may provoke a further increase in hindfoot valgus (**Fig. 1**). Thus, the bones move, but in the wrong direction, guided by the "memory" of the "abnormal" soft tissues. Normal mechanics are, therefore, not restored, abnormal loading of the joints continues, and degenerative changes may progress.

All these may explain why excision of coalitions in younger children's feet can yield relatively good results, whereas older adolescents and adults do not respond in the same way.

CLINICAL PRESENTATION AND EXAMINATION

After failed excision of a tarsal coalition, patients may present complaining of pain and often stiffness, saying that the arch of their foot has dropped even more. At this point, it is incumbent on the treating physician to determine whether the patient's primary complaint is pain, deformity, lack of movement or, a combination of all three. The source of pain has to be accurately identified because this will guide the decisions regarding further management. Nevertheless, to diagnose what the affected structures are, given the patient has had surgery before, may not be a task for the inexperienced.

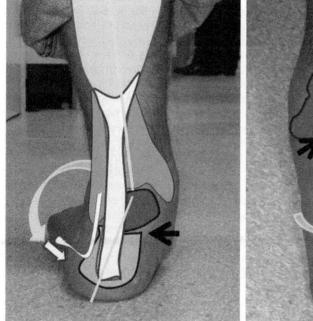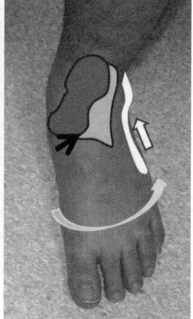

Fig. 1. When a medial facet talocalcaneal coalition is excised (*black arrow*), the peroneal tendons on the lateral side can act as a deforming force (*white arrow*), resulting in eversion of the subtalar joint and foot pronation (*yellow arrow*). Furthermore, the relatively tight Achilles tendon is "pulling" the heel into valgus.

Careful history taking is essential. How was the condition affected by surgery and what is the timescale of events (eg, whether there was initial improvement, but then gradual deterioration, or whether they felt immediate worsening of symptoms)? The examiner should enquire about factors aggravating pain (certain activities, type of shoes) and has to determine the character of any pain. If available, the records of the previous status of the foot should be taken into consideration (operation records, preoperative examination findings, diagnosis).

Patients can not normally tolerate walking long distances or sports participation. They report that post-activity swelling and pain is an issue and it may take a few days for them to recover after any type of strenuous activity involving walking.

Certain types of footwear, like boots, that support the hindfoot from side to side, may help, whereas walking barefoot or on uneven ground (eg, sand, certain types of outdoor terrain), usually aggravates their symptoms. Certain activities, like repetitive use of the foot when driving, may aggravate symptoms too and are related to the peroneal tendons.

The patient should be asked to point out the source of their symptoms on the surface of his/her foot. At this stage, the examiner can begin relating the pain to specific structures of the foot (eg, medial, lateral, or posterior structures related to the symptoms).

Clinical examination of the ankle and foot will follow, after the patient is asked to expose both his/her lower legs below the knee. Alignment should be assessed, observing the patient from the front, side, and back. Observation includes assessment for surgical scars and presence of bony or soft tissue prominences. Gait observation is essential, as well as checking the patient's shoes for increased wear in specific areas of the sole (eg, medial heel region in valgus feet). With the patent standing, eversion and inversion are assessed asking patients to turn on the outside and then inside edges of their feet, respectively. This assessment may reveal hindfoot joint stiffness. Difficulty walking on the heels may indicate tight calf muscles, whereas difficulty walking on tiptoes may indicate posterior impingement, Achilles tendinopathy, or degenerative joint disease. The patient is then observed from behind while asked to "single heel raise" (raising his/her heel off the floor on one side, while the other foot is off the floor), if possible. In a normal foot the heel inverts (rotates into varus), indicating normal subtalar motion. Inability to perform the test may reveal insufficiency of tibialis posterior. If single heel raising is possible, but the heel remains in valgus, subtalar joint stiffness is the reason (**Fig. 2**).

The patient is then asked to sit, with his/her legs hanging off the examination couch. The foot and ankle are first observed closely for areas of swelling, surgical scars, or deformity. Then the Silfverskiöld test can be performed to assess tightness of the gastrocnemius muscle.[21] The Silfverskiöld knee flexion test has now been adapted to distinguish between isolated gastrocnemius contracture and combined shortening of the gastrocnemius-soleus complex by measuring ankle dorsiflexion with the knee extended or flexed. Subtalar joint movement is assessed, with the examiner grasping the heel, while stabilizing the tibia with his/her other hand and moving it medially and laterally. The feet are gently palpated, starting from areas that are not expected to cause discomfort. The tender "spots" are identified. The examiner has to correlate any tender areas on the surface with the underlying structures (eg, ankle joint – medial vs lateral, Achilles tendon – insertional vs noninsertional portion, subtalar joint – medial vs lateral side, peroneal tendons on lateral side, tibialis posterior on the medial side, calcaneocuboid joint, sinus tarsi, calcaneo-navicular interspace, tarsometatarsal joints, forefoot joints). Any surgical scar sensitivity should be documented. Normal skin sensation is assessed and any lack of sensation should be documented. The

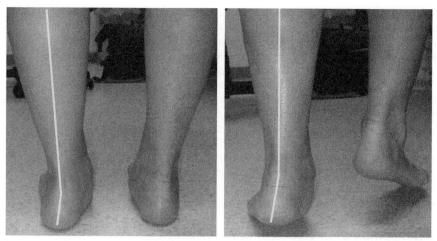

Fig. 2. The valgus aligned heel does not invert during single heel rise. This indicates a stiff subtalar joint.

sural, superficial peroneal, and saphenous nerves are assessed using the Tinel sign. The presence of palpable pulses (dorsalis pedis and tibial arteries) is checked for.

IMAGING

Appropriate imaging is essential for those patients presenting with deterioration of symptoms after previous surgery for tarsal coalition.

Weight bearing (WB), anteroposterior (AP), and lateral radiographs of the ankle and foot are essential. The ankle/foot lateral WB view reveals how flat the foot is but is also useful for identifying degenerative changes of the hindfoot joints. The talocalcaneal axis and talonavicular joint congruity (affected in planovalgus feet) are checked on the foot AP WB radiograph. Ankle AP WB and mortise views may indicate subfibular impingement in valgus-aligned feet (**Fig. 3**). Oblique views of the foot are also needed. Oblique

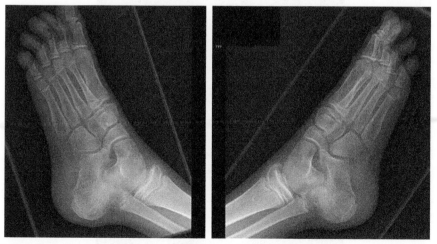

Fig. 3. Bilateral calcaneonavicular coalitions, in a 11-year-old boy, revealed on oblique foot radiographic views.

radiographs are used for assessing the calcaneonavicular interspace (**Fig. 4**). Many foot and ankle surgeons advocate the use of the hindfoot alignment radiograph as proposed by Saltzman.[22] If gross deformity is present or if the source of the valgus hindfoot alignment is not certain, long-leg standing views may be needed (not routinely).

Further imaging is often needed, depending on the examination findings. A computed tomography (CT) scan could reveal the details of osseous anatomy (eg, recurrence of bone growth at the resection site of a synostosis) or joint degenerative changes. Often, the physician may choose to combine the CT scan with a radionuclide bone scan (single-photon emission computed tomography-CT) to detect the "hot spots" that cause pain. If soft tissue abnormalities (eg, peroneal, Achilles, or tibialis posterior tendinopathy; deltoid and spring ligament integrity; sinus tarsi scar tissue) are expected at the same time, magnetic resonance imaging (MRI) is superior. Depending on available expertise, ultrasound scanning can be used to detect tendon problems or nerve entrapment in scar tissue.

INTERPRETATION OF FINDINGS AND DECISION MAKING

Interpretation of clinical examination and imaging findings is an important part of the decision-making process. The physician has spent time with the patient, listened carefully taking notes, asked key questions to highlight the problem, examined the patient, and reviewed imaging studies; these should be taken into consideration, together with the background knowledge of the pathomechanics described earlier. Now, the key questions that need to be answered are

- What is the patient's primary problem (appearance/deformity, pain, stiffness)?
- Is there recurrent coalition formation?
- What are the patient's age, level of activity, and expectations?
- Is the foot flexible? Are the joints mobile?
- Do joints degenerate, causing pain?
- Which joint(s) is/are causing pain?
- Are the tendons/ligaments affected?

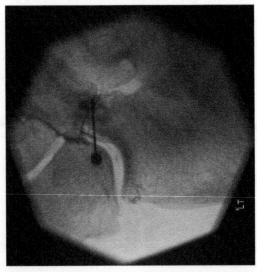

Fig. 4. Image-guided steroid injection into the calcaneonavicular interspace/synchondrosis.

If the physician cannot answer any of these questions, he/she should not proceed to interventional management. Re-examination may be essential or more imaging studies may be needed. One may have to obtain an MRI in addition to a CT scan or vice versa. Alternatively, consider whether a bone scan or ultrasound scan may be helpful. Often, image-guided steroid and local anesthetic injections may be helpful to detect the painful site in the foot. Furthermore, they may offer pain relief that may last.

The treating surgeon has to then decide whether nonoperative management options have been exhausted. Surgery for these conditions, as will be discussed in the following sections of this article, is fairly invasive and recovery time is long. Therefore, the symptoms must be bad enough to justify further surgical intervention. Furthermore, there is no clear evidence to suggest that correcting the shape of the valgus foot will lead to improved function or will prevent further deterioration of symptoms in the future. The presence of pain is the crucial parameter that justifies surgical management. Nevertheless, patients' expectations have to be managed accordingly, whatever the decision regarding further management is. This is especially the case if one of the patients' principal concerns is hindfoot stiffness. Because, if on examination the hindfoot is rigid, it is very unlikely that mobility will be restored with revision surgery and so, both patient and surgeon must be realistic about this. The investigators would advise allowing a "trial period" of nonoperative management first (injection, rest, insoles, physiotherapy) for 3 to 6 months, before offering revision surgery.

Young patients (children, adolescents, young adults) with flexible feet and no arthritic changes in the hindfoot joints may suffer from muscle spasm and tightness. They would probably benefit from physiotherapy and insole treatment. If the problem persists, they are candidates for joint preserving surgery (eg, corrective calcaneal osteotomy) combined with soft tissue procedures (tendon/muscle releases) and, occasionally, an arthroreisis procedure.

Older patients with stiff feet may be candidates for joint fusions, once nonoperative management has failed.[12] Steroid injections may postpone surgical management.

NONOPERATIVE MANAGEMENT

Nonoperative management should not mean "no treatment". It should be offered to patients as a means of actively improving their symptoms.

As mentioned earlier, peroneal and calf muscle tightness is often an issue, leading to a vicious cycle resulting in more valgus. At the same time, the patient may be troubled by pain related to peroneal and Achilles tendinopathy. Physiotherapy is therefore a valuable tool to improve hindfoot flexibility in these patients. Other patients who may benefit from physiotherapy are those suffering from tibialis posterior tendinopathy, secondary to the planovalgus alignment.

Accommodative orthotics should be tried to stabilize the hindfoot, offering pain relief. Corrective insoles (eg, medial heel wedge-type) are more likely to increase discomfort as the hindfoot is usually stiff. Corrective insoles could be tried after resection of the coalition, to neutralize hindfoot alignment; this would off-load the medial structures (eg, tibialis posterior, spring ligament, talonavicular joint) and improve the mechanics of the foot, bringing the peroneal tendons into a more favorable position, biomechanically.

Image-guided steroid injections (see **Fig. 4**) are both of therapeutic and diagnostic value, as mentioned earlier. They do not change the alignment of the foot, but offer pain relief, the longevity of which is unpredictable.

Modification of activities may often be required to control patients' symptoms. Although it may not be easily accepted by all patients, the surgeon should clarify that even corrective surgery may not allow them to participate in certain sports or other strenuous activities.

SURGICAL MANAGEMENT

When previous surgery has failed, any further intervention could be considered as a salvage procedure. Even an inadequate previous bone bar resection is not an exception, because the foot "is now even flatter". The type of surgery (joint preserving vs joint sacrificing) largely depends on the age, the condition of the joint surfaces, and the flexibility of the foot. Soft tissue procedures, tailored to the needs of the individual patient, may be needed to accompany bony corrective surgery.

The aim of joint preserving surgery for the planovalgus foot after previous resection of a tarsal coalition is to

- Neutralize the hindfoot axis to improve the mechanics
- Relieve any abnormal loading of joints
- Release soft tissue structures (muscles, tendons, ligaments) to avoid secondary effects of tissue tightness
- Re-excise any "recurrence" of coalition

These operations usually necessitate a calcaneal osteotomy.[23,24] The calcaneal tuberosity is slid medially (heel brought into varus) and fixed with one large screw (**Figs. 5** and **6**). Some investigators advocate the use of staples or lateral plates. In skeletally immature patients, Kirschner wires can be used instead. Some investigators may sometimes use an arthroreisis device in children/adolescents. Others advocate use of a lateral column lengthening osteotomy which, in turn, may necessitate a cuneiform osteotomy to correct any secondary forefoot supination (varus) that may result as a consequence of the lateral column lengthening procedure. A gastrocnemius muscle slide or percutaneous Achilles tendon lengthening procedure may be needed. Peroneal tendons may require lengthening if a true contracture has developed. One

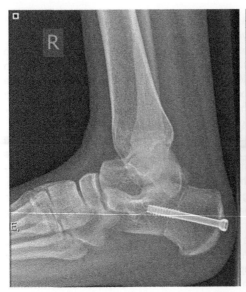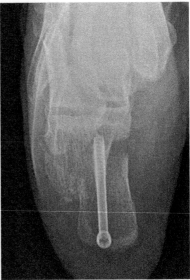

Fig. 5. Calcaneal osteotomy. The calcaneal tuberosity was shifted medially.

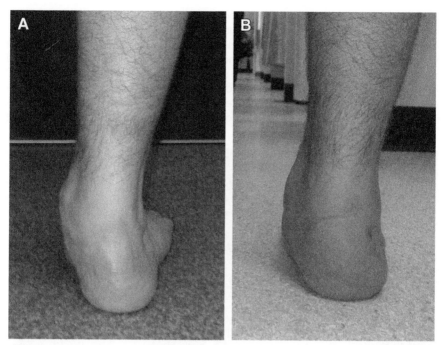

Fig. 6. The valgus heel alignment (*A*) was corrected to neutral (*B*) by performing a calcaneal osteotomy.

has to differentiate between peroneal muscle spasm and true shortening of the tendons. If a pre-operative botox injection does not result in relief of any peroneal spasm, it means a contracture is present and formal lengthening may well be needed. Tibialis posterior tendon reconstruction may be performed (using flexor digitorum longus tendon transfer) in cases where the tendon has been secondarily affected by chronic valgus alignment. In cases of advanced tendinopathic change, tibialis posterior is better sacrificed. Care should be taken to repair the spring ligament, as well.

Post-operatively, the patient remains non–weight bearing for 6 weeks, immobilized in a below knee back slab for 2 weeks (until wound check/suture removal), followed by a bivalved below knee cast or boot for another 4 to 6 weeks (to allow some early ROM exercises). Then, partial–weight bearing mobilization in a removable boot is recommended. At the same time, physiotherapy, hydrotherapy, and further gentle joint range of movement exercises can be commenced. It usually takes 3 months for patients to be able to safely bear full weight. Full recovery is not expected before 6 months. Certain sports that involve running and turning are not recommended for 9 to 12 months after surgery.

Joint sacrificing—arthrodesis procedures are aimed at:
- Elimination of pain arising from degenerate joints
- Restoration of neutral foot/ankle alignment

Depending on the pathology, arthrodesis of several joints may be required.[12] A triple (subtalar, talonavicular, calcaneocuboid) arthrodesis is advocated by many investigators, especially after a failed calcaneonavicular bar resection. It is important to aim to correct the hindfoot valgus deformity at the same time. Currently, there is the tendency for more "selective" fusion procedures. For the consequences of a failed talocalcaneal coalition excision, an isolated subtalar fusion may be all that is needed (**Figs. 7–9**). Care should be taken to resect more bone from the medial side while preparing the joint surfaces, to allow varization of the heel. Calcaneonavicular coalitions may lead to degeneration of the talonavicular and subtalar joints. In these cases, a "double" or "triple" arthrodesis might be required (depending on the status of the calcaneocuboid joint). Any major hindfoot valgus correction may require release of the gastrocsoleus complex to avoid post-operative equinus contracture. Either a percutaneous

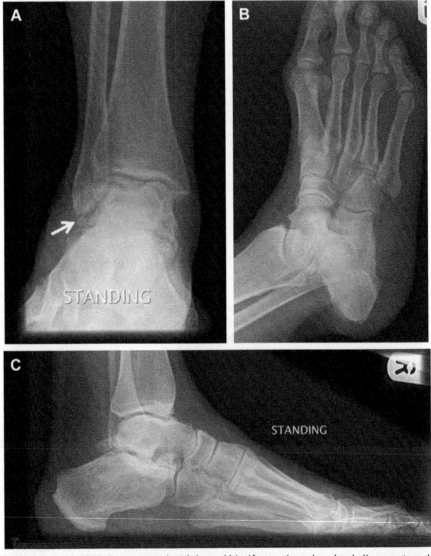

Fig. 7. A 41-year-old lady presented with lateral hindfoot pain, valgus heel alignment, and a stiff subtalar joint (clinical pictures shown in **Fig. 2**). Some years previously she had undergone resection of a medial facet talocalcaneal coalition. Radiographs (*A*) show subfibular impingement (*white arrow*) and raise suspicion of subtalar joint degeneration (*C*).

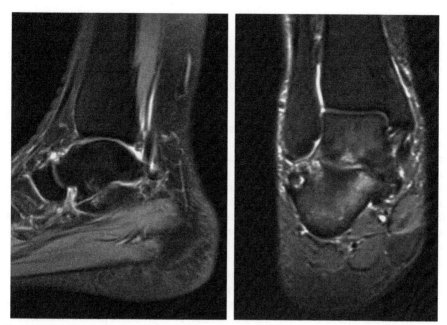

Fig. 8. MRI confirmed subtalar joint degeneration.

Achilles tendon release or a gastrocnemius muscle slide (at the musculotendinous junction) may be needed.

Patients undergoing fusion procedures are immobilized in a below knee cast for 3 months. They should remain non–weight bearing for 6 weeks, then start to bear weight partially, in a cast, for another 6 weeks. In cases of delayed union, progression to a full-weight bearing status may be delayed. Full recovery is not expected before 6 months. It is unlikely that these patients will be able to participate in sports requiring running and turning (eg, tennis).

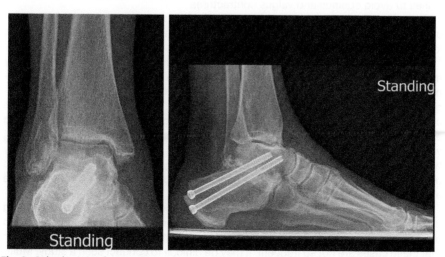

Fig. 9. Subtalar joint fusion was performed. The patient was pain free and satisfied with the outcome a year later.

DISCUSSION

When considering primary or revision surgery for coalitions, the surgeon must consider what the goals of surgical intervention are. It must be borne in mind that the principal goal is to abolish/improve pain and, in so doing, improve function. This goal can be achieved by not only aiming to resect the coalition but also by aiming to correct any pre-existing valgus deformity with a combination of bony and soft tissue procedures; this is because simple resection (with or without soft tissue interposition) may not be adequate for patients with tarsal coalition and a valgus deformity.[15] Often, their pain recurs and the planovalgus deformity increases due to the secondary effects of soft tissue contractures "pulling" the foot into more valgus. This issue needs to be addressed when treating these patients either primarily, or in the revision situation. Assessment of flexibility of the hindfoot and of the subtalar joint in particular, is probably key, when considering further intervention because restoring flexibility to a hindfoot that is already rigid is difficult, if not unrealistic. Also, there is a lack of high-level evidence to safely identify those suitable for joint preserving procedures and clear indications do not exist. Younger patients though, with flexible subtalar joints, are candidates for joint preserving surgery.

When the subtalar joint is not mobile (even after soft tissue releases), even if not clearly degenerate on imaging studies, there is little, if any benefit, in preserving the joint that is likely to cause pain in the future. Performing an image-guided subtalar joint injection before intervention may aid the clinician in appropriate patient selection. In the authors' experience, patients who undergo isolated corrective subtalar joint arthrodesis for progressive planovalgus deformity, secondary to tarsal coalition resection, were very satisfied with the outcome and had no reservations regarding the fusion procedure (see **Figs. 7–9**). These patients, irrespective of age, do not notice the lack of eversion/inversion after the fusion, as their hindfoot "has always been stiff". They will be satisfied if their pain has resolved and their foot and ankle are not "tilted outwards". Arthrodesis procedures are probably more predictable with regard to outcome compared with joint preserving operations. Careful patient selection is therefore a precursor to success. The authors are in favor of selective fusions (a triple fusion is not always needed) and would like to highlight the need for calf muscle/tendon releases to avoid equinus and valgus contractures.

Given the complexity of the pathology in these feet, to ensure a good post-operative outcome, preoperative planning is key and this mandates a careful examination to identify all elements of the problem.

Patients with tarsal coalitions and pronounced hindfoot valgus may be better treated with resection of the coalition and simultaneous corrective surgery (eg, calcaneal varization osteotomy). There is some level IV evidence to suggest that these procedures are successful when performed in children.[15,22] Resection of the coalition alone is likely to increase their hindfoot valgus alignment, for reasons described earlier. As such, young patients with relatively flexible deformities and hindfoot valgus are probably candidates for resection of the coalition, done simultaneously with a calcaneal varization osteotomy and possibly an arthroreisis procedure, to restore more normal foot mechanics and prevent deterioration of the heel valgus alignment.

The authors are not aware of any studies reporting on the success of joint preserving corrective surgery in the long term. Furthermore, comparative studies (eg, coalition resection alone vs combined with corrective osteotomy) are not available. Given that these cases are not so frequent, it may be difficult to conduct such a study. Multicentre collaboration may give evidence-based answers in the future.

For the patient to give informed consent, these procedures should be clearly offered as salvage procedures in that, they could help improve symptoms and foot function and not as a cure to the primary problem.

REFERENCES

1. Hefti F. Pediatric orthoapedics in practice. Springer Verlag; 2007. p. 394–6.
2. Stormont DM, Peterson HA. The relative incidence of tarsal coalition. Clin Orthop 1983;181:28–36.
3. Sakellariou A, Sallomi D, Janzen DL, et al. Talocalcaneal coalition. Diagnosis with the C-sign on lateral radiographs of the ankle. J Bone Joint Surg Br 2000;82(4): 574–8.
4. Kawashima T, Uhthoff HK. Prenatal development around the sustentaculum tali and its relation to talocalcaneal coalitions. J Pediatr Orthop 1990;10: 232–7.
5. Bohne WH. Tarsal coalition. Curr Opin Pediatr 2001;13(1):29–35.
6. Cowell HR, Elener V. Rigid painful flatfoot secondary to tarsal coalition. Clin Orthop 1983;177:54–60.
7. Zaw H, Calder JD. Tarsal coalitions. Foot Ankle Clin 2010;15(2):349–64.
8. Kulik SA Jr, Clanton TO. Tarsal coalition. Foot Ankle Int 1996;17(5):286–96.
9. Gonzalez P, Kumar SJ. Calcaneonavicular coalition treated by resection and interposition of the extensor digitorum brevis muscle. J Bone Joint Surg Am 1990;72(1):71–7.
10. Mubarak SJ, Patel PN, Upasani VV, et al. Calcaneonavicular coalition: treatment by excision and fat graft. J Pediatr Orthop 2009;29(5):418–26.
11. Scott AT, Tuten HR. Calcaneonavicular coalition resection with extensor digitorum brevis interposition in adults. Foot Ankle Int 2007;28(8):890–5.
12. Thorpe SW, Wukich DK. Tarsal coalitions in the adult population: does treatment differ from the adolescent? Foot Ankle Clin 2012;17(2):195–204.
13. Bonasia DE, Phisitkul P, Saltzman CL, et al. Arthroscopic resection of talocalcaneal coalitions. Arthroscopy 2011;27(3):430–5.
14. Bauer T, Golano P, Hardy P. Endoscopic resection of a calcaneonavicular coalition. Knee Surg Sports Traumatol Arthrosc 2010;18(5):669–72.
15. Lisella JM, Bellapianta JM, Manoli A 2nd. Tarsal coalition resection with pes planovalgus hindfoot reconstruction. J Surg Orthop Adv 2011;20(2):102–5.
16. Wright DG, Desai SM, Henderson WH. Action of the subtalar and ankle-joint complex during the stance phase of walking. J Bone Joint Surg Am 1964;46: 361–82.
17. Piazza SJ. Mechanics of the subtalar joint and its function during walking. Foot Ankle Clin 2005;10:425–42.
18. Kitaoka HB, Wikenheiser MA, Shaughnessy WJ, et al. Gait abnormalities following resection of talocalcaneal coalition. J Bone Joint Surg Am 1997;79(3): 369–74.
19. Mosier KM, Asher M. Tarsal coalitions and peroneal spastic flat foot. A review. J Bone Joint Surg Am 1984;66(7):976–84.
20. Hetsroni I, Nyska M, Mann G, et al. Subtalar kinematics following resection of tarsal coalition. Foot Ankle Int 2008;29(11):1088–94.
21. Singh D. Nils Silfverskiöld (1888–1957) and gastrocnemius contracture. Foot Ankle Surg 2013;19(2):135–8.
22. Saltzman CL, el-Khoury GY. The hindfoot alignment view. Foot Ankle Int 1995; 16(9):572–6.

23. Mosca VS, Bevan WP. Talocalcaneal tarsal coalitions and the calcaneal lengthening osteotomy: the role of deformity correction. J Bone Joint Surg Am 2012; 94(17):1584–94.
24. Malerba F, De March F. Calcaneal osteotomies. Foot Ankle Clin 2005;10: 523–40.

Osteomyelitis of the Foot and Ankle

Diagnosis, Epidemiology, and Treatment

Benjamin J. Lindbloom, MD[a], Eric R. James, MD[b],
William C. McGarvey, MD[a,b],*

KEYWORDS

- Osteomyelitis • Diabetic foot • Imaging • Surgical treatment • Laboratory studies
- Adjuvant therapies

KEY POINTS

- Osteomyelitis of the foot and ankle is a common, potentially devastating condition with diagnostic and treatment challenges.
- History and physical examination, laboratory studies, vascular studies, histologic and microbiologic analyses, and various imaging modalities contribute to the diagnosis and treatment.
- Treatment should take a multidisciplinary approach to optimize patient factors, ensure eradication of the infection, and restore function.
- Surgical treatment needs to consider the physiology of the infection and the patient, must be extensive, and may use multiple techniques to achieve successful outcomes.
- Adjuvant therapies and novel laboratory markers may enhance outcomes as they are further studied and used.

INTRODUCTION

Osteomyelitis of the foot and ankle can be extremely debilitating to patients and a management challenge to the orthopedic surgeon. In the preantibiotic era, acute staphylococcal osteomyelitis carried a mortality rate of 50%.[1] Osteomyelitis of the foot and ankle can arise from multiple etiologies, and one of the most frequently encountered clinical scenarios is in the context of diabetic foot infections. The incidence of diabetic

Disclosures: The authors of this article received no external funding for this material. None of the authors have a relationship that might pose a conflict of interest, such as a paid consultancy, stock ownership or other equity interest, or patent-licensing agreements.
[a] Department of Orthopaedic Surgery, University of Texas Health Science Center at Houston, 6431 Fannin Street, Room MSB 6.140, Houston, TX 77030, USA; [b] Foundation for Athletic and Reconstructive Research, 6410 Fannin Street, Suite 1535, Houston, TX 77030, USA
* Corresponding author. University of Texas, 23920 Katy freeway, Suite 160, Katy, TX 77494
E-mail address: William.C.McGarvey@uth.tmc.edu

Foot Ankle Clin N Am 19 (2014) 569–588
http://dx.doi.org/10.1016/j.fcl.2014.06.012
foot.theclinics.com

foot infections is 36.5 per 1000 persons per year, with a lifetime incidence of patients with diabetes developing a diabetic foot ulcer of 25%.[2–5] Underlying osteomyelitis is present in 20% to 68% of diabetic foot ulcers.[6–9] The presence of osteomyelitis in diabetic foot infections has an amputation rate of up to 66%.[9,10] In-hospital mortality associated with osteomyelitis in one study was 1.6%.[11] The economic burden of osteomyelitis is severe, with a median length of stay of 7 hospital days, mean hospital charges $19,000, and the direct costs of amputation associated with osteomyelitis exceeding $34,000.[2,3,11] Understanding how to accurately diagnose and effectively treat osteomyelitis is critical for the foot and ankle surgeon.

CLASSIFICATION AND PATHOPHYSIOLOGY OF OSTEOMYELITIS

Several classifications of osteomyelitis and diabetic foot wounds exist. Classification of osteomyelitis popularized by Waldvogel focused on the duration and mechanism of infection.[12] The duration of osteomyelitis is classified as acute, subacute, or chronic. Acute osteomyelitis refers to inflammatory bone changes caused by pathogens with symptoms manifesting within 2 weeks of infection.[12,13] Histologic findings of acute osteomyelitis include microorganisms, neutrophil infiltration, and congested or thrombosed nutrient blood vessels.[10,14] Chronic osteomyelitis is defined by the presence of necrotic bone and the absence of osteocytes, and symptoms may not occur until 6 weeks of infection.[10,12–14] Mechanisms of infection in osteomyelitis include hematogenous or exogenous spread. Hematogenous osteomyelitis involves bacteremia and seeding of the bone with an organism from a remote source.[12] Hematogenous osteomyelitis is primarily seen in pediatric patients, patients with chronic indwelling catheters, and intravenous drug abusers.[15] It generally occurs in bones with rich blood supply, such as the metaphases of long bones in children and the vertebral bodies of adults.[12,16] Exogenous osteomyelitis occurs from direct inoculation of the bone caused by contiguous spread from adjacent tissue, open fractures, penetrating trauma, or iatrogenic postsurgical contamination.[12,15,16] In diabetic foot osteomyelitis, there typically is contiguous spread from adjacent soft tissue infection or ulcer.

The pathophysiology of osteomyelitis begins as the infection spreads through the periosteum or is seeded hematogenously and extends within the medullary canal. The increased intramedullary pressure secondary to inflammation leads to bone necrosis and the overlying periosteal reaction begins the formation of new bone, creating an involucrum.[1] Inflammatory factors and leukocytes further contribute to bone necrosis and destruction. Local vascular channels are compressed and obliterated by the inflammatory process, creating areas of necrosis and sequestra where antibiotic penetration is insufficient.[1] At the edge of the infarcted microvascular channels, there is relative hyperemia, which causes bone dissolution and localized osteoporosis secondary to increased osteoclastic activity.[1] Osteoclastic activity is further stimulated by inflammatory factors, such as interleukin (IL)-1 and tumor necrosis factor released by inflammatory cells in response to bacterial antigens, leading to further attempts at remodeling because of dissolution.[6]

The Cierny classification of chronic osteomyelitis uses the anatomic location and extent of infection and also considers the physiologic factors of the patient.[17] There are four anatomic types: medullary (I), superficial (II), localized (III), and diffuse (IV). Based on the comorbidities and clinical status of the patient, the physiologic class of the host is defined as normal (A host), compromised (B host), or prohibitive (C host). This classification is presented in **Table 1**.

Consideration of surrounding soft tissues or staging of diabetic foot wounds is also important in foot and ankle osteomyelitis. The Wagner classification of diabetic foot

Table 1
Cierny and Mader system for chronic osteomyelitis

Anatomic type		
I	Medullary	Nidus is medullary; endosteal disease
II	Superficial	Infection limited to cortical surface infected because of coverage defect
III	Localized	Localized infection involving a stable, well-demarcated lesion with full-thickness cortical sequestration and cavitation Complete excision/debridement does NOT lead to instability
IV	Diffuse	Diffuse osteomyelitic lesion with mechanical instability that requires complex reconstruction
Physiologic class		
A host	Normal	Immunocompetent with good local vascularity; will have normal immune response to infection and healing response to surgery
B host	Compromised	Local or systemic factors that compromise immunity or healing potential
C host	Prohibitive	Results of treatment are potentially more damaging than the presenting condition

wounds consists of six grades: high-risk foot without ulcer (grade 0), superficial noninfected ulcer (grade 1), deep infected ulcer with limited cellulitis (grade 2), very deep infected ulcer with tendon/fascial and/or bone involvement (grade 3), limited gangrene (grade 4), or extensive gangrene and tissue necrosis (grade 5).[18] This classification is presented in **Table 2**.

EPIDEMIOLOGY

Many cases (11%–55%) of osteomyelitis in diabetic foot infections are polymicrobial, with an average of 2.3 organisms isolated per patient.[19–22] The most frequently isolated organism in osteomyelitis is *Staphylococcus aureus* (up to 49.2% of cases).[21,23] *S aureus* adheres to multiple components of the bone matrix, including fibrinogen, fibronectin, laminin, bone sialoglycoprotein, and clumping factor A via bacterial surface protein adhesins known as microbial surface components recognizing adhesive matrix molecules.[1,16,24,25] *S aureus* also has several mechanisms to resist host defenses. Staphylococcal protein A is expressed on the cell wall and binds to IgG via Fc-reactive sites, defending against phagocytosis.[1] The surface proteins of *S aureus* induce the release of tumor necrosis factor-α, prostaglandins, and IL-1 from immune

Table 2
Wagner classification of diabetic foot wounds

Wagner Grade 0	Wagner Grade 1	Wagner Grade 2	Wagner Grade 3	Wagner Grade 4	Wagner Grade 5
High-risk foot, no ulcerations	Superficial, noninfected ulcer	Deep, infected ulcer Limited cellulitis	Deep, infected ulcer with tendon, fascia, and/or bone involvement	Limited gangrene	Extensive gangrene

cells, which increase osteoclast activity and cause osteolysis.[6,26] *S aureus* forms a polysaccharide pseudocapsule "biofilm" that further secures it to bone or surgical implants and interferes with opsonization, phagocytosis, and antibiotic penetration.[1,25] *Staphylococcus epidermidis*, group A streptococcus, and *Pseudomonas aeroginosa* can also form biofilms in osteomyelitis.[1]

Methicillin-resistant *S aureus* (MRSA) prevalence is increasing and accounts for 15.3% of osteomyelitis in diabetic foot infections.[23,27] MRSA and other multidrug-resistant organism infections are more common in institutionalized patients or patients with a history of recurrent or recent hospitalization.[28] MRSA infections are associated with a higher body temperature and white blood cell count than methicillin-sensitive *S aureus* osteomyelitic infections.[29] Patients with MRSA osteomyelitis of the foot and ankle have been shown to undergo a greater number of surgical procedures to achieve eradication of the infection, but there is not a statistically significant difference in amputation rate or healing time when early aggressive treatment is initiated between MRSA and methicillin-sensitive *S aureus* osteomyelitis.[6,28–30] The rise in prevalence of MRSA infections has prompted many clinicians to include empirical broad-spectrum antibiotic treatment as part of early, aggressive treatment and later tailor antibiotic therapy according to culture and sensitivity data.[29,30]

P aeruginosa is isolated in 2.5% to 14.6% of foot osteomyelitic infections.[21,23] *Pseudomonas* is a common infecting organism in hematogenous osteomyelitis associated with intravenous drug abuse.[31] A history of a puncture wound to the foot is another common etiologic factor in *Pseudomonas* osteomyelitis.[23] *P aeruginosa* osteomyelitis of the foot is associated with a significantly higher recurrence rate and more strongly correlated with amputation than *S aureus* osteomyelitis.[32]

Other common organisms include gram-negative bacteria (7.0%–33.7%), *Streptococcus* (15.4%), coliforms (8.5%), and anaerobes (11.5%).[21,23] Enterobacteriacae are the most common gram-negative bacteria isolated.[21] *Enterococcus* is a gram-positive bacteria commonly found in patients who have received prior treatment with cephalosporins, because *Enterococcus* has inherent resistance to these antibiotics.[21,22] Group B streptococcus is the most likely organism in otherwise healthy 2- to 4-week old infants with osteomyelitis and is also a common contaminant in patients with a history of skin ulceration or surgery.[31] Fungal infections are seen in patients receiving prolonged intravenous therapy or parental nutrition for chronic illnesses.[31,33] These are often attributed to specimen contamination, but fungal osteomyelitis is a real entity and must be addressed if identified because of difficulty with complete eradication. Anaerobic infections are more likely to be present in cases of infections that are severe, long-standing, resistant to antibiotic therapy, and accompanied by foul odor and necrotic tissue debris.[21,34] *Salmonella* is a common organism in osteomylitic infections in patients with sickle cell or sickle trait hemoglobinopathies.[31]

DIAGNOSING OSTEOMYELITIS
History and Physical Examination

The history and physical examination can be very informative when approaching suspected osteomyelitis. Pertinent historical information includes the timing, duration, nature, and quality of symptoms, such as swelling, fevers, chills, myalgias, diaphoresis, drainage, pain, and redness.[1] Symptoms are often vague, highly variable, and lack specificity when used in isolation. History of trauma, travel, or environmental exposures is essential. A comprehensive past medical history should focus on current or chronic illnesses, the history and management of comorbid conditions, surgical history, functional and ambulatory status, age, overall health, and nutritional status. In diabetic patients, the duration of disease, current and past medications, history of glycemic control, and presence of microvascular or macrovascular complications, especially neuropathy or peripheral vascular disease, should be documented.[1,4,13] Factors significantly associated with the presence of osteomyelitis include increased duration of diabetes, history of previous foot ulcer, prior lower-extremity amputation, lower-extremity vascular procedure, Charcot-type foot fracture, or history of recurrent foot infections.[5]

On physical examination, it is important to note any contractures, foot deformities, or gait abnormalities. The Silfverskiöld knee flexion test is used to distinguish between isolated gastrocnemius contracture and combined shortening of the gastrocnemius-soleus complex in nonspastic contracture by measuring the range of ankle dorsiflexion with the knee flexed and the knee straight.[35] Increased dorsiflexion with the knee flexed indicates isolated gastrocnemius contracture. Semmes-Weinstein monofilament testing with a 4.5-g should be performed to evaluate for neuropathy.[36] Examination and documentation of the vascular status of the extremity, including pulses, skin, and presence or absence of swelling, is critical.[6] The presence and location of skin callouses on the foot should be noted because these indicate sites of pressure. In a nonneuropathic foot, pressure most commonly occurs in the plantar forefoot at the metatarsal heads, especially the first and second toes or the fifth metatarsophalangeal joint.[10,14] Accordingly, the metatarsal heads are the most common location of osteomyelitis in diabetic feet.[6] In neuropathic feet, callous can also predominate over the posterior plantar calcaneus.[10,14] In neuropathic feet with mid-foot prominence and a rocker-bottom foot deformity, callous is most prominent under the cuboid.[10] Local signs of inflammation including the classic redness (rubor), tenderness (dolor), heat (calor), and swelling (tumor) all alert the clinician to maintain a high suspicion for infection.[1] In delineating erythema secondary to neuro-osteoarthropathy, the erythema tends to be dependent and resolve with elevation of the extremity, whereas the erythema is less likely to resolve with elevation in cases of infection.[6] One highly suggestive clinical finding of pedal osteomyelitis is the "sausage toe" deformity: the toe is swollen and erythematous with obliteration of the normal toe contour in addition to a local ulceration of the toe or adjacent metatarsophalangeal joint.[10,37]

Documentation of the size, depth, location, drainage, and a detailed probe examination should be included when an ulcer or sinus tract is present. A greater than 2 cm^2 diabetic foot ulcer has a sensitivity of 56% and specificity of 92% in diagnosing underlying osteomyelitis.[8] Ulcer depth greater than 3 mm is also highly suggestive of underlying osteomyelitis, with a univariate odds ratio (OR) of 10.4.[3] The "probe-to-bone" test is performed at bedside and has a sensitivity of 56% to 66%, specificity of 85% to 92%, positive predictive value of 89%, and OR 5.0 in the diagnosis of osteomyelitis.[3,7,38–40] The "probe-to-bone" test is performed by probing the wound with a sterile, blunt, stainless steel probe; a positive test is indicated if a hard, gritty structure (bone) is encountered.[7] Exposed bone has a positive likelihood ratio (LR) of 9.2 for osteomyelitis in diabetic foot wounds.[3] One study calculated the pooled diagnostic OR for exposed bone or a positive probe-to-bone test to be 49.45, indicating that these tests when positive have excellent power to determine the presence of osteomyelitis.[40]

Laboratory Studies

Laboratory markers are useful in diagnosis and trending therapeutic efficacy in osteomyelitis. A complete blood cell count with differential is indicated in patients with a suspected infection or inflammatory conditions. White blood cell count greater than $11.0 \times 10^3/\mu L$ (OR, 6.3) and a neutrophil percentage greater than 70% (OR, 3.8) are suggestive of osteomyelitis.[3] The white blood cell count may be normal, however, and is only elevated in 35% of patients.[4,41,42] A basic or comprehensive metabolic panel contains useful markers of the physiologic status of the patient. The calcium, phosphorus, and alkaline phosphatase levels are elevated in malignancy and metabolic disorders, whereas they are normal in osteomyelitis.[43] The nutritional status can be assessed on values of serum proteins (malnutrition is defined as albumin <3.5 mg/dL; prealbumin <15 mg/dL; transferrin <200 mg/dL), nitrogen balance, cholesterol, and creatinine.[44] The measure of glycosylated hemoglobin (HbA_{1c}) is a useful marker of compliance and glucose control in diabetic patients. Patients with higher HbA_{1c} values have longer healing times and higher rates of amputation in patients with lower-extremity ulcers and osteomyelitis.[40,45,46]

The erythrocyte sedimentation rate (ESR) is a marker of inflammation that is elevated in osteomyelitis within 24 hours of the onset of symptoms, returning to normal after 3 to 4 weeks of adequate treatment.[25] An ESR of greater than or equal to 70 mm/h has a sensitivity of 89%, specificity of 100%, and positive LR of 11 (95% confidence interval, 1.6–79.0), making it highly suggestive of osteomyelitis.[3,39,47] In 70% of cases with osteomyelitis, however, the ESR is less than 70 mm/h.[10] An ESR less than 70 has a summary LR of 0.34 (95% confidence interval, 0.06–1.90).[39] ESR greater than 60 mm/h in addition to clinical indicators (ulcer depth >3 mm) has an accuracy of 88% in the prediction of osteomyelitis.[3]

C-reactive protein (CRP) is a measure of the acute phase response to inflammation and is highly sensitive in the diagnosis of osteomyelitis. CRP is elevated within 6 hours of onset of symptoms, peaks within 48 hours of infection, and begins to normalize within 1 week of disease resolution.[25] CRP greater than 3.2 mg/dL has a sensitivity of 85%, specificity of 77%, negative LR of −0.23, OR of 10.8, and accuracy of 88%.[3] The CRP normalizes more rapidly than the ESR value; both should be monitored weekly to monitor the course of treatment in osteomyelitis.[25]

Novel markers of bone turnover are being investigated, and may have utility in the diagnosis and monitoring of treatment of patients with osteomyelitis. One study compared two such markers, serum amino-terminal telopeptides and bone alkaline phosphatase, in patients with diabetes with and without osteomyelitis but failed to note a difference.[48] Other antimicrobial peptides and biomarkers, such as IL-1 and IL-6, are being studied in orthopedic periprosthetic joint infections, and may have further utility in osteomyelitis.[49] Further investigation is required to determine the clinical application of such tests.

Imaging Modalities

Plain radiographs are an appropriate and indicated first step in the evaluation of a patient with suspected osteomyelitis. Initial radiographs may be negative or show only soft tissue swelling, which typically develops 1 to 3 days after the onset of infection. The radiographic signs of osteomyelitis include periosteal reaction, sequestra, loss of trabecular pattern, or cortical destruction and typically are not seen until 10 to 14 days after the onset of infection.[6,16,50–52] Bone mineral loss of 30% to 50% is required before positive radiographic findings are evident on plain radiographs.[51,53–55] Therefore, radiographs should be repeated within 2 to 4 weeks when clinical suspicion of osteomyelitis persists.[4,10,56] In addition, plain radiographs provide valuable information on foot alignment, joint congruency, and bony architecture. In chronic osteomyelitis with a draining sinus tract, sinography performed by injecting radiopaque liquid into the sinus tract can aid in localizing the focus of infection.[53]

Computed tomography (CT) provides excellent definition of cortical bone. Because of this, it is extremely useful in identifying sequestra, periosteal reaction, extent of bony erosion, and cortical destruction.[53,57] CT also visualizes small foci of gas within the medullary canal, foreign bodies, soft tissue changes, and the full extent of sinus tracts.[57] When MRI is unavailable because of patient factors or contraindications, CT is the study of choice to localize osteomyelitis.[57]

Nuclear medicine studies are useful in the diagnosis of osteomyelitis.[58–60] Three-phase technetium-99m methylene diphosphate (MDP) bone scan can confirm the diagnosis of osteomyelitis within 24 to 48 hours of onset.[53,61] A normal three-phase Tc-99m MDP bone scan nearly entirely excludes the diagnosis of osteomyelitis.[55,62] Three-phase bone scintigraphy uses a radiotracer and images at three phases: (1) nuclear angiogram/blood flow phase (immediately after injection), (2) blood pool phase (within 5 minutes of injection), and (3) a bone phase (3 hours after injection).[63] Cellulitis is characterized by high uptake in the blood flow and blood pool phases, with normal intake in the bone phase. In contrast, osteomyelitis has increasing uptake over all three phases throughout the course of the study.[63] The pooled sensitivity and specificity for three-phase bone study is 81% and 28%, respectively, with a diagnostic OR of 2.10 and summary measure of accuracy (Q*) of 0.60.[40] The limited specificity is caused by the uptake of the radiotracer at all sites of bone metabolism, irrespective of the underlying cause.[64] In patients with early high uptake intensity, further delayed images are not needed to make an accurate diagnosis of osteomyelitis.[10] In patients with early, mild uptake intensity, many advocate the addition of a fourth phase at 24 hours because this increases the overall accuracy of the test from 80% to 85%.[10,55,65]

Gallium scan is slightly more specific than bone scanning, but false-positives can occur in areas of bone healing, neuropathic fractures, neoplasm, or noninfected prostheses.[1,66] Gallium scans use gallium-67 citrate, which binds to acute phase reactants, such as transferrin and lactoferrin as they travel in the bloodstream to areas of infection where the metabolism of iron by bacteria, chemotaxis, and uptake by leukocytes cause focal accumulation of the isotope.[1,51] Imaging is performed 24 hours after the injection of the isotope.[1] Normal gallium scan virtually excludes the presence of osteomyelitis and can be useful as a follow-up examination postoperatively to confirm eradication of the focus of osteomyelitis.[31] The reported sensitivity ranges from 25% to 80% with a specificity of 67% for gallium-67 scans.[1]

Indium-111–labeled leukocyte scans are extremely useful in differentiating acute osteomyelitis from neuro-osteoarthropathy in the diabetic foot.[31,51] Indium-111–labeled leukocytes accumulate at the site of infection by chemotaxis, then cross capillary walls (diapedesis). Leukocyte scans have a high sensitivity and specificity even in the face of coexisting fractures, adjacent cellulitis, and neuro-osteoarthropathy.[51] Chronic infections are not well imaged with indium-111, because the labeled leukocyte preparation consists primarily of neutrophils, whereas monocytes and lymphocytes predominate in chronic infection.[4,67] Leukocyte scans have a reported sensitivity of 89%, diagnostic OR of 10.7, and Q* of 0.59.[40] Combining Tc-99m MDP and indium-111 increases the ability to detect osteomyelitis, with a 100% sensitivity and 89% specificity reported.[4] This combination is useful, because the Tc-99m MDP scan localizes the anatomic site of infection and the indium-111 labels the infected bone.[68] Indium-111–labeled leukocyte scan combined with Tc-99m MDP scintigraphy is the imaging of choice in posttraumatic and nonunion site osteomyelitic infections.[64,69]

Fluorodeoxyglucose-labeled positron emission tomography (FDG-PET) uses 18-FDG, a marker of increased intracellular glucose metabolism, and monitors its accumulation in areas of inflammation and infection.[57,70] FDG-PET has the highest accuracy of confirming or excluding the diagnosis of chronic osteomyelitis, with a pooled sensitivity of 96% and specificity of 91%.[66,67,71] Standardized uptake values in regions of sterile neuro-osteoarthropathy tend to be lower (0.7–2.4) and located in the midfoot, whereas the standardized uptake values associated with osteomyelitis are higher (2.9–6.2) and more likely located in the forefoot or calcaneus.[72] In cases with equivocal MRI findings or adjacent metal hardware complicating imaging, FDG-PET is a useful adjuvant.[64,67] FDG-PET alone has low spatial resolution compared with other imaging modalities, but this is easily overcome to achieve excellent anatomic detail and localization with the combined FDG-PET/CT study.[64,67,72]

Magnetic resonance imaging (MRI) is considered to be the imaging study of choice for the diagnosis and treatment of osteomyelitis.[50,57,67,73,74] MRI is useful in detecting intraosseous and subperiosteal abscesses, provides clear anatomic detail, does not expose the patient to ionizing radiation, and is rapidly completed and readily available in most centers.[31,75] The addition of gadolinium contrast improves the result and gives better anatomic detail of soft tissue involvement.[57] In acute osteomyelitis, the diagnosis on MRI is made based on altered bone marrow signal and signs of edema and inflammation in adjacent soft tissues. In chronic osteomyelitis, MRI may demonstrate a well-defined rim of high signal intensity surrounding a focus of active disease, known as the "rim sign."[57] On T1-weighted images, bone marrow becomes low signal intensity in acute osteomyelitis because there is a loss of fat in the bone marrow.[6,57] T2 and short-tau inversion recovery images demonstrate high signal intensity in the bone marrow, sinus tracts, and areas of soft tissue inflammation and cellulitis.[6,14,76] Osseous extent is best determined on T1 images, because T2 images can overestimate the amount of infected bone in preoperative planning.[14,77] Both osteomyelitis and bone marrow edema have high signal on T2 and short-tau inversion recovery MRI images; bone marrow edema has a normal T1 image, whereas osteomyelitis has a low signal density.[14,78] Soft tissue abscesses demonstrate low to intermediate signal on T1-weighted images and high signal on T2 images.[14] The pooled sensitivity of MRI in the diagnosis of osteomyelitis is 90%, specificity 79%, and diagnostic OR of 24.36, indicating excellent discriminatory power.[40] An overview of imaging studies useful in the diagnosis and treatment of osteomyelitis is found in **Table 3**.

Perfusion Studies

Arterial perfusion is an important clinical parameter to consider in the evaluation and treatment of osteomyelitis. Peripheral vascular disease contributes to ulceration and impaired wound healing, and decreases the ability to fight infection by disrupting the delivery of immune cells, oxygen, nutrients, and antibiotics to the affected extremity.[79] Diabetic peripheral vascular disease preferentially affects the tibial and peroneal arteries, and also the microvascular system.[79] Other risk factors for peripheral vascular disease include a positive family history, hypertension, tobacco use, hyperlipidemia, obesity, and hyperhomocystinemia.[79] Ankle brachial index is a noninvasive test that can be a useful objective measure of limb perfusion. A systolic ankle pressure of less than 50 mm Hg or ankle brachial index less than 0.6 suggests critical limb ischemia.[79] An absolute toe pressure of less than 30 mm Hg is considered inadequate for wound healing.[79,80] Ankle brachial index can be falsely elevated because of medial arterial calcinosis.[4,79] Another minimally invasive perfusion study is the arterial Doppler waveform or pulse volume recordings. Normal arterial waveforms are triphasic with good amplitude, reflective of the elasticity and recoil of healthy arterial wall musculature. Hemodynamically significant calcinosis or stenosis is demonstrated by blunting of the amplitude and biphasic or monophasic waveforms on the pulse volume recordings.[79] Transcutaneous oxygen tension is another minimally invasive test to quantify tissue ischemia. Normal transcutaneous oxygen tension is defined as greater than or equal to 55 mm Hg. Tension of 30 mm Hg or greater suggests the arterial blood supply may be adequate for healing; less than 30 mm Hg prompts further vascular studies and possibly vascular interventions because wound healing is questionable.[4,79]

Arteriography is the gold standard for defining the anatomic location and extent of atherosclerotic occlusive disease of the lower extremities.[79] Angiography, although invasive, may allow for diagnosis and endovascular interventions, such as balloon angioplasty and stenting, in one procedure for the patient.[38] In patients with contraindications (especially renal) to angiography, MR angiography may be a useful alternative.[79]

Microbiology Studies

The gold standard diagnostic test for osteomyelitis is to obtain a biopsy specimen for histologic and microbiologic evaluation.[1,4,5,20,81] Culture and sensitivity data establish a definitive diagnosis and are invaluable in implementing an appropriate antibiotic regimen. Samples taken from an ulcer or sinus tract drainage are not sufficient to identify and isolate the causative organism in osteomyelitis, with concordance rates reported of 26% to 44%, a false-negative rate of 52%, and a false-positive rate of 36%.[1,16,81–84] When obtaining open biopsy specimens intraoperatively, it is necessary for the surgeon to send soft tissue and bone specimens for microbiologic evaluation, because only 36% of soft tissue cultures accurately identify the bone pathogen.[20] Intraoperative frozen sections can be useful. Greater than 5 to 10 neutrophils per high power field is highly suggestive of acute deep infection.[4] Blood cultures can identify the causative organism in up to 50% of cases of hematogenous osteomyelitis.[16]

Percutaneous bone biopsy may be considered to obtain bacteriologic culture and sensitivity data when prolonged medical treatment is indicated. To accurately interpret these data, antibiotic therapy must be discontinued for 2 to 4 weeks prior (to avoid a false-negative result) and the needle must be inserted through normal skin, avoiding all ulcers or areas of soft tissue infection, to obtain the bone sample.[10] Percutaneous biopsy under CT guidance may be helpful in accurate anatomic localization over fluoroscopic guidance. The current recommendation of the Infectious Diseases Society of America is that percutaneous bone biopsy only be considered in the following circumstances: (1) uncertainty regarding the diagnosis of osteomyelitis despite clinical and imaging evaluations, (2) absent or unclear culture data from soft tissue specimens, (3) failure of empiric antibiotic therapy, and (4) a desire to use antibiotic agents that may be especially effective for osteomyelitis but have a high potential for selecting resistant organisms.[54]

TREATMENT OF OSTEOMYELITIS

Effective management of osteomyelitis is best achieved with a multifaceted approach involving medical optimization of the patient's physiologic status; infectious disease consultation for targeted antibiotic therapies and treatment durations; and surgical specialists for debridement, revascularization, wound care, and soft tissue or limb reconstruction when necessary. Antibiotic suppression is most effective when broad-spectrum empiric antibiotics are initiated early and therapies are then tailored with the help of an infectious disease specialist as culture and sensitivity data become available.[6,19,33,85] Collaboration with a primary care provider to optimize the patient's physiology and comorbid conditions is essential for successful management of

Table 3
Summary of imaging modalities, characteristic findings, and clinical application in osteomyelitis

Imaging Modality	Findings of Osteomyelitis	Clinical Application
Plain radiographs	Periosteal reaction, sequestra, cortical destruction, loss of trabecular organization, soft tissue swelling	Appropriate initial imaging study Provides information on foot alignment, joint congruency, and bony architecture Repeat radiographs in 2–4 wk when clinical suspicion persists
CT	Periosteal reaction, sequestra, cortical destruction, soft tissue swelling, sinus tracts, intramedullary gas foci, foreign bodies	Provides excellent anatomic definition of cortical bone Study of choice to localize infection when MRI is unavailable
Tc-99m MDP bone scan	Increasing uptake in affected area over all three phases: blood-flow phase, blood-pool phase, and bone phase (in cellulitis, high uptake only seen during blood-flow and blood-pool phases)	Findings evident within 24–48 h of symptom onset Limited specificity because of uptake of radiotracer at all sites of increased bone metabolism May add fourth phase at 24 h in patients with early, mild intensity uptake to increase accuracy
Gallium-67 citrate scan	Increased accumulation of isotope in affected areas (gallium binds to acute-phase reactants, taken up by leukocytes and used by bacteria for iron metabolism)	Normal gallinium scan virtually excludes osteomyelitis, therefore useful postdebridement to confirm eradication False-positives may occur in areas of bone healing, neoplasms, neuro-osteoarthropathy, and around prostheses

Indium-111–labeled leukocyte scan	Neutrophils accumulate at areas of acute infection by chemotaxis and diapedesis	Useful when coexisting fractures, cellulitis, or osteoarthopathy is present Chronic infections not well imaged, because monocytes and lymphocytes predominate Indium-111 leukocyte scan combined with Tc99m bone scan is the modality of choice in posttraumatic and nonunion site osteomyelitis
FDG-PET	Increased accumulation in areas with increased intracellular glucose metabolism	Highest accuracy imaging study in chronic osteomyelitis Poor spatial resolution, therefore combined with CT scan (PET/CT) for excellent anatomic detail PET/CT is imaging study of choice when MRI is equivocal or hardware scatter complicates imaging
MRI	In acute osteomyelitis T1: low signal intensity in bone marrow, determine osseous extent T2/short-tau inversion recovery: high signal intensity in bone marrow, sinus tracts, and soft tissue inflammation In chronic osteomyelitis "Rim sign," well-defined rim of high signal intensity surrounding active disease focus	Imaging study of choice in osteomyelitis Gadolinium contrast improves anatomic detail of soft tissues

osteomyelitis. These include tight glycemic control, tobacco cessation, treatment of hepatic and/or renal dysfunction, and optimization of the patient's nutritional status.[1,5,23,31,86–89] When indicated, aggressive arterial reconstruction of the limb results in improved wound healing and a five-fold increase in limb salvage.[11] The foot and ankle surgeon must consider optimization of foot biomechanics, including tendoachilles lengthening, correction to a plantigrade foot, appropriate footwear or orthoses, and preservation of the soft tissue envelope with avoidance of bony pressure or contact points.[90]

Surgical Management

Key principles of surgical treatment of osteomyelitis involve complete debridement of all devitalized tissue, stabilization of the bone and soft tissues, appropriate specimen collection and antibiotic delivery, and a well-vascularized soft tissue envelope covering contact points. Surgical debridement is indicated in the presence of an abscess, necrotic tissue, systemic indicators of sepsis, or failure to improve despite adequate antibiotic therapies.[1,31] Numerous factors including site and extent of infection, physiologic status of the patient, and surgeon preference formulate the surgical treatment. Surgical debridement and antibiotic therapy historically achieved success rates nearing 70%.[91–93] Advances over the past 40 years including the use of antibiotic cement, advances in soft tissue procedures, improved bone grafting techniques, and multiplanar external fixator techniques have led to success rates greater than 90%.[94–102]

Surgical debridement removes all nonviable tissue in an expansive manner with a focus on preserving blood supply to the area. Bony debridement should remove necrotic, sclerotic, and avascular bone while minimizing periosteal stripping. Bone resection proceeds until pinpoint bleeding bone (Paprika sign) is encountered.[17] Wide debridements, with serial debridements when necessary, are preferable to leaving nonviable tissue behind despite the size of defect created.[17,31]

Bony stability must be assessed and restored. External fixation is frequently used to provide stabilization while keeping the infected area free of surface implants that may become colonized. A newer technique that has shown effectiveness in small studies is the use of antibiotic coated intramedullary nails.[99,100,103] Although this technique provides for some stabilization of the bone, it is typically supplemented with additional procedures or methods to address the tissue and bony dead space.

There are multiple options for the management of bony defects. Antibiotic cement beads are often used to provide high local antibiotic concentrations (up to 200 times higher than systemic antibiotic levels) with lower systemic toxicity and fill dead space.[31,104] Antibiotic beads made of polymethylmethacrylate and clindamycin, vancomycin, and/or tobramycin have been shown to have the highest local bioavailability and elution.[97] Bacteriocidal levels of antibiotics are maintained for 2 to 4 weeks, at which time the beads can be removed and replaced with cancellous bone graft or vascularized bone graft. This technique and its many variations have success rates near 90%.[101,102,105,106] Autograft cancellous grafts can be harvested from the calcaneus, proximal tibia, and iliac crest. Novel techniques allow harvest of autograft cancellous bone graft from the intramedullary canal using the Reamer/Irrigator/Aspirator device (DePuy Synthes, Paoli, PA). Allograft cancellous graft is widely commercially available. Structural (corticocancellous) grafts can be obtained with or without a vascular pedicle from the iliac crest, fibula, ribs, and scapula. The utility and efficacy of osteoinductive and osteoconductive materials, such as bone morphogenic proteins, demineralized bone matrix, and various calcium scaffold complexes for management of bone defects in the setting of osteomyelitis, are currently being explored.

In certain situations of extensive bone loss, the Ilizarov technique of external fixation with distraction osteogenesis has the benefit of stabilizing the bone and providing a mechanism for managing the bony defect.[107–109] In this technique, the bony defect is eliminated by bone transport or acute shortening of the limb followed by distraction osteogenesis at a distant corticotomy site to regain the lost length. This technique can also be combined with intentional deformity, which is frequently used to allow for closure of the soft tissues overlying the site of the defect without the need for muscle flap or free flap coverage.[110] In this technique, the deformity is then slowly corrected allowing for tissue stretching after healing of the wound.

An essential component of the treatment of osteomyelitis is closure or coverage of any soft tissue defects to allow for adequate blood flow to the area. Consultation with a reconstructive plastic surgeon or an orthopedic surgeon familiar with management of soft tissue defects may be necessary. Multiple options exist for coverage of defects including rotational muscle flaps, free muscle, and fasciocutaneous flaps.[111–113]

Indications for amputation include arterial insufficiency, major nerve paralysis or paresthesias, and severe joint contractures or stiffness that renders the limb nonfunctional.[31,90,114] Patient factors associated with amputation include previous ulceration (OR, 0.23), HgA$_{1c}$ greater than 7.4 (OR, 5.9), soft tissue infection accompanying osteomyelitis (OR, 5.9), peripheral arterial disease (OR, 6.2), and skin necrosis (OR, 12.2).[45]

Adjunctive Therapies

Several adjunctive therapies may be considered. Hyperbaric oxygen therapy affects the microenvironment of wounds and has been shown to promote healing in diabetic wounds through its antiedema, antibacterial, and neovascularization effects.[115,116] In hyperbaric conditions, wound tissue oxygen tension can be increased 10- to 15-fold, which stimulates fibroblast proliferation, collagen production, neovascularization, and epithelialization, and has direct lethal effects on anaerobic organisms.[1,116,117] Hyperbaric oxygen therapy may prove useful as an adjunctive therapy in the treatment of osteomyelitis.[31,116,118] Growth factors, such as bone morphogenic proteins, enhance bone healing and callous formation at infection sites.[119] Platelet-rich plasma and leukocyte- and platelet-rich plasma gel have demonstrated faster healing times, eradication of infection, positive synergy with antibiotic therapy, and antimicrobial effects in several animal models and case studies.[120–123] Some studies using pulsed electromagnetic fields and ultrasound suggest these physical energy modalities may directly interfere with biofilm formation, increase bone formation and maturation, accelerate soft tissue healing, and work synergistically with antibiotic therapies to increase their efficacy.[124–128] Further research is needed on the efficacy and application of these adjunctive therapies for clinical use in osteomyelitis of the foot and ankle.

SUMMARY

Osteomyelitis of the foot and ankle is a common, potentially devastating condition with diagnostic and treatment challenges. An understanding of the epidemiology and pathogenesis of osteomyelitis can raise clinical suspicion and guide further testing and treatments. History and physical examination, laboratory studies, vascular studies, histologic and microbiologic analyses, and various imaging modalities contribute to the diagnosis and treatment. Treatment should take a multidisciplinary approach to optimize patient factors, ensure eradication of the infection, and restore function. Empiric broad-spectrum antibiotic treatment should be included in early, aggressive treatment, with later antibiotic regimens tailored according to culture and sensitivity data. Surgical treatment needs to consider physiologic factors of the infection and patient, must be extensive, and may use multiple techniques to achieve successful outcomes. Optimization of vascular status, soft tissues, limb biomechanics, and the physiologic state of the patient must all be considered to accelerate and ensure healing. Adjuvant therapies and novel laboratory markers may enhance outcomes as they are further studied and applied clinically.

REFERENCES

1. Chihara S, Segreti J. Osteomyelitis [Systematic review or meta-analysis]. Dis Mon 2010;56(1):5–31.
2. Tennvall GR, Apelqvist J, Eneroth M. Costs of deep foot infections in patients with diabetes mellitus. Pharmacoeconomics 2000;18(3):225–38.
3. Fleischer AE, Didyk AA, Woods JB, et al. Combined clinical and laboratory testing improves diagnostic accuracy for osteomyelitis in the diabetic foot. J Foot Ankle Surg 2009;48(1):39–46.
4. Frykberg RG, Zgonis T, Armstrong DG, et al. Diabetic foot disorders. A clinical practice guideline (2006 revision) [Systematic review or meta-analysis]. J Foot Ankle Surg 2006;45(Suppl 5):S1–66.
5. Lavery LA, Peters EJ, Armstrong DG, et al. Risk factors for developing osteomyelitis in patients with diabetic foot wounds. Diabetes Res Clin Pract 2009;83(3): 347–52.
6. Shank CF, Feibel JB. Osteomyelitis in the diabetic foot: diagnosis and management [Systematic review or meta-analysis]. Foot Ankle Clin 2006;11(4):775–89.
7. Grayson ML, Gibbons GW, Balogh K, et al. Probing to bone in infected pedal ulcers. A clinical sign of underlying osteomyelitis in diabetic patients. JAMA 1995;273(9):721–3.
8. Newman LG, Waller J, Palestro CJ, et al. Unsuspected osteomyelitis in diabetic foot ulcers. Diagnosis and monitoring by leukocyte scanning with indium in 111 oxyquinoline. JAMA 1991;266(9):1246–51.
9. Balsells M, Viade J, Millan M, et al. Prevalence of osteomyelitis in non-healing diabetic foot ulcers: usefulness of radiologic and scintigraphic findings. Diabetes Res Clin Pract 1997;38(2):123–7.
10. Hartemann-Heurtier A, Senneville E. Diabetic foot osteomyelitis [Systematic review or meta-analysis]. Diabetes Metab 2008;34(2):87–95.
11. Henke PK, Blackburn SA, Wainess RW, et al. Osteomyelitis of the foot and toe in adults is a surgical disease: conservative management worsens lower extremity salvage. Ann Surg 2005;241(6):885–92 [discussion: 892–4].
12. Waldvogel FA, Medoff G, Swartz MN. Osteomyelitis: a review of clinical features, therapeutic considerations and unusual aspects (second of three parts) [Systematic review or meta-analysis]. N Engl J Med 1970;282(5):260–6.
13. Hatzenbuehler J, Pulling TJ. Diagnosis and management of osteomyelitis [Systematic review or meta-analysis]. Am Fam Physician 2011;84(9):1027–33.
14. Chatha DS, Cunningham PM, Schweitzer ME. MR imaging of the diabetic foot: diagnostic challenges [Systematic review or meta-analysis]. Radiol Clin North Am 2005;43(4):747–59, ix.
15. Wald ER. Risk factors for osteomyelitis. Am J Med 1985;78(6B):206–12.
16. Skolnik NS, Albert RH. Essential infectious disease topics for primary care [Systematic review or meta-analysis]. Totowa (NJ): Humana Press; 2008.
17. Cierny G III, Mader JT, Penninck JJ. A clinical staging system for adult osteomyelitis. Clin Orthop Relat Res 2003;(414):7–24.

18. Wagner FW Jr. The diabetic foot [Systematic review or meta-analysis]. Orthopedics 1987;10(1):163–72.
19. Ge Y, MacDonald D, Hait H, et al. Microbiological profile of infected diabetic foot ulcers. Diabet Med 2002;19(12):1032–4.
20. Lavery LA, Sariaya M, Ashry H, et al. Microbiology of osteomyelitis in diabetic foot infections. J Foot Ankle Surg 1995;34(1):61–4.
21. Crouzet J, Lavigne JP, Richard JL, et al. Diabetic foot infection: a critical review of recent randomized clinical trials on antibiotic therapy [Systematic review or meta-analysis]. Int J Infect Dis 2011;15(9):e601–10.
22. Lipsky BA. Evidence-based antibiotic therapy of diabetic foot infections [Systematic review or meta-analysis]. FEMS Immunol Med Microbiol 1999;26(3–4): 267–76.
23. Acharya S, Soliman M, Egun A, et al. Conservative management of diabetic foot osteomyelitis. Diabetes Res Clin Pract 2013;101:e18–20.
24. Foster TJ, Hook M. Surface protein adhesins of Staphylococcus aureus. Trends Microbiol 1998;6(12):484–8.
25. Adcock PM, Marshall GS. Osteomyelitis of the axial skeleton and the flat and small bones [Systematic review or meta-analysis]. Semin Pediatr Infect Dis 1997;8(4):234–41.
26. Littlewood-Evans AJ, Hattenberger MR, Luscher C, et al. Local expression of tumor necrosis factor alpha in an experimental model of acute osteomyelitis in rats. Infect Immun 1997;65(8):3438–43.
27. Dang CN, Prasad YD, Boulton AJ, et al. Methicillin-resistant Staphylococcus aureus in the diabetic foot clinic: a worsening problem. Diabet Med 2003;20(2):159–61.
28. Hartemann-Heurtier A, Robert J, Jacqueminet S, et al. Diabetic foot ulcer and multidrug-resistant organisms: risk factors and impact. Diabet Med 2004; 21(7):710–5.
29. Aragon-Sanchez J, Lazaro-Martinez JL, Quintana-Marrero Y, et al. Are diabetic foot ulcers complicated by MRSA osteomyelitis associated with worse prognosis? Outcomes of a surgical series. Diabet Med 2009;26(5):552–5.
30. Richard JL, Sotto A, Jourdan N, et al. Risk factors and healing impact of multidrug-resistant bacteria in diabetic foot ulcers. Diabetes Metab 2008;34(4 Pt 1):363–9.
31. Canale ST, Beaty JH, Campbell WC. Campbell's operative orthopaedics. 12th edition. St Louis (MO); London: Mosby; 2012.
32. Tice AD, Hoaglund PA, Shoultz DA. Risk factors and treatment outcomes in osteomyelitis. J Antimicrob Chemother 2003;51(5):1261–8.
33. Cunha BA. Antibiotic selection for diabetic foot infections: a review [Systematic review or meta-analysis]. J Foot Ankle Surg 2000;39(4):253–7.
34. Lipsky BA, Berendt AR, Deery HG, et al. Diagnosis and treatment of diabetic foot infections [Systematic review or meta-analysis]. Plast Reconstr Surg 2006;117(Suppl 7):212S–38S.
35. Singh D. Nils Silfverskiold (1888-1957) and gastrocnemius contracture. Foot Ankle Surg 2013;19(2):135–8.
36. Saltzman CL, Rashid R, Hayes A, et al. 4.5-gram monofilament sensation beneath both first metatarsal heads indicates protective foot sensation in diabetic patients. J Bone Joint Surg Am 2004;86A(4):717–23.
37. Rajbhandari SM, Sutton M, Davies C, et al. Sausage toe: a reliable sign of underlying osteomyelitis. Diabet Med 2000;17(1):74–7.
38. Besse JL, Leemrijse T, Deleu PA. Diabetic foot: the orthopedic surgery angle [Systematic review or meta-analysis]. Orthop Traumatol Surg Res 2011;97(3): 314–29.

39. Butalia S, Palda VA, Sargeant RJ, et al. Does this patient with diabetes have osteomyelitis of the lower extremity? [Systematic review or meta-analysis]. JAMA 2008;299(7):806–13.
40. Dinh MT, Abad CL, Safdar N. Diagnostic accuracy of the physical examination and imaging tests for osteomyelitis underlying diabetic foot ulcers: meta-analysis [Systematic review or meta-analysis]. Clin Infect Dis 2008;47(4):519–27.
41. Armstrong DG, Lavery LA, Sariaya M, et al. Leukocytosis is a poor indicator of acute osteomyelitis of the foot in diabetes mellitus. J Foot Ankle Surg 1996; 35(4):280–3.
42. Eneroth M, Apelqvist J, Stenstrom A. Clinical characteristics and outcome in 223 diabetic patients with deep foot infections. Foot Ankle Int 1997;18(11):716–22.
43. Lew DP, Waldvogel FA. Osteomyelitis [Systematic review or meta-analysis]. Lancet 2004;364(9431):369–79.
44. Kavalukas SL, Barbul A. Nutrition and wound healing: an update [Systematic review or meta-analysis]. Plast Reconstr Surg 2011;127(Suppl 1):38S–43S.
45. Aragon-Sanchez J, Lazaro-Martinez JL. Impact of perioperative glycaemia and glycated haemoglobin on the outcomes of the surgical treatment of diabetic foot osteomyelitis. Diabetes Res Clin Pract 2011;94(3):e83–5.
46. Lepore G, Maglio ML, Cuni C, et al. Poor glucose control in the year before admission as a powerful predictor of amputation in hospitalized patients with diabetic foot ulceration. Diabetes Care 2006;29(8):1985.
47. Kaleta JL, Fleischli JW, Reilly CH. The diagnosis of osteomyelitis in diabetes using erythrocyte sedimentation rate: a pilot study. J Am Podiatr Med Assoc 2001; 91(9):445–50.
48. Nyazee HA, Finney KM, Sarikonda M, et al. Diabetic foot osteomyelitis: bone markers and treatment outcomes. Diabetes Res Clin Pract 2012;97(3):411–7.
49. Gollwitzer H, Dombrowski Y, Prodinger PM, et al. Antimicrobial peptides and proinflammatory cytokines in periprosthetic joint infection. J Bone Joint Surg Am 2013;95(7):644–51.
50. Croll SD, Nicholas GG, Osborne MA, et al. Role of magnetic resonance imaging in the diagnosis of osteomyelitis in diabetic foot infections. J Vasc Surg 1996; 24(2):266–70.
51. Harvey J, Cohen MM. Technetium-99-labeled leukocytes in diagnosing diabetic osteomyelitis in the foot. J Foot Ankle Surg 1997;36(3):209–14 [discussion: 256].
52. Wheat J. Diagnostic strategies in osteomyelitis [Systematic review or meta-analysis]. Am J Med 1985;78(6B):218–24.
53. Boutin RD, Brossmann J, Sartoris DJ, et al. Update on imaging of orthopedic infections [Systematic review or meta-analysis]. Orthop Clin North Am 1998;29(1):41–66.
54. Game FL. Osteomyelitis in the diabetic foot: diagnosis and management [Systematic review or meta-analysis]. Med Clin North Am 2013;97:947–56.
55. Hochhold J, Yang H, Zhuang H, et al. Application of 18F-fluorodeoxyglucose and PET in evaluation of the diabetic foot [Systematic review or meta-analysis]. PET Clin 2006;1(2):123–30.
56. Poirier JY, Garin E, Derrien C, et al. Diagnosis of osteomyelitis in the diabetic foot with a 99mTc-HMPAO leucocyte scintigraphy combined with a 99mTc-MDP bone scintigraphy. Diabetes Metab 2002;28(6 Pt 1):485–90.
57. Pineda C, Vargas A, Rodriguez AV. Imaging of osteomyelitis: current concepts [Systematic review or meta-analysis]. Infect Dis Clin North Am 2006;20(4):789–825.
58. van der Bruggen W, Bleeker-Rovers CP, Boerman OC, et al. PET and SPECT in osteomyelitis and prosthetic bone and joint infections: a systematic review [Systematic review or meta-analysis]. Semin Nucl Med 2010;40(1):3–15.

59. Palestro CJ, Torres MA. Radionuclide imaging in orthopedic infections [Systematic review or meta-analysis]. Semin Nucl Med 1997;27(4):334–45.
60. Palestro CJ, Love C, Miller TT. Infection and musculoskeletal conditions: imaging of musculoskeletal infections [Systematic review or meta-analysis]. Best Pract Res Clin Rheumatol 2006;20(6):1197–218.
61. Remedios D, Valabhji J, Oelbaum R, et al. 99mTc-nanocolloid scintigraphy for assessing osteomyelitis in diabetic neuropathic feet. Clin Radiol 1998;53(2): 120–5.
62. Yuh WT, Corson JD, Baraniewski HM, et al. Osteomyelitis of the foot in diabetic patients: evaluation with plain film, 99mTc-MDP bone scintigraphy, and MR imaging. AJR Am J Roentgenol 1989;152(4):795–800.
63. Schauwecker DS. The scintigraphic diagnosis of osteomyelitis [Systematic review or meta-analysis]. AJR Am J Roentgenol 1992;158(1):9–18.
64. Dioguardi P, Gaddam SR, Zhuang H, et al. FDG PET assessment of osteomyelitis: a review [Systematic review or meta-analysis]. PET Clin 2012;7(2):161–79.
65. Alazraki N, Dries D, Datz F, et al. Value of a 24-hour image (four-phase bone scan) in assessing osteomyelitis in patients with peripheral vascular disease. J Nucl Med 1985;26(7):711–7.
66. Guhlmann A, Brecht-Krauss D, Suger G, et al. Fluorine-18-FDG PET and technetium-99m antigranulocyte antibody scintigraphy in chronic osteomyelitis. J Nucl Med 1998;39(12):2145–52.
67. Basu S, Zhuang H, Alavi A. Imaging of lower extremity artery atherosclerosis in diabetic foot: FDG-PET imaging and histopathological correlates. Clin Nucl Med 2007;32(7):567–8.
68. Schauwecker DS, Park HM, Burt RW, et al. Combined bone scintigraphy and indium-111 leukocyte scans in neuropathic foot disease. J Nucl Med 1988; 29(10):1651–5.
69. Strobel K, Stumpe KD. PET/CT in musculoskeletal infection [Systematic review or meta-analysis]. Semin Musculoskelet Radiol 2007;11(4):353–64.
70. Palestro CJ. FDG-PET in musculoskeletal infections [Systematic review or meta-analysis]. Semin Nucl Med 2013;43(5):367–76.
71. Basu S, Zhuang H, Alavi A. FDG PET and PET/CT imaging in complicated diabetic foot [Systematic review or meta-analysis]. PET Clin 2012;7(2):151–60.
72. Basu S, Chryssikos T, Moghadam-Kia S, et al. Positron emission tomography as a diagnostic tool in infection: present role and future possibilities [Systematic review or meta-analysis]. Semin Nucl Med 2009;39(1):36–51.
73. Weinstein D, Wang A, Chambers R, et al. Evaluation of magnetic resonance imaging in the diagnosis of osteomyelitis in diabetic foot infections. Foot Ankle 1993;14(1):18–22.
74. Wang A, Weinstein D, Greenfield L, et al. MRI and diabetic foot infections. Magn Reson Imaging 1990;8(6):805–9.
75. Heiba SI, Kolker D, Mocherla B, et al. The optimized evaluation of diabetic foot infection by dual isotope SPECT/CT imaging protocol. J Foot Ankle Surg 2010; 49(6):529–36.
76. Roug IK, Pierre-Jerome C. MRI spectrum of bone changes in the diabetic foot. Eur J Radiol 2012;81(7):1625–9.
77. Morrison WB, Schweitzer ME, Batte WG, et al. Osteomyelitis of the foot: relative importance of primary and secondary MR imaging signs. Radiology 1998; 207(3):625–32.
78. Schweitzer ME, Morrison WB. MR imaging of the diabetic foot. Radiol Clin North Am 2004;42(1):61–71, vi.

79. Gibbons GW. Lower extremity bypass in patients with diabetic foot ulcers [Systematic review or meta-analysis]. Surg Clin North Am 2003;83(3):659–69.
80. Morrison WB, Ledermann HP. Work-up of the diabetic foot [Systematic review or meta-analysis]. Radiol Clin North Am 2002;40(5):1171–92.
81. Zuluaga AF, Galvis W, Jaimes F, et al. Lack of microbiological concordance between bone and non-bone specimens in chronic osteomyelitis: an observational study. BMC Infect Dis 2002;2:8.
82. Elamurugan TP, Jagdish S, Kate V, et al. Role of bone biopsy specimen culture in the management of diabetic foot osteomyelitis. Int J Surg 2011;9(3):214–6.
83. Senneville E, Melliez H, Beltrand E, et al. Culture of percutaneous bone biopsy specimens for diagnosis of diabetic foot osteomyelitis: concordance with ulcer swab cultures. Clin Infect Dis 2006;42(1):57–62.
84. Mackowiak PA, Jones SR, Smith JW. Diagnostic value of sinus-tract cultures in chronic osteomyelitis. JAMA 1978;239(26):2772–5.
85. Bessman AN, Sapico FL. Infections in the diabetic patient: the role of immune dysfunction and pathogen virulence factors. J Diabetes Complications 1992; 6(4):258–62.
86. Hill SL, Holtzman GI, Buse R. The effects of peripheral vascular disease with osteomyelitis in the diabetic foot. Am J Surg 1999;177(4):282–6.
87. Bamberger DM, Daus GP, Gerding DN. Osteomyelitis in the feet of diabetic patients. Long-term results, prognostic factors, and the role of antimicrobial and surgical therapy. Am J Med 1987;83(4):653–60.
88. Vardakas KZ, Horianopoulou M, Falagas ME. Factors associated with treatment failure in patients with diabetic foot infections: an analysis of data from randomized controlled trials [Systematic review or meta-analysis]. Diabetes Res Clin Pract 2008;80(3):344–51.
89. Lewis S, Raj D, Guzman NJ. Renal failure: implications of chronic kidney disease in the management of the diabetic foot. Semin Vasc Surg 2012;25(2):82–8.
90. Coughlin MJ, Saltzman CL, Anderson RB. Mann's surgery of the foot and ankle. 9th edition.
91. Burri C, Passler HH, Henkemeyer H. Treatment of posttraumatic osteomyelitis with bone, soft tissue, and skin defects. J Trauma 1973;13(9):799–810.
92. Kelly PJ, Martin WJ, Coventry MB. Chronic osteomelitis. II. Treatment with closed irrigation and suction. JAMA 1970;213(11):1843–8.
93. Shannon JG, Woolhouse FM, Eisinger PJ. The treatment of chronic osteomyelitis by saucerization and immediate skin grafting. Clin Orthop Relat Res 1973;(96):98–107.
94. Anthony JP, Mathes SJ, Alpert BS. The muscle flap in the treatment of chronic lower extremity osteomyelitis: results in patients over 5 years after treatment. Plast Reconstr Surg 1991;88(2):311–8.
95. May JW Jr, Jupiter JB, Gallico GG III, et al. Treatment of chronic traumatic bone wounds. Microvascular free tissue transfer: a 13-year experience in 96 patients. Ann Surg 1991;214(3):241–50 [discussion: 250–2].
96. Klemm KW. Antibiotic bead chains. Clin Orthop Relat Res 1993;(295):63–76.
97. Adams K, Couch L, Cierny G, et al. In vitro and in vivo evaluation of antibiotic diffusion from antibiotic-impregnated polymethylmethacrylate beads. Clin Orthop Relat Res 1992;(278):244–52.
98. Green SA. Skeletal defects. A comparison of bone grafting and bone transport for segmental skeletal defects. Clin Orthop Relat Res 1994;(301):111–7.
99. Thonse R, Conway J. Antibiotic cement-coated interlocking nail for the treatment of infected nonunions and segmental bone defects. J Orthop Trauma 2007; 21(4):258–68.

100. Pawar A, Dikmen G, Fragomen A, et al. Antibiotic-coated nail for fusion of infected Charcot ankles. Foot Ankle Int 2013;34(1):80–4.
101. Donegan DJ, Scolaro J, Matuszewski PE, et al. Staged bone grafting following placement of an antibiotic spacer block for the management of segmental long bone defects. Orthopedics 2011;34(11):e730–5.
102. Apard T, Bigorre N, Cronier P, et al. Two-stage reconstruction of post-traumatic segmental tibia bone loss with nailing [Systematic review or meta-analysis]. Orthop Traumatol Surg Res 2010;96(5):549–53.
103. Wasko MK, Borens O. Antibiotic cement nail for the treatment of posttraumatic intramedullary infections of the tibia: midterm results in 10 cases. Injury 2013; 44(8):1057–60.
104. Roeder B, Van Gils CC, Maling S. Antibiotic beads in the treatment of diabetic pedal osteomyelitis. J Foot Ankle Surg 2000;39(2):124–30.
105. Calhoun JH, Henry SL, Anger DM, et al. The treatment of infected nonunions with gentamicin-polymethylmethacrylate antibiotic beads. Clin Orthop Relat Res 1993;(295):23–7.
106. Cierny G III. Chronic osteomyelitis: results of treatment. Instr Course Lect 1990; 39:495–508.
107. Marsh JL, Prokuski L, Biermann JS. Chronic infected tibial nonunions with bone loss. Conventional techniques versus bone transport. Clin Orthop Relat Res 1994;(301):139–46.
108. Morandi M, Zembo MM, Ciotti M. Infected tibial pseudarthrosis. A 2-year follow up on patients treated by the Ilizarov technique. Orthopedics 1989;12(4):497–508.
109. Paley D, Catagni MA, Argnani F, et al. Ilizarov treatment of tibial nonunions with bone loss. Clin Orthop Relat Res 1989;(241):146–65.
110. Nho SJ, Helfet DL, Rozbruch SR. Temporary intentional leg shortening and deformation to facilitate wound closure using the Ilizarov/Taylor spatial frame [Systematic review or meta-analysis]. J Orthop Trauma 2006;20(6):419–24.
111. Fitzgerald RH Jr, Ruttle PE, Arnold PG, et al. Local muscle flaps in the treatment of chronic osteomyelitis. J Bone Joint Surg Am 1985;67(2):175–85.
112. Weiland AJ, Moore JR, Daniel RK. The efficacy of free tissue transfer in the treatment of osteomyelitis. J Bone Joint Surg Am 1984;66(2):181–93.
113. Christy MR, Lipschitz A, Rodriguez E, et al. Early postoperative outcomes associated with the anterolateral thigh flap in Gustilo IIIB fractures of the lower extremity. Ann Plast Surg 2014;72:80–3.
114. Shojaiefard A, Khorgami Z, Larijani B. Septic diabetic foot is not necessarily an indication for amputation. J Foot Ankle Surg 2008;47(5):419–23.
115. Duzgun AP, Satir HZ, Ozozan O, et al. Effect of hyperbaric oxygen therapy on healing of diabetic foot ulcers. J Foot Ankle Surg 2008;47(6):515–9.
116. Chen CE, Ko JY, Fong CY, et al. Treatment of diabetic foot infection with hyperbaric oxygen therapy. Foot Ankle Surg 2010;16(2):91–5.
117. LaVan FB, Hunt TK. Oxygen and wound healing [Systematic review or meta-analysis]. Clin Plast Surg 1990;17(3):463–72.
118. Rose D. Hyperbaric oxygen therapy for chronic refractory osteomyelitis. Am Fam Physician 2012;86(10):888 [author reply p: 888–9].
119. Southwood LL, Frisbie DD, Kawcak CE, et al. Evaluation of Ad-BMP-2 for enhancing fracture healing in an infected defect fracture rabbit model. J Orthop Res 2004;22(1):66–72.
120. Li GY, Yin JM, Ding H, et al. Efficacy of leukocyte- and platelet-rich plasma gel (L-PRP gel) in treating osteomyelitis in a rabbit model. J Orthop Res 2013;31(6): 949–56.

121. Sakata J, Sasaki S, Handa K, et al. A retrospective, longitudinal study to evaluate healing lower extremity wounds in patients with diabetes mellitus and ischemia using standard protocols of care and platelet-rich plasma gel in a Japanese wound care program. Ostomy Wound Manage 2012;58(4):36–49.

122. Wang HF, Gao YS, Yuan T, et al. Chronic calcaneal osteomyelitis associated with soft-tissue defect could be successfully treated with platelet-rich plasma: a case report. Int Wound J 2013;10(1):105–9.

123. Yuan T, Zhang C, Zeng B. Treatment of chronic femoral osteomyelitis with platelet-rich plasma (PRP): a case report. Transfus Apher Sci 2008;38(2):167–73.

124. Emara KM, Ghafar KA, Al Kersh MA. Methods to shorten the duration of an external fixator in the management of tibial infections [Systematic review or meta-analysis]. World J Orthop 2011;2(9):85–92.

125. Perez-Roa RE, Tompkins DT, Paulose M, et al. Effects of localised, low-voltage pulsed electric fields on the development and inhibition of *Pseudomonas aeruginosa* biofilms. Biofouling 2006;22(5–6):383–90.

126. Pickering SA, Bayston R, Scammell BE. Electromagnetic augmentation of antibiotic efficacy in infection of orthopaedic implants. J Bone Joint Surg Br 2003; 85(4):588–93.

127. Kasimanickam RK, Ranjan A, Asokan G, et al. Prevention and treatment of biofilms by hybrid- and nanotechnologies. Int J Nanomedicine 2013;8:2809–19.

128. Voigt J, Wendelken M, Driver V, et al. Low-frequency ultrasound (20-40 kHz) as an adjunctive therapy for chronic wound healing: a systematic review of the literature and meta-analysis of eight randomized controlled trials [Systematic review or meta-analysis]. Int J Low Extrem Wounds 2011;10(4):190–9.

Index

Note: Page numbers of article titles are in **boldface** type.

Foot Ankle Clin N Am 19 (2014) 589–601
http://dx.doi.org/10.1016/S1083-7515(14)00074-6
1083-7515/14/$ – see front matter © 2014 Elsevier Inc. All rights reserved.

foot.theclinics.com

Moving?

Make sure your subscription moves with you!

To notify us of your new address, find your **Clinics Account Number** (located on your mailing label above your name), and contact customer service at:

Email: journalscustomerservice-usa@elsevier.com

800-654-2452 (subscribers in the U.S. & Canada)
314-447-8871 (subscribers outside of the U.S. & Canada)

Fax number: 314-447-8029

Elsevier Health Sciences Division
Subscription Customer Service
3251 Riverport Lane
Maryland Heights, MO 63043

*To ensure uninterrupted delivery of your subscription, please notify us at least 4 weeks in advance of move.

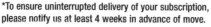